Health policy implications of unemployment

ACKNOWLEDGEMENTS

Thanks are due to Jane Welsh, Carole Munro, Jane Bailey and Jane Thompson for preparing the manuscript and to the Director of the Nuffield Centre, Keith Barnard for his role in facilitating the workshop at which these papers were presented.

World Health Organization
Regional Office for Europe
Copenhagen

Health policy implications of unemployment

Edited by

G. Westcott

Nuffield Centre for Health Services Studies
WHO Collaborating Centre for
the Managerial Process for Health Development
Leeds

P.-G. Svensson

Scientist, Health Research
WHO Regional Office for Europe

H.F.K. Zöllner

Regional Officer for Health Economics
WHO Regional Office for Europe

This publication has been reproduced by photo-offset from the original typescript, and has not received such detailed revision as is normally accorded to Regional Office publications.

ISBN 92 890 1029 0

PRINTED IN DENMARK

CONTENTS

Page

FOREWORD

The World Health Organization, Regional Office for Europe has sought for many years to encourage research into the effects of economic processes and economic instability on health. The papers in this volume were originally presented to a workshop held for WHO by the Nuffield Centre for Health Services Studies, Leeds University in December 1982. This was the third in a series of workshops on this topic falling within the programme of Social Equity and Health (formerly known as Unemployment, Poverty and Health).

Previous workshops in Copenhagen in 1980 and in Munich in 1981 had gathered research reports and proposals from participant countries. On this occasion a number of reviews of the growing literature on unemployment, recession and health were presented as well as reports on individual research projects and studies in progress. For the first time it was also felt appropriate to build on this body of findings with a discussion of their implications for health policy.

The reviews and research reports presented from seven European countries and the USA clearly indicate the presence of marked and sometimes severe health hazards caused by unemployment in the community. It is hoped that the differences in approach and design of the various projects as well as the findings will assist those continuing research in this field, and that the material presented will be of use to those formulating and evaluating policy interventions to prevent and to ameliorate these hazards, both in the economic sphere and in the health sector. Regrettably, the health impact of unemployment is likely to remain a policy issue for the foreseeable future.

J. E. Asvall, M.D.
Regional Director

INTRODUCTION

Per-Gunnar Svensson and Herbert Zöllner

THE PROBLEM

It is estimated that, in the major industrialized countries, 35 million persons are out of work. In the coming years, the labour force is calculated to grow by 18-20 million persons, with a corresponding need for additional jobs (OECD, 1983).

The International Labour Office (ILO) puts the global need for new employment up to the year 2000 (i.e. in the next 15 years) at one billion jobs (ILO, 1983).

This is being accompanied by industrialization and agricultural mechanization in the developing, and computerization in the developed countries, which might add up to fewer job opportunities than at present. In other words: a likelihood of persistently high and possibly rising unemployment in many places.

Experience from many countries indicates that insecurity at work, unemployment and under-employment can seriously affect social functioning, health and well-being.

In the present climate of low or zero economic growth, following a period of rapid replacement of man by machine, there is less opportunity of meaningful work. In some countries, the economic recession manifests itself in high overt unemployment; and in other societies where unemployment is ideologically unacceptable, there are a rising number of persons working in jobs beneath their levels of skill and competence. Again other countries experience economic instability, in the form of, e.g., rapid labour turnover and migration. Unemployment and/or the other forms of lack of meaningful work and of economic instability have grown to alarming rates in many European countries and are hitting the weakest groups most severely: the young entering the labour market and trying to lay a foundation for adult life; workers near retirement age who are laid off or relegated to less satisfactory work; middle-aged women trying to take up work after rearing their children; migrant workers coming from other regions or countries; and all types of less well educated and unskilled workers. The psychological, economic and social consequences of unemployment, less meaningful work and/or economic instability can lead to a broad spectrum of health problems in the long term such as depression, alcohol addiction, drug abuse and other chronic health and social conditions leading to chronic vulnerability.

In summary, there is a vicious circle of poverty, unemployment (and other forms of lack of meaningful work), other social and economic symptoms of inequality, discrimination, social vulnerability and chronic illness. The socioeconomically disadvantaged are less likely to attain health, while the chronically ill are less likely to fulfil their socioeconomic roles and may thereby become impoverished.

THE DEBATE

A number of solutions to the above-mentioned problems - especially overt unemployment - have been advocated.

The most obvious solution of interest to the health authorities consists in identifying the ways in which unemployment etc. does in fact cause ill health, in whom, under what circumstances, and through what mechanisms, and in directing health action at these mechanisms and targets.

A second approach of interest to the health sector is to promote the expansion of the service sector of the economy, including public and private health services, for example by promoting voluntary work and the setting up of cooperative and other small-scale enterprises.

The following approaches aim at creating more opportunities for work and at distributing the existing opportunities more equitably: the creation of new jobs through appropriate economic and industrial policies; more effective job placement than at present; appropriate employment policies to offset any remaining deviations from full employment; the fairer distribution of access to paid employment and to its economic benefits; the more optimal distribution of paid employment over the life cycle, e.g. by reducing working hours for parents with young children, for persons approaching retirement age, and for persons who care for sick or old relatives at home.

A further approach is to extend the concept of "work" to denote not just paid employment but any socially and economically productive and satisfying work. This would, e.g. also include unpaid activities in the family, in family enterprises and family-occupied farms, work for voluntary organizations such as pensioners' Red Cross and child welfare societies, caring for persons in one's social network of relatives, neighbours, etc., and personal care in the widest sense. This implies that this work is accorded the same social status as paid employment and that those who undertake it are guaranteed an equitable living standard. In this way unemployed and under-employed persons could at least obtain or retain the content that gives to life a goal and meaning, to the day a purpose and a structure, and to the individual an identity, self-assurance, access to a social network, and an acceptable standard of living.

REVIEW OF EXISTING RESEARCH

Research on the experience of unemployed individuals (i.e. at the micro level) has consistently shown that unemployment of more than a few weeks' duration causes physiological stress. This in turn may lead to an increase in blood pressure and heart disease.

In addition to the worsened affective state among the unemployed, with corresponding changes in body chemistry, there is also a greater tendency to exhibit psychiatric symptoms as shown by an increase in admissions to psychiatric hospitals at times of high unemployment and by a higher than average proportion of suicides and para-suicides. It seems likely that this is caused by the financial strain and the breakdown in close relationships that occur in periods of sustained unemployment.

Research on the national and cross-sectional levels (i.e. at the macro and intermediate levels) provides additional evidence that the unemployed suffer excess morbidity and mortality.

At the same time, the health of those at work suffers too, be it because the work content becomes less meaningful, the work load increases due to fewer workers on the job, the stress increases because of the need to service new types of machines, workers are afraid to assume sick roles even when appropriate - for fear of losing their job, or because team work and social support at work becomes more difficult in assembly lines. This in turn may imply that it will be increasingly difficult to detect great differences in the health status of the unemployed and underemployed on the one hand and the employed on the other. In addition, an increasing number of young people are suffering directly from the effects of economic depression and instability and experiencing the corresponding increase in risk of mental illness, suicide or parasuicide; however any resulting physiological health effects are more likely to appear in their old age rather than immediately.

Moreover, those outside the labour force, such as infants and the elderly, are likely to be effected by the impact of unemployment on the family and the rundown of social services and social support networks. It increases in recessions and with economic stability.

A large body of research shows, therefore, that high levels of unemployment and economic instability cause a significant increase in the levels of mental ill health and also have adverse effects on the physical health not only of the unemployed but also of their families and the community in general.

Policy formulation is usually based on the over simplistic assumption that the process of vulnerability can be represented as in figure 1. However, the reality is far more complex: an important system of multivariate interaction overshadows any simple explanation based on unemployment per se. Even through figure 2 is still simplified, it serves to indicate the complexity of the subject under discussion.

Fig. 1

FALLACIOUS PROBLEM FORMULATIONS

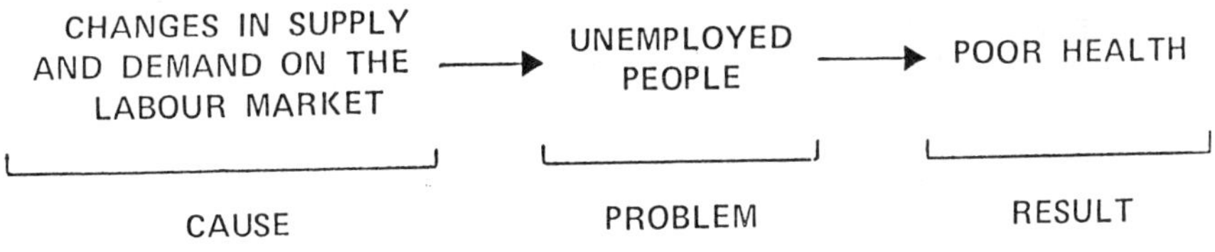

Source: Spruit, 1983

Fig. 2

THE PROCESS FROM UNEMPLOYMENT TO DISEASE

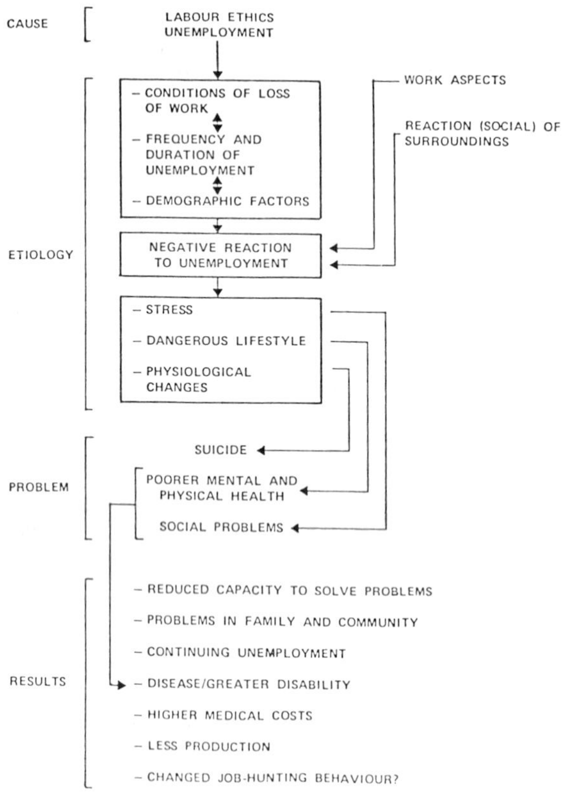

It may help to understand why, e.g., the same amount of unemployment may be related to different results.

Further epidemiological cross-sectional and longitudinal studies are required at the community level especially, in order to elucidate the ways in which economic change has the observed effects, especially as regards the relative importance of income loss, poverty and psychological impact due to becoming and being unemployed. On the policy level, emphasis should be given to those social and demographic groups that are most vulnerable to disruptive effects, by linking socioeconomic, demographic and health information and action.

Within the recently established programme on Social Equity and Health, the Regional Office for Europe of the World Health Organization is putting its emphasis on the issues raised above. Regarding unemployment this includes the following research activites:

- to study health effects of short and long-term employment
- to undertake cohort studies of the long-term unemployed
- to carry out specific (case study) interventions in order to determine effective approaches to health and social services (ranging from lay to specialized)
- to study the underlying process of becoming socially vulnerable through longitudinal studies following cohorts.

All these research efforts will result in health-related recommendations regarding social vulnerability and unemployment to governments, politicians, health professionals, health policy makers and social workers.

POLICY IMPLICATIONS OF RESEARCH FINDINGS

Economic policy Economic decisions can be made socially more relevant by taking full account of social costs, such as the erosion of working capacity and the costs to the health and social services that unemployment and economic instability entail. It must at the same time be stressed that not all types of employment are preferable to unemployment: work has its own hazards and social costs, particularly when health and safety conditions and environmental standards are relaxed in the name of promoting employment.

Employment policy In so far as there are limits to the possible scope of employment creation, there are advantages in sharing out of the existing employment opportunities rather than concentrating additional work hours and stress on those already employed. In addition, socially useful work can be devised to use temporarily spare capacity. The employment of workers below their skill levels, and other forms of underemployment, may look better than overt unemployment but they are not satisfactory solutions.

Social policy Health damage caused by unemployment can be limited by reducing poverty among the unemployed and other groups suffering from economic instability, and by ensuring that public decisions do not break networks of social support. There is the dual - sometimes conflicting - need to encourage, especially in children, the dependence of self-esteem on having a job, and to diminish the scope of self-blame among the unemployed. Agencies responsible for counselling the unemployed in a number of countries need additional capacity in times of recession because of the increased demands on them to attend to cash payments.

Health service policy Health services can be planned to meet the additional health needs resulting from recession. Better identification and quantification of the burdens on health services caused by disruptive economic events can help improve the relevance and cost-effectiveness of these services. The activities of nongovernmental agencies, such as self-help groups, labour unions and churches, can play a constructive role both in health and social policy.

Many other sectors of society are also of high relevance, e.g. education and industry.

These thoughts are preliminary; the programme on Social Equity and Health will at a later stage make a determined effort to identify strategies which can serve to stimulate other sectors of the economy and society to take measures capable of reducing unemployment and poverty and the resulting negative effects on health.

CONCLUSION - A SYSTEMS APPROACH

The lines of approach described above, taken singly, are not likely to achieve the desired results. The chance of success will be greater if approaches are combined and integrated in practice, and if action is simultaneously planned and implemented at different levels, regardless of any scientific, administrative, professional and political boundaries, namely at the supra-national level, at the national, county, municipal and company levels and by individual persons and their relatives and friends.

We may know less than we would like to, in relation to the effect of these actions. This modest report indicates where further research would be of benefit and where, by contrast, action should already be considered and initiated by decision-makers on the strength of the scientific evidence.

REFERENCES

ILO Yearbook of Labour Statistics, 1983

John, J., Schwefel, D. & Zöllner, H. (eds). Influence of economic instability on health. Springer-Verlag, 1983.

OECD Labour Force Statistics, Quarterly Labour Force Statistics, 1983

Spruit, I.P. Unemployment, employment and health. Leiden University, 1983.

Medium-term programme on social equity and health. Copenhagen, WHO Regional Office for Europe, 1982 (unpublished document ICP/SPM 050 (2)).

WHO Regional Office for Europe. Health policy in relation to unemployment in the community: summary report on a WHO Workshop, 1983 (unpublished document ICP/RPD 804 (3)(S)).

Part I

Reviews

UNEMPLOYMENT AND HEALTH

Urban Janlert

In the present sense of the word, there was no unemployment in Sweden during most of the 19th century. Agriculture and forestry were the main occupational fields. Special Swedish legislation made unemployment a punishable offence. The last of these special laws was repealed in 1885. The 1870 Royal Commission on Poverty noted that unemployment was the fault of the individual.

'It must be extremely rare for anyone having made serious attempts to procure work to fail in this venture or to fail to such a degree that he is unable to obtain at least the bare essentials of life'.[1]

It was obvious that illness at this time led to unemployment. Any person who was ill for any length of time ran the risk of losing his job. Good health improved the chances of obtaining work. Many companies refused to hire people who suffered from certain disorders or who were disabled. The emergence of the industrialised society resulted in the identification of new disabilities.

If the relationship between unemployment and illness is examined, (perhaps up to the time of the First World War) it was observed that illness led to unemployment up to the time of the First World War (arrow A in Fig. 1).

Most of the research into the correlation between unemployment and ill health was carried out during the Depression years of the 1930's.[2] Research in this decade clearly showed how unemployment led to a sharp decline in the standard of living, starvation, malnutrition and premature death. Poverty was the cause of this (arrow B in Fig. 1 below).

Fig. 1
Several different correlations between unemployment and poor health

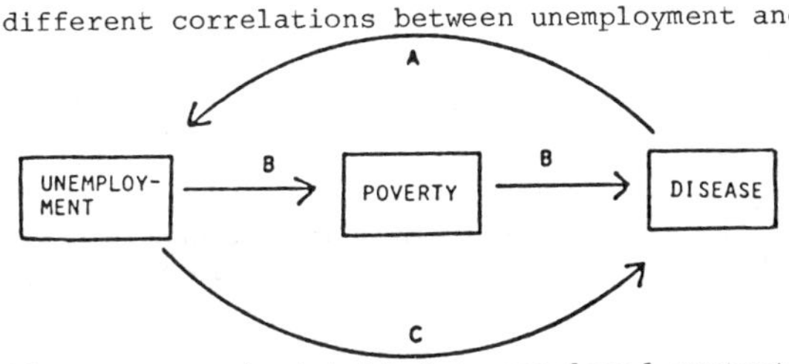

Entries in a literature contest held for unemployed contestants in Poland of the 1930's dealt mainly with the effects of unemployment, effects such as poverty, hunger, begging and general privation.[3] A large-scale study of unemployed in Montreal in the 1930's disclosed in increased level of morbidity.[4]

The accepted view, confirmed, it was felt, by this study, was that the low income situation caused the illness and poor health among the unemployed, not the unemployment itself.

This view led to the conclusion that efforts should primarily be made to improve economic compensation to the unemployed. With adequate unemployment compensation, unemployment would not have to lead to ill health.

CORRELATION BETWEEN UNEMPLOYMENT AND MORBIDITY

To summarise, new research in this field shows that the hypothesis of the 1930's about poverty eliciting the effects of unemployment on healh is inadequate.

Most western countries currently have comprehensive unemployment insurance programmes which do not force unemployed people into poverty, even if unemployment still leads to a decline in the standard of living. But despite this insurance, unemployment can still be shown to cause ill health.

M. Harvey Brenner at Johns Hopkins University in the U.S. is at the forefront of work being done to create a model of the way unemployment affects health.

In a study of the incidence of first admissions to psychiatric hospitals in New York City from 1861 to 1967, he found that the rate of admissions displayed co-variance with unemployment during the same period. Admissions increased when unemployment was high and declined during economic booms.[5] No other indicators out of a number tested (e.g. the concentration of doctors and consumption of medication) yielded anything like the same degree of correlation.

Studies in other fields disclosed, for example, that suicides increased within a few years after a rise in unemployment.[6]

A study of the mortality for a number of chronic disorders suggested increased mortality from cardiovascular disease with a peak two to three years after peak unemployment.[7]

These and several other studies were based on advanced statistical analysis of comprehensive material. Long periods of observation, ie. 20 to more than 100 years, were used to make it possible to follow variations in the state of the economy. The most important independent variable was an indicator of unemployment. The dependent variables were various indicators of morbidity and mortality (eg. mental illness, infant mortality, death from cardiovascular disease, death from cirrhosis of the liver, suicide etc.).

The analysis technique employed in these studies was based upon comparisons of the way morbidity varied with the state of the economy (usually recorded as unemployment). No consideration was paid to long-term changes in health.

If we take an indicator of morbidity - line A in Fig. 2 - we can see how this indicator slowly changes in the course of time at the same time as the line displays heavy undulation. Line C is the line obtained when the trend line (line B) is removed. The C line was the line employed in the analyses.

Fig. 2
Examples of a curve analysis which was the basis of studies by Brenner et al.

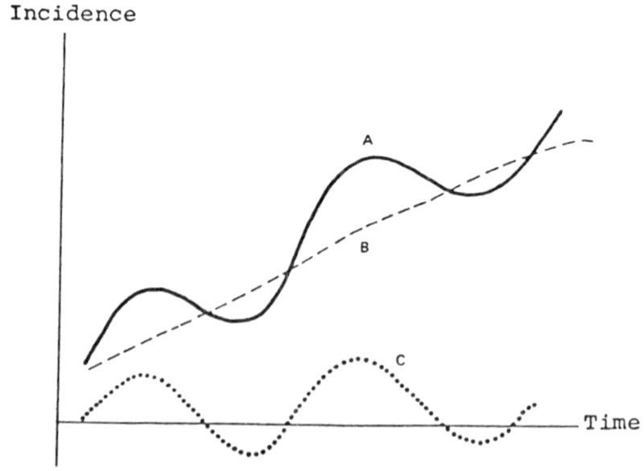

The results presented by Brenner in various papers could be schematically rendered as in Fig. 3. This is a somewhat simplified presentation since the figure utilises a diagram in describing the results of several different studies carried out using slightly different methods.

Fig. 3
Correlations between unemployment and morbidity due to cardiovascular disease and mental illness according to Brenner.

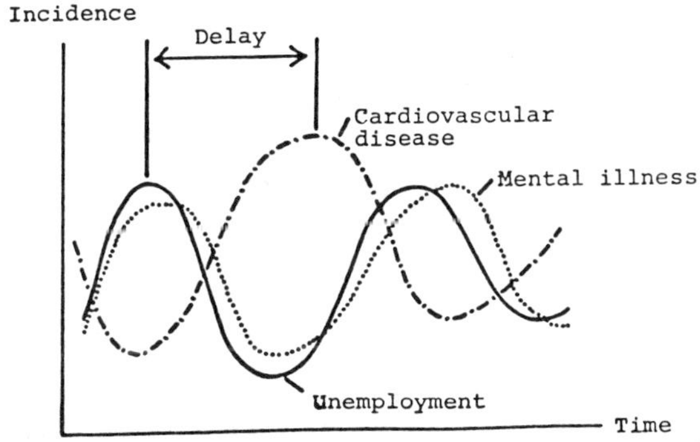

The Figure shows that there is a simultaneous increase in mental illness (the dotted line) in times of high unemployment (the solid line). This morbidity was measured as the number of admissions to psychiatric hospitals and as the rate of suicide.

Other indicators which parallel variations in unemployment are the consumption of hard liquor and infant mortality. On the other hand, the prevalence of cardiovascular disease (the dashed and dotted line) displays a peak about two years after peak unemployment (the delay is designated with arrows in the Figure). The term "disease" is somewhat misleading here since the indicator employed was mortality due to cardiovascular disease. Death due to cirrhosis of the liver also displayed the same pattern as the variation in cardiovascular disease.

One criticism made of Brenner's study is the circumstance that death due to cardiovascular disease appears to decline in periods of high unemployment and rise during economic booms.[8] Could the heavy demand for labour, the influx of many new and workers unaccustomed to work increased overtime and a faster work pace be the reasons for this increase in mortality?

In a later and more sophisticated model, Brenner was able to show that several factors must be taken into consideration when considering the effect of the state of the economy on health. He obtained extremely close correlation in one multi-variable analysis model between these economic indicators and various indicators of health. Several different independent variables were employed, including indicators of economic growth, unemployment and the rate of inflation, and in which it was possible to work with varying time intervals between dependent and independent variables.[9]

The model was used with data from the US, England, and Wales and shows that the long-term increase in income per capita was correlated with improved health at the same time as cyclical fluctuations produced increased morbidity in the goods and services sectors most heavily hit by recession, people with limited education , people unemployed for long periods of time, and people whose vocational skills are no longer needed because of rationalisation and the introduction of new technology.[10]

In brief, Brenner's model can be explained in the following way:

1. A recession leads to increased unemployment. People who lose their jobs become less competitive on the labour market than people who retain their jobs and become therefore more sensitive to future shifts in the economy.

2. Unemployment can have virtually an immediate effect on health (eg. mental health) but also appears to initiate long-range processes which can lead to chronic disease which take many years to cause death.

3. Taken as a whole, a recession with increased unemployment causes an interaction between chronic disease processes and increased susceptibility to economic pressure.

Australian studies of mortality from cardiovascular disease have disclosed a similar pattern.[11] The fact that the same hypothesis has been confirmed in many different societies is a strength.

The statistical analysis can be translated into concrete figures to make the picture clear.

In one study conducted on behalf of the US Congress, an attempt to estimate the social costs of national economic policy, Brenner found that the number of deaths in the US would rise by nearly 37,000 (more than 20,000 of which because of cardiovascular disease, 900 suicides, 650 murders, and 500 deaths due to liver cirrhosis) if unemployment in the country rose by one percentage point and the rise persisted for six years. It would also lead to 4,200 admissions to psychiatric departments, and 3,300 admissions to prisons.[12]

Translating these findings into equivalent figures for Sweden is difficult. But we will attempt to do so anyway just to provide some idea of the magnitude of the figures. If the findings obtained by Brenner were applied to Swedish conditions and population size, although without considering any differences in mortality patterns, age structure and so forth, the corresponding increase in unemployment would lead to an increase in the number of deaths over a six year period by 1,500.

Added to this are a number of less grave, but still important changes. Australian studies have shown that the number of visits to a doctor increases, as well as the consumption of medicine, when unemployment rises.[11]

Brenner's pioneering work has been described by leader writers in magazines such as the Journal of the American Medical Association (JAMA) and the Lancet as both interesting and warranting further research.[13] [14]

However, the studies have not gone unopposed. One type of criticism concerned the reliability of the medical data employed over long periods of time.[15] Other critics question the wisdom of bothering about analyses of statistical correlations of this kind in which macroeconomic factors are linked to individual biological phenomena.[16]

No matter how people view the criticism, it is obvious that these statistical correlations can only suggest causal relationships. We require more detailed studies on the individual level in order to detect mechanisms capable of explaining the relationship between phenomena such as unemployment and illness.

STRESS THEORIES

One of the explanatory models most frequently used in contemporary unemployment research is the "stress model." In this context, the term "stress" usually refers to genetically-governed, stereotype and non-specific responses by an organism exposed to changes in or demands from its environment. These changes and demands are usually referred to as "stressors." Stressors may be anything from simple physical stimuli, such as cold or heat, to complex social situations calling for advanced interpretations, such as losing a promotion to someone else. Job loss and unemployment are probably stressors.

The effect of stress can be roughly divided into effects on the body's immunity system and effects on the cardiovascular system. Special behavioural patterns such as excess smoking, large alcohol consumption and weight gain due to overeating must be added. Effects on the cardiovascular system may be in the form of elevated blood pressure and high levels of serum lipids, factors which increase the risk of ischaemic heart disease and strokes.

Kasl et al. worked on the basis of these stress concepts in a careful study.[17] [18] [19] [20] [21] [22] They kept track of the effects following the closure of two factories and compared events at these companies with events at two factories which remained in business. One of the closed factories was located in a large urban area and the other in a small rural community.

Participants in the study were examined on five occasions. The first occasion was immediately prior to closure during the period referred to as the "anticipatory phase," ie. the phase in which the employees still retained their jobs but knew that the factory was about to close. This first study was conducted from one to two months before closure. Subsequent examinations took place 1-2 months, 6 months and about 1 year after closure.

By then, most of the subjects had found permanent employment. A fifth investigation was made about a year after the fourth.

The investigations were all made in the homes of the subjects. A project nurse visited the subjects, took samples, conducted interviews and carried out certain measurements.

The control groups in the urban and rural areas did not display any significant changes in blood pressure during the period of observation. However, a definite increase was found in the blood pressure of workers from the two closed factories even at the first examination. This rise in blood pressure persisted throughout the period of unemployment and probationary employment. Blood pressures did not return to normal until permanent employment was obtained. The blood pressure of subjects who viewed unemployment as difficult (ie. felt that it took a long time for them to get back to normal living habits after losing their jobs) tended to return to normal less frequently than the blood pressure of others. The greater the anxiety felt about the closure, the greater the rise in blood pressure.[20]

Another feature of the examination was determination of the stress hormone level during the period of observation. Here, the excretion of norepinephrine in urine was measured.[21] Norepinephrine is a stress hormone which, among other things, increases the heart rate, triggers the release of blood sugar, heightens metabolism and sets the body up to deal with danger or changes in the environment. Fig. 4 lists the average levels on different occasions.

Fig. 4
Norepinephrine excretion in the study group immediately prior to and at different times after factory closure. The bars designated with * show a statistical significant increase compared to the control group.

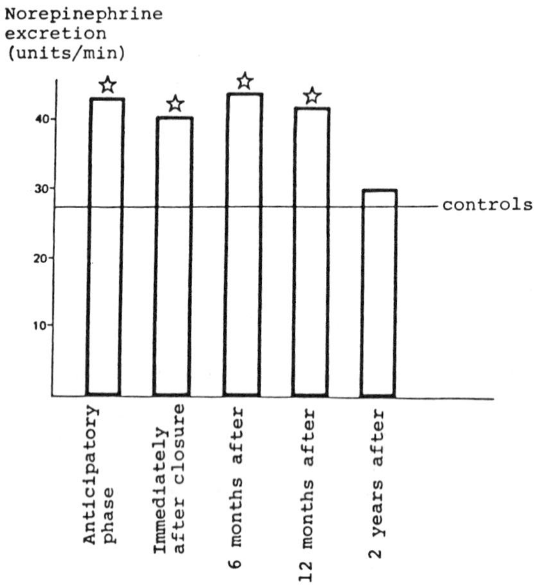

The level of stress hormones was raised in the study group from the anticipatory phase until one year after closure. The level was found to have dropped to normal values only at the examination two years after closure. On the other hand, the values of the control group remained constant during the corresponding period of time. A greater rise was found among subjects from the factory in the large town than those from the factory in the small town. The large urban environment apparently contains components which aggravate the response to unemployment (or the more rural environment may somehow exert an alleviating effect.)

Other biochemical changes were checked in a corresponding way.[19] Blood cholesterol levels were not affected during the anticipatory phase but rose sharply in subjects forced into unemployment. Their values did not return to normal until the subjects got new jobs.

The results obtained by Kasl et al. strongly support the view that unemployment and the threat of unemployment is a major stress factor. The physiological findings shed some light on eg. the correlation found by Brenner between unemployment and cardiovascular disease. The stress response as such (ie. with elevated blood pressure, elevated blood lipid levels etc.) plus stress-related behaviour (eg. weight gain, smoking etc.) are both risk factors in the pathogenesis of cardiovascular disease.

UNEMPLOYMENT AND HIGH BLOOD PRESSURE

The relationship between unemployment and high blood pressure has attracted considerable interest. In 1977, Gronqvist published a report, "Hypertonins sociala orsaker" (Eng. = The social causes of hypertension 1977.)[23] He studied the prevalence of hypertension by measuring sales of anti-hypertensive drugs. Geographic differences in drug sales were tested against a large number of variables, such as age, sex, prevalence of certain disorders (eg. diabetes), unemployment, alcohol consumption, municipal tax increases etc. A total of more than 40 different variables were tested.

His analysis disclosed that geographic differences in respect to the prevalence of high blood pressure could be explained by ten factors. The most important factor was "unemployment." It explained more than 32% of the variation in the spread of hypertensive disease. The factor "percentage of people employed in industry" was in second place and accounted for more than 14%. In other words, the greater the level of unemployment and the more people employed in industry, the greater the consumption of anti-hypertensive drugs in the area. About 72% of the variation, a remarkably high figure for this technique, was ascribable to these and a further five factors - all related to "a changing society" or "changes in working life."

A Norwegian study reported on blood pressure measurements made on the same group of employees in a small company in Oslo on three occasions.[24] The first and last measurements displayed the same results. However, a significant rise in systolic blood pressure was recorded in the intermediate examination. A subsequent check revealed that the employees had discovered, just prior to the second examination, that the company was in financial straits and that there was a real risk of bankruptcy and closure. Subsequently, ie. after the second examination, the economic difficulties were resolved and the company was able to continue as before.

The ability of unemployment and the threat of unemployment to elicit hypertension has been confirmed. However, controversy remains regarding the relationship between this symptom and persistent hypertensive disease. It seems likely that protracted stress may accelerate the development of hypertensive disease in predisposed individuals.[25]

UNEMPLOYMENT AFTER COMPANY CLOSURES

Studies of the effects of unemployment on individuals have been made primarily in conjunction with company closures.

In 1968, a very broad study was started in Sweden of company closures in the Billerud Group. An attempt was made to shed light on the consequences of company closure on employees and their families as regards working conditions, other living conditions and health. The study pursued a pronounced inter-disciplinary approach and included experts in sociology, psychology, medicine and cultural geography.[26]

The position of people out of work for a long period of time was the subject of a special report. It was found that the social and psychological consequences of unemployment are highly complicated. A number of adaptation patterns were found - from passive submission to unemployment to positive response to the experience it provided. The fact that personal identity is undermined by unemployment was stressed. From having been a productive, profitable worker, the unemployed person becomes a non-productive recipient of benefits and a burden on the society. The world's new view of him conflicts with his previous perception of self and the need to preserve his identity. Leisure pursuits, hobbies, club activities and membership in a family with fixed roles enabled some of the unemployed to maintain a strong personal identity long after the loss of work. The relationship between spouses often deteriorated when the husband attempted to take over duties traditionally carried out by the wife. People who viewed unemployment as something positive were invariably people very close to the normal retirement age.[26] Complementary attitude studies showed that people who had been unemployed for long periods of time lost their sense of personal merit more often than people who had remained employed. Unemployed people also displayed more psychosomatic symptoms and their faith in the world declined.[27]

The medical part of the study has not been published as yet.

In a sociomedical study of the unemployed in Vestlandet, Norway (when a sardine factory was closed) it was found found that factory closure led to widespread unemployment.[28] Between 40-50% of the people who lost their jobs were "chronically unemployed" one year after the factory closed. A few months before the closure, a rather high level of morbidity was found in the group, but more of the subjects were still healthy enough to do their work at the factory. A new examination conducted one year after factory closure disclosed that the heath of the group had changed.

As Table 1 shows, just under 30% had contracted new disorders in the period since the previous examination, whereas the health of just under 20% had actually improved. The improvements were mainly with regard to somatic disorders such as joint disease.

Table 1. Heath improvements and deterioration in the study group one year after job loss.

	% Yes				% No	Total	No.
	Mental	Somatic	Both	Total			
New disease or complaint in past year.	14	11	4	29	70	100	95
Improved health the past year.	1	15	2	18	82	100	95

This should be viewed in the light of the fact that the health of the workers was relatively poor. Improvement in their health after the closure points to serious shortcomings in the old work environment. The new disorders were largely mental complaints.

The report points out that there was a clear correlation between the uncertainty which arose after the factory closure and the mental disorders.

These were mainly mild mental disorders. But serious mental disease and severe alcoholism were found in a few cases. The consumption of medication also increased sharply, but these figures are difficult to interpret since the group which conducted the medical screenings also prescribed medication for subjects in need of it.

Following comprehensive medical and work environment examinations at a shipyard in Copenhagen, an unexpected decision to close the yard was announced later that year. This provided an unusual opportunity to study what happened to workers who lost ther jobs.

A study made about four months after the closure disclosed that there had been a decline in health after that closure.[29] About half of the previous work force of about 100 people was still out of work at that time. The health impairment was found primarily in this category. The impairment was especially striking as regards nervous disorders. Twenty-eight percent of the unemployed reported a decline here. The corresponding percentage for people with jobs was 5%. People who had succeeded in finding a new job after the closure displayed an increased incidence of back complaints and fatigue but a reduced incidence of stomach disorders. The consumption of medicine increased sharply, but this increase was not confined to the unemployed. Results from a new examination made 15 months after the closure is currently being processed and not yet available.

EARLY RETIREMENT

The number of people who were retired prematurely increased sharply at the start of the 1970's. This was the result of legislative changes making early retirement easier on medical grounds with a view to the prevailing situation on the labour market. Demands for rehabilitation measures also became less stringent than was previously the case. The number of prematurely retired people rose to more than 300,000 by the middle of the 1970's. Fig. 5 shows the percentage of males in different age brackets who were prematurely retired in various years. In 1975 more than a third of Swedish men from 65-66 had been prematurely retired on medical grounds. The figure was lower for other age brackets but displayed the same rising tendency throughout the 1970's.

Fig. 5
Early retirements as a percentage of the average population in each age bracket

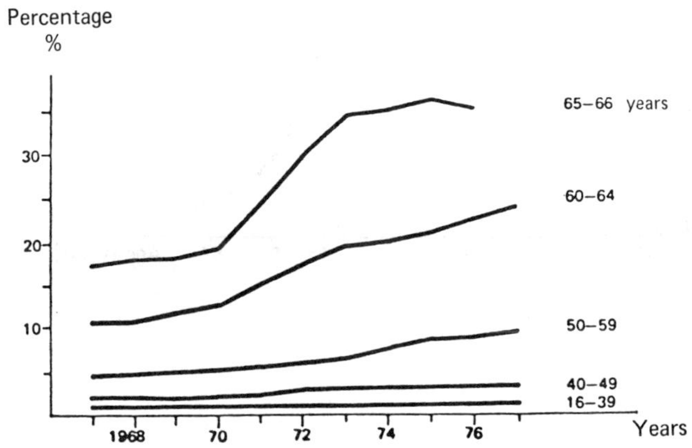

The percentage of early retirements varied considerably from one part of the country to another.

A special report from a commission on employment made an attempt to analyse the causes of the variations in the population's early retirement patterns.[30]

The main results are quite clear: unemployment is the overriding explanation. This is also the case in younger age brackets, even though the objective of the legislation was to facilitate early retirement of older people. Large numbers of early retirements have continued too. The labour market problems were just not susceptible to quick solution with the aid of early retirement.

Nevertheless, early retirement does take place largely on medical grounds. The category referred to as the "A group", which receive early retirements without a medical certificate because of special labour market circumstances, is comparatively small. The commission on employment suggested that early retirement is only slightly related to the health of the individual but is actually more indicative of the health of the labour market.

An interesting study designed to shed light on this aspect was conducted by Lars Dahlberg.[31] He scrutinized every case of early retirement granted in 1971 on the diagnosis of scoliosis. Here, it was possible to utilise the circumstance that scoliosis is measurable, ie. it can be objectively assessed by an impartial observer. Fig. 6 shows the relationship between the degree of lumbar scoliosis, in people granted a full early retirement pension in 1971, and the main diagnosis of "scoliosis."

Fig. 6
Correlation between the degree of spinal curvature and age in cases of early retirement.

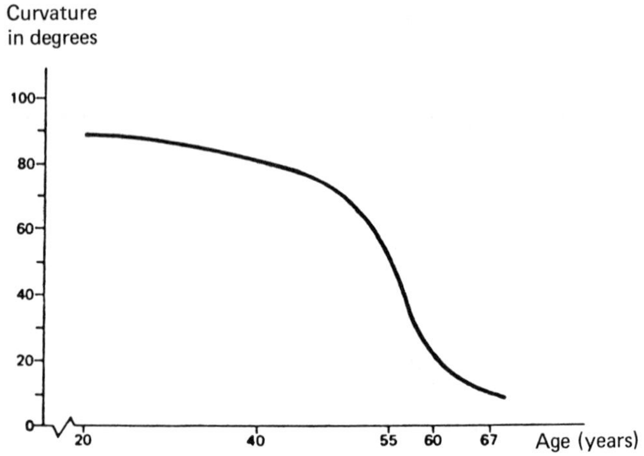

The Figure shows that the older the pensioner, the less the degree of spinal curvature, ie. the less severe the disorder has to be for a diagnosis of "scoliosis". In people over the age of 55, the curvature was so slight that it could be regarded as more or less normal. Here, it should be remembered that the majority of the early retirements granted belong to this category (more than 70%).

The conclusion drawn by Dahlberg in his report is that doctors have become an important factor on the labour market.

Even if the mechanisms for the way unemployment leads to early retirement via genuine or formal disease are fairly well known, we still know very little about the way early retirement affects health. On the basis of the available literature, the following summary can be made of the factors which probably have a favourable or adverse effect in early retirement.[32] [33] [34] [35] [36] [37] [38] [39]

Unfavourable factors	Favourable factors
Deterioration in finances - poor pension	Acceptable income - relatively good pension
Poorly developed social contact network	Social contacts with relatives and friends outside the job
Non-membership of clubs	Active in clubs, political organisations etc.
Few interests outside of work	Instrumental view of work
No family	Family
Relatively young	Relatively old
Good health	Somatic or mental disorders, so unable to work
Brief transition time (retirement comes rather suddenly)	Long transition time (aware of retirement a long time in advance)

This listing should be viewed as assumptions rather than facts. The medical consequences of the expanded form of early retirement seen in the 1970's cannot be foreseen.

YOUTH UNEMPLOYMENT

There is a remarkable lack of modern research on the relationship between youth unemployment and health.

At the beginning of this century, one of the arguments put forward in Sweden [40] and eg. Great Britain [41] in favour of reducing the retirement age was that it would reduce unemployment among young people, an unemployment that was regarded as being particularly unsatisfctory.

Even though there have been a number of studies of the effects of unemployment on the health of the adult population, no equivalent medical study has been conducted on unemployment among young people. When the Swedish society of sociomedicine planned a symposium to be held in conjunction with the annual meeting of the Swedish Medical Association, it was unable to find a scientist who could represent the field of youth unemployment.

Nevertheless, many people - both scientists and laymen feel that unemployment among young people is especially serious.[42]

Encountering unemployment as their first experience of the labour market after leaving school - a time when young people are particularly sensitive and impressionable - may not lead to sickness directly. But there is a major risk of the unemployment establishing patterns which have an adverse effect on health. This is currently an important but neglected field of research.

At the Public Health Institute of Jyvaskyla, Finland, Kannas and Hietaharju have studied unemployment among young people and the ways of life and habits which could have an influence on future health.[43] A questionnaire survey of 19-year old men in which unemployed youths were compared to employed contemporaries disclosed clear differences between the groups (see Table 2).

Table 2. Health behaviour of 19-year old boys with and without jobs.

	Unemployed % yes	With job % yes
Eats at irregular hours	14	10
Drinks regular milk instead of low-fat milk	48	42
Drinks more than 6 cups of coffee/day	33	24
Smokes daily	66	52
Has tried narcotics on some occasion	23	9
Uses alcohol every week	60	41
Gets drunk every week	31	16
Showers or takes a bath no more than once/week	35	18
Does not brush teeth daily	35	18
Has not visited a dentist the past two years	45	37
Irregular sleeping habits	28	19
Exercises less than once a week	70	49
No. of subjects	97	475

It was shown that the unemployed do not eat as well, use more intoxicants and neglect their personal hygiene and physical condition more than contemporaries with jobs.

In summarising, the study noted that young unemployed people are "worn out" more rapidly than others and expressed the belief that the unemployed young people of today are likely to be the sick, middle-aged men of tomorrow. They differ in fields in which we already know that the choice of life styles has major importance (smoking, alcohol consumption, dental hygiene etc.)

As in many other studies, it is difficult to know what is cause and effect. Is physical neglect the result of unemployment or are people who neglect their bodies people who neglect opportunities to obtain employment? No definite answer can be provided to this question.

In the original questionnaire survey, people who had reported illness or some complaint which reduced their possibility of getting a job were deleted from the material (about 8% of the respondents).

Both studies were concluded with the same "prescription": jobs and health information.

In their view, most unemployment is involuntary, even if the same mechnisms of selection which govern the ability to obtain work also govern health behaviour. Having work appears to create more stringent demands on certain routines, including the care of personal health. In the long run, having a job should promote health.

UNEMPLOYMENT IN CERTAIN RISK GROUPS

It has been clearly shown that certain groups are hit by unemployment more than others. There is a marginal labour force which is the first to become unemployed in a recession and the last to get new jobs when the demand for labour again rises.

A large proportion of the variation in the population's health which is ascribable to the state of the economy is probably to be found in this group. This has been shown in the aforementioned studies by Brenner.[19]

British, American and French research reports with the same findings show that health gaps in the society have widened in the present century. Even though public health services have been greatly expanded and the previous wide variations in access to health care have declined.[44]

The average life span is increasing less rapidly (or even declining) in the lowest social categories but still rising in the upper social categories.

Fig. 7 shows age-standardised mortality (whose mean value for each year is 100) for the five social groups described in British statistics on causes of death. Social category 1 covers people with the highest education and social category 2 workers without any particular education. The curve shows the gap is increasing between the social categories.[45]

Fig. 7
Age-standardised mortality figures for males, 15-64 years, in England and Wales

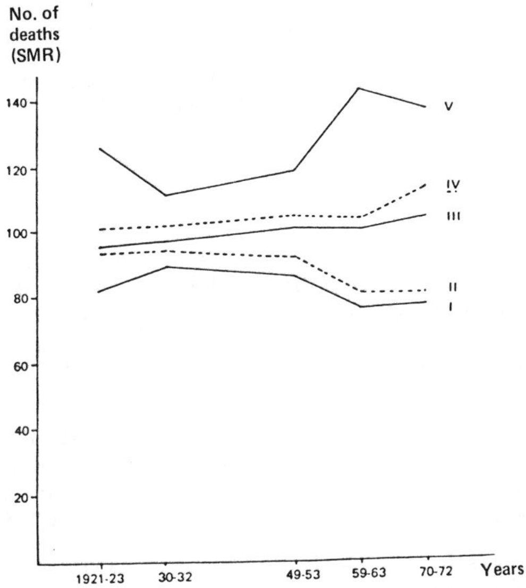

Source: Occupational Mortality (1970)

Interpreting these data is a difficult task. Is social category 1 of today comparable to social category 5 from eg. 1920? It is probably reasonable to assume that social group 5 is currently a more selected group than before and that it probably corresponds to the aforementioned "marginal labour force" to a greater degree. However, the fact remains that the gap is apparently widening. Even if the data present considerable methodological and interpretive problems, the unanimous findings from reports from various countries pointing to increasing differences between the health of different population groups represent an ominous observation.

Swedish records on mortality in alcohol misusers shed some light on Swedish conditions. Dahlgren showed that in the 1940's there was no significant difference between the mortality of the normal population and that of registered alcoholics.[46] However, figures published by the Central Bureau of Statistics from the 1970's show that the mortality of alcoholics during a five-year period was about four times higher than for other Swedish males of the same age.[47] In recent years in Sweden, there has been a stagnation in the increase in average life span (the average life span has even begun to decline for certain groups, such as middle-aged and older men.) The reason for this is unclear. No equivalent change has been noted for women. We know that this is the group most badly hit by unemployment, early retirement and protracted illness.[30] In view of the aforementioned research on the medical aftermath of unemployment, part of the explanation may be found here.[48]

Housewives are another interesting group. The commission on low income found insomnia, depression, an extremely negative correlation between nervous complaints and the scope of both housework and employment. None of the full-time employed women with a great deal of housework reported any mental disorders and none consumed any tranquilizers or hypnotics. At the other end of the scale were housewives with only a little household work to do. No fewer than 33% of the women reported nervous disorders, and 28% reported the use of tranquilizers.[49]

The position of housewives has not been studied extensively. The group does not appear to have attracted much reseach interest. This is regrettable since so much data on record which are used for other groups cannot be used in this context. Neither sickness registration nor early retirement is subdivided into this category in a manner making it possible to compare this group to others.

THE IMPORTANCE OF WORK

According to one Buddhist proverb, work has three functions: First of all, work provides the company of others. This is the most important component of work. Secondly, work enables you to do something meaningful in the society. And thirdly, work provides food for the day.

In man's attitudes to work, distinctions are usually made between two different views.[65]

One view is that man only works in order to procure material advantages. This is usually referred to as an <u>instrumental</u> attitude to work. Work is not necessary as these advantages can be obtained in some other way. You can live as conveniently on a lottery prize as on salaried labour.

And then there is the <u>expressive</u> attitude to work. In addition to giving us material advantages, work also incorporates us into the society. Work gives us prestige and status. It enables us to make contributions to the society's development. We can at least feel as if we are doing something useful. We make friends and acquaintances and acquire new interests. These aspects cannot be compensated for with money. Work contains so many components that there is just no way to compensate for it.

From the expressive point of view, work is irreplaceable.

The literature on unemployment and suicide (see Chapter 4) particularly the finding that economic compensation for unemployment does not reduce the risk of suicide (Vigterhous and Fishman 1978) support a view of work as being a highly complex activity which cannot be replaced with money. It is possible that people with unqualified assembly line work would be afflicted less. Their attitude to work is probably highly instrumental. However, data from eg. Brenner's studies suggest a completely different picture. The effects of unemployment are most striking in the lowest social categories.[66]

The fact that work is an extremely central feature in man's life has been demonstrated in many ways. One example is the study in which a group of people were asked what they would do if they suddenly inherited enough money to live a carefree life for the rest of their days. Eighty percent replied that they would keep on working. But only 9% reported that they had an interesting job. [67]

Another example is a study in which attempts were made, employing prospective, longitudinal techniques, to predict life span. The factor which proved to be best at predicting how long a person would live was by no means genetic factors, smoking habits or a medical assessment of the state of health. The factor was simply the answer to the question: "Do you like your job" The greater the degree of job satisfaction, the longer the life span.[68]

In this context, it should be noted that unemployment is not always a bad thing from the health point of view. There are work environments more hazardous than the risk presented by not having any work environment. But this can never be an argument in favour of unemployment. It merely directs attention to the problems of the work environment.

THE RESPONSIBILITY AND ROLE OF PUBLIC HEALTH

How does unemployment affect public health? While it is perfectly clear that labour market policy is not a medical issue, the fact remains that a person's ability to obtain work is of major importance to that person's health. Public health authorities apparently share this view. In 1976, a pair of students on a course for public health administrators in Umeå (Sweden) conducted a questionnaire survey among district medical officers and district nurses in Lycksele public health district, Västerbotten County.[69] Out of a total of 48 participants, more than 70% of the doctors and 52% of the nurses were of the opinion that unemployment leads to certain disease symptoms. No one replied in the negative but some did select the "sometimes" alternative. Seventy-six percent of the doctors and 68% of the nurses supported the assertion that the employment situation was important to the demand for medical care. In reply to the question: "Where do you think investments and efforts should be mainly made in order to improve the general state of health in Sweden?", measures to defeat unemployment were assigned to highest priority, much higher priority than eg. increased physical activity, reduced tobacco and alcohol consumption or environmental improvements. The answers disclosed that unemployment is a practical everyday problem for public health staff, even if labour market issues are viewed with particular interest in that part of Sweden where unemployment is high.

We now know that structural unemployment is likely to be one of the major problems of the 1980's and 1990's. The issue was discussed in a Spring 1979 issue of the medical journal The Lancet.[10] [14] [66] [70-74] The loss of jobs caused by computerisation was an example cited. Reports from West Germany show that certain companies feel that they would be able to reduce their staff numbers by 40% within 15 years.[70] Even if our current knowledge about the consequences of unemployment to health is both limited and fragmentary, we already know enough to realise that this development will be of major importance to the population's state of health and public health demands.

In view of this, we feel that the public heath authorities should urgently address themselves to the problems of unemployment. Several issues which merit particular attention in this sector are as follows:

1. To a greater degree than ever before, the routine activities of public health must be cognizant of and devote greater attention to a person's work situation. The issue of unemployment or the threat of unemployment is currently only considered sporadically in public health. In most instances, no note is made as to whether a patient is unemployed or not. The phenomenon must first be noted and recorded before public health will be able to take any effective steps.

2. Information on the correlation between work/unemployment and health available to public health must somehow be fed back to the authorities responsible for and dealing with labour market issues. The fund of information which public health represents must be utilised better than before.

3. The fact that work opportunities have definite medical consequences must be considered on a more overall basis, eg. in social planning programmes. One of the main tasks of public health is to bring these facts to the fore so they can be utilised in regional and employment policy planning.

4. As noted above, our knowledge of these issues is still fragmentary and inadequate. Public health must accept responsibility for initiating and stimulating research in important fields, such as research into unemployment among young people and sensitive groups.

REFERENCES

1 Underdånig betänkande den 5 December 1870 med förordning angående fattigvården i riket m m (Eng = Humbly submitted report of 5 December 1870 on provisions etc for the country's poor). Stockholm 1871 (pp. 38-38).

2 Janlert U, Arbetslöshet och ohälsa. En litteratur-översikt. Rapport från socialmedicinska föreningen i Luleå (Eng = Unemployment and ill health. A revew of the literature by the society of social medicine in Lulea) 1979.

3 Zawadski, B and Lazarsfeld, P, The psychological consequences of unemployment, Journal of Social Psychology, 1935, 6, 244-251.

4 Marsh, L, Fleming, A G, and Blackler C F, Health and unemployment. Some studies of their relationships. New York, Oxford 1938.

5 Brenner, M H, Mental Illness and the economy. Cambridge, Mass 1973.

6 Brenner, M H, Time series analysis of relationships between selected economic and social indicators. US National Technical Information Service, Springfield, Virginia 1971.

7 Brenner, M H, Economic changes and health disease mortality. American Journal of Public Health, 1971, 61, 606-611.

8 Eyer, J, Prosperity as a cause of death. International Journal of Health Services, 1977, 7, 125-150.

9 Brenner, M H, Health costs and benefits of economic policy. International Journal of Health Services, 1977, 7, 581-623.

10 Brenner, M H, Mortality and the national economy. A review and the experience of England and Wales 1936-76. Lancet 1979, 2, 568-573.

11 Bunn, A R, Ischaemic heart disease mortality and the business cycle in Australia. American Journal of Public Health 1979, 69, (8) 772-781.

12 Brenner, M H, US Congress, Joint Committee: Estimating the social costs of national economic policy: Implications for mental and physical health and criminal aggression. US Government Printing Office, Washington DC, 1976.

13 Unemployment and health (editorial). Journal of American Medical Association (JAMA) 1977, 237 (18), 1965.

14 Does Unemployment Kill? (editorial) Lancet, 1979, 1, 708-709.

15 Lew, E A, Mortality and the business cycle: how far can we push an association. American Journal of Public Health, 1979, 69, (8) 782-783.

16 Kasl, S V, Mortality and the business cycle: some questions about research strategies when utilising macro-social and ecological data. American Journal of Public Health 1979, 69 (8), 784-788.

17 Cobb, S, and Kasl S V, Termination. The consequences of job loss, DHEW (NIOSH) Publication no 77-244, Cincinnati, Ohio, 1977.

18 Cobb, S, Brooks, G W, Kasl, S V, and Connelly, W E, The health of people changing jobs: A description of a longitudinal study. American Journal of Public Health, 1966, 56, (9) 1476-1481.

19 Kasl, S V, Cobb, S, and Brooks, G W, Changes in serum uric acid and cholesterol levels in men undergoing job loss. Journal of American Medical Association (JMA) 1968, 206, (7) 1500, 1507.

20 Kasl, S V, and Cobb, S, Blood pressure changes in men undergoing job loss: A preliminary report. Psychosomatic Medicine, 1970, 32, (1), 18-38.

21 Cobb, S, Physiological changes in men whose jobs were abolished. Journal of Psychosomatic Research, 1974, 18, (4), 245-258.

22 Kasl, S V, Gore, S, and Cobb S, The experience of losing a job: Reported changes in health, symptoms, and illness behaviour. Psychosomatic Medicine 1975, 37, (2), 106-122.

23 Hypertonins sociala orsaker (Eng - Social Causes of Hypertension). Låkartidningen (Eng - Journal of Swedish Medical Society), 1977, 74, (45), pp. 3968-3970.

24 Erikssen, J, Rognum, T, and Jervell, J, Unemployment and health. Lancet, 1979, 1, 1189.

25 Stress i patogenesen av hypertoni (Eng = Stress in the pathogenesis of hypertension). Läkartidningen 1977, 74, (45), pp. 3963-3964.

26 Backlund, A, Företagsnedläggningars konsekvenser för personalen. Läget för de anställda vid Jössefors Bruk ca ett ar efter nedlägggningen. Delrapport 5: Specialstudie av de långtidsarbetslösa. Rapport nr 52 från PA-rådet. (Eng = Consequences for employees of company closures. The position for the employees at Jossefors Bruk about a year after closure. Interim report no. 5: Special study of long-term unemployment. Report no. 52 from the Swedish Council for Personnel Administration) Stockholm, 1973.

27 Andersson, I, Backhans, C, and Keisu, L, Foretagsned laggningars konsekvenser for personalen. Laget for de anstallda vid Jossefors Bruk ca ett ar efter nedlaggningen. Delrapport 7: Forandringar i individens sjalvuppfattning/ sjalvvardering vid en krissituation. Rapport nr 82 fran PA-radet (Eng = Consequences for employees of company closures. The position of employees at Jossefdors Bruk about a year after closure. Interim report no. 7: Changes in the individual's perception and evaluation of self during a crisis. Report no. 82 from PA-radet). Stockholm 1975.

28 Westin, S and Norum D, Nar sardinfabrikken nedlegges. En sosialmedisinsk undersokelse omkring arbeidsledighet i en Vestlandsbygd. Bergen 1977.

29 Klausen, H, and Iverson, L, Beskaeftigelsemaessige og helbredsmaessige konsekvenser af en virksomhedslukning. Socialmedicinsk Tidskrift. (Forthcoming).

30 Berglin, H, Fortidspension eller arbete? En studie av utveckling och regionala variationer. I Fortidspensionering. (Eng = Early retirement or Work? A study of development and regional variations. In 'Early retirement'). SOU 1977: 88. Stockholm 1977, pp. 7-102.

31 Dahlberg, L, Tack nasta (Eng - Next, Please). Ekonomisk Debatt 1975, 1, pp. 65-68.

32 Allander, B, Okar eller minskar pensioneringen vid reumatiska sjukdomar? (Eng = Does retirement increase or decline in rheumatic disorders?) Lakartidningen, 1973, 70, --. 3695-3697.

33 Dalhanm, T, and Lindgren, C, Sjukpensioneringen bland de kommunalanstallda i stockholms stad (Eng = Retirement due to illness among employees of the city of Stockholm). Nordisk Hygienisk Tidskrift 1958, 39, pp. 65-68.

34 Helander, E, Har vi fatt fri fortidspensionering? (Eng = Are there no longer any restraints on early retirement?). Lakartidningen, 1972, 69, pp. 3577-3583.

35 Klareskog, L, Smedby, B, and Ostenson, C-G, Fortidspensionerade i Tierp. Kort rapport fran Tierpsprojektet 5. (Eng = People granted early retirement in Tierp. Brief Report from the Tierp Project 5). National Board of Health and Welfare, Stockholm, 1977.

36 Kristenson, H, Kugelberg, G, and Medhus, A, Man med sjukbidrag och fortidspension. (Eng = Men with partial pensions due to illness and early retirement pensions). Lakartidningen 1977, 74, pp. 1837-1839.

37 Olson-Frick, H, Fortidspensionarernas situation. I Fortidspensionering. (Eng = The position of people with early retirement pensions. In 'Early Retirement'). SOU 1977: 80. Stockholm 1977.

38 Proje, J G, and Ekstrom, N A, Fortidspensionering eller arbete - svara avvagningsproblem vid hjart karlsjukdomar. (Eng = Early retirement or work - a complicated choice in cardiovascular disease). Socialmedicinska tidskrift, 1967, 44, pp. 190=198.

39 Westerlund, G, and Marke, S, De fortidspensionerades anpassningsproblem. En sociologisk undersokning inom SCA. (Eng = The adaptation problems of people with early retirement pensions. A sociological study in SCA).

40 Ålderdomskommittén: I Betänkande och förslag angående allmän pensionsförsäkring. (Eng = Committee on the aged. In reports and proposals on general pension insurance). Stockholm 1912.

41 Roebuck, J, When does old age begin? Journal of Social History 1979, 12, (3), 416-428.

42 Ungdomens problem på arbetsmarknaden. Rapport från ett symposium i Lerum den 20-28 Oktober 1976 under redaktion av Inga Hellberg. Monografier utgivna av Sociologiskia Institutionen vid Göteborgs universitet. Nr 11. (Eng = The problems of young people on the labour market. Report from a symposium in Lerum 20-28 October 1976. Edited by Inga Hellberg. Monographs published by the Department of Sociology, University of Göteborg. no. 11). Göteborg 1977.

43 Kannas, L, and Hietarharju, M, Työttömistä Nourista sairaita keski-ikäisiä. Sosiaalinen aikakauskirja 1979, 1, 37-45.

44 Kitagawa, E M, On mortality. Demography 1977, 14, 381-389.

45 Occupational mortality. The Registrar Generals Decenial Supplement for England and Wales 1979-72. London 1978.

46 Dahlgren, K G, On death rates and causes of death in alcohol addicts. Acta Psyciatrica Scandinavia 1951, 26, 297-311.

47 Uppföljningsstatistik inom nykterhetsväsendet 1971-1976. (Eng = Follow-up statistics on programmes for the care of alcoholics from 1971-1976). SCB, Stockholm 1977, SM:S 1977:34.

48 Syme, S L, and Berkman, L F, Social Class, susceptibility and sickness. American Journal of Epidemiology, 1976, 104, (1), 1-8.

49 Kompendium om låginkomstutredningen. (Eng = Compendium on the Commission on low incomes). Stockholm 1973.

50 Dublin, L I, and Bunzel, B, To be or not to be, New York, 1933.

51 Henry, A F, and Short, F, Jr, Suicide and homicide, New York, 1954.

52 Sainsbury, P, Suicide in London, London 1955.

53 MacMahon, B, Johnson, S, and Pugh T F, Relation of suicide rates to social conditions. Public Health Reports 1963, 78, 285-293.

54 Walbran, B, MacMahon, B, and Bailey A E, Suicide and unemployment in Pennsylvania, 1954-1961. Archives of Environmental Health 1965, 10, 11-15.

55 Wallis, C P and Maliphand, R, Delinquent areas in the county of London. Ecological factors. British Journal of Criminology, 1967, 7, 250.

56 Pierce, A, The economic cycle and the social suicide rate. American Sociological Review, 1967, 32, 457-462.

57 Whitlock, E A, and Schapira, A, Attempted suicide in Newcastle upon Tyne. British Journal of Psychiatry, 1967, 113.

58 Tuckman, J, and Youngman W, Scale for Assessing suicide risk of attempted suicide. Journal of Clinical Psychology, 1968, 24, 17-19.

59 Lester, D, Suicide and unemployment. Archives of Environmental Health, 1970, 20, 277-278.

60 Begley, C, Jacobson, S, and Palmer, C, Social structure and the ecological distribution of mental illness, suicide and delinquency. Psychological Medicine, 1973, 3, 177.

61 Hjortsjö, T, Suicider och konjunkturer. (Eng = Suicides and the state of the economy). Communicatons from the Department of Anatomy no. 13, Lund 1973.

62 Hamermesh, D S, and Soss, N M, An economic theory of suicide. Journal of Political Economy, 1974, January-February 83-98.

63 Buglass, D, and Duffy, J C, The ecological pattern of suicide and parasuicide in Edinburgh. Social Science and Medicine, 1978, 12, 241-253.

64 Vigderhous, G, and Fishman G, The impact of unemployment and familial integration on changing suicide rates in the USA 1920-1969. Social Psychiatry, 1978, 13, (4), 239-248.

65 Tausky, C, and Piedmont, E B, The meaning of work and unemployment: Implications for mental health. International Journal of Social Psychiatry 1967/68, 14, (1) 44-59.

66 Brenner, M H, Unemployment, economic growth, and mortality. The Lancet, 1979, 1, 672.

67 Morse, N C, and Weiss, R S, The function and meaning of work and the job. American Sociological Review, 1955, 20, 191-198.

68 Palmore, E, The relative importance of social factors in predicting longevity. In Palmore, E (ed) Prediction of Life Span. Massachusetts, 1971.

69 Lindgren, G, and Linder V, Arbetslöshet - ohälsa. Synpunkter och erfarenheter bland distriktpersonalen inom Lycksele sjukvårdsdistrikt. (Eng = Unemployment - ill health. Views and experience of district medical staff in Lycksele Public Health Distirct). Umeå University. Halso- och sjukvårdsadministration. 1978, Mimeo.

70 Draper, P O A, Micro-processors, macro-economic policy, and public health, Lancet, 1979, 1, 373-375.

71 Draper, P O A, Unemployment and Health, Lancet, 1979, 1, 558.

72 Loraine, J A, Unemployment and Health, Lancet, 1979, 1, 558.

73 Scott-Samuel, A, Unemployment and Health, Lancet, 1979, 1, 498.

74 Jobling, R G, Unemployment and Health, Lancet 1979, 1, 1189.

RECESSION AND HEALTH - A LITERATURE REVIEW

Stephen Watkins

SCIENCE AND POLICY

Scientists, especially social scientists, often complain that decision makers, especially politicians, pay inadequate attention to scientific findings which are relevant to policy. Unfortunately, styles of scientific discourse are not such as to fit easily into the decision making machinery. Decision makers seek scientific facts, whereas science deals predominantly in uncertainties, and scientific method attaches considerable importance to scepticism.

Many scientists carry their legitimate academic scepticism into the decision making machinery, thereby leaving the politicians with the view that nothing ever seems to be proved and that all scientists ever seem to recommend is more research. To those who wish to prevent change a recommendation for more research is a godsend. Other scientists apply their scientific knowledge to the polemic of politics, marshalling the scientific arguments in favour of the political position to which they subscribe. Such scientists are popular with the politicians to whom they give support, but not with their scientific colleagues. Since their advice tends to conflate their scientific conclusions with the value judgements which lead them on to political conclusions, their approach tends to turn political disagreements, which the decision making machinery can handle, into scientific disagreements, which it can't handle at all well.

If we understand that decisions must often be made in conditions of uncertainty, and should not always await the final settlement of every niggling academic doubt, it should be possible to devise a method of conveying to decision makers the best possible conclusion and the degree of uncertainty attached to it.

I propose the following definitions, which I shall use in this paper, but which I think could have a much wider use:

"almost certain" — the evidence is extremely strong. There are a few doubts, but if the doubts proved true we would need to restructure a number of well established theoretical frameworks. Decision makers should accept this conclusion as true.

"highly probable" — the evidence is extremely strong, but there are a few niggling doubts which are not incompatible with established theoretical frameworks. Decision makers should accept this conclusion as true, but keep at the back of their mind the possibility that it may be disproved.

"probable" — the evidence is strong, but there are quite definite doubts. It is safer to regard the conclusion as true, but caution should be demonstrated when major expenditure or major policy changes are required. In such circumstances a decision should be deferred if no harm is thereby caused. However if consequences of deferring a decision are as great as consequences of making one, this conclusion should be used as the basis for the decisons.

"highly plausible"	the best explanation available for the data, but derived mainly from theoretical frameworks with rather limited evidence. Has the same implications for the decision maker as "probable".
"plausible"	evidence is suggestive, but far from strong. The decision maker should work on the assumption that to accept or reject this conclusion is equally likely to be wrong. The decision to take is the one which has the most beneficial consequences if right and the least harmful consequences if wrong, and any decison made should be reviewed in the light of further research developments.
"possible"	this point of view could be right but the evidence is against it, although far from strong. Decisions should not be made on the basis of this suggestion, except where major harm can be averted by very minor precautions. This is the reverse of "probable" or "highly plausible".
"unlikely"	this is the reverse of "highly probable". For decision making purposes it should be regarded as untrue.
"highly unlikely"	this is the reverse of "almost certain". For decision making purposes it should be regarded as untrue.

I suspect that if scientists are compelled to draw conclusions rather than merely describe doubts, and to fit their conclusions into the above framework, scientific disagreement in policy related areas will be easier to cope with. I suspect, for example, that much of the heated debate abut occupational hazards turns on the company's scientific adviser using the category "plausible" and combining it with value judgements which attach a high premium to undisturbed production, whilst the scientific advisers of the workforce have used the category "highly plausible" and combined it with value judgements which attach a high premium to the health of workers. If it was appreciated that the scentific disagreement is quite limited, political and collective bargaining machineries would find it easier to digest the value conflicts which actually underlie the debate.

In this paper I shall follow the approach which I have advocated above. I shall first review the literature on recession and health critically, with the intention of seeing what conclusions can be drawn and with what degree of certainty. I shall then set out those conclusions using the definitions which I have proposed above.

In Chapter 16 I shall contribute to the discussion of the policies which flow from those conclusions. There is considerable debate as to the extent to which scientists should contribute to political discussion. This is especially true of doctors since their legitimation as medical advisers rests upon the presumed impartiality of their advice. Scientific integrity demands that scientific and political contributions to debate should not be conflated. But often the best contribution that can be made to debate is made by combining the two. They can be combined without being conflated. This conflict has always faced public health doctors who must weigh the advantages of campaigning against the disadvantage of being labelled a campaigner.

THE EVIDENCE

Does recession cause ill health?

We know that economically developed countries are healthier than they were when they were less developed and are healthier than the developing countries of today. We also know that within economically developed countries the richer sections of the community enjoy better health than the poorer sections (Black Report 1980). It would therefore be plausible, even without any evidence at all, to conclude that temporary disturbances in economic success will harm health. On the other hand we know that about 20 000 deaths a year in the United Kingdom are probably occupational (Fox and Adelstein 1978) and that there are a wide range of occupational hazards (Kinnersley 1973; Stellman and Daum 1971), so it would also be plausible, if we had no evidence, to suppose that to reduce industrial activity would improve health.

The earliest analysis of the effects of recession and health, by Thomas (1925) seemed to bear out the hypothesis that recessions improved health. Since this seems anomalous in view of the beneficial effects of economic growth on health it became referred to as the "Thomas anomaly".

Thomas's findings need only be anomalous if it is presumed that industry is good for people. Reverse that proposition (for the sake of argument) so that industry is considered to be bad and the following proposition emerges. In the 18th and early 19th centuries, the Agricultural Revolution achieved substantial improvements in health, but these were overwhelmed by the damage to health caused by industrialisation and urbanisation. As the productive capacity of industry increased, some of that potential growth was diverted by social reformers and by the growing strength of the trade union movement into controls on environmental and working conditions. At the same time the public health movement was beginning to correct the most harmful consequences of urbanisation. As the health damage caused by industry was controlled the underlying health improvement produced by the Agricultural Revolution was able to express itself. Since industry was able to concede improvements in environmental and working conditions only as a consequence of increasing productive capacity and since that same increasing capacity was also used to increase production, the unveiling of these health benefits went hand in hand with industrial growth and came to be ascribed to it. However, the true relationship can be seen in recession when the fall in industrial activity revealed the health benefits, even though industrial growth fell.

The indicator used by most investigators has been the unemployment rate. This has led to the assumption that unemployment mediates the health effects of recession. That assumption need not be true, and the question of whether unemployment is good for people is a different question from the question of whether the unemployment rate, as an indicator of recession, is associated with improvements or deterioration in health. Unemployment could be bad for people and yet the unemployment rate could still be associated with improved health if recession improved the health of the rest of the community and this outweighed the harm caused by unemployment. Conversely unemployment could be good for health and yet the unemployment rate could be associated with deteriorating health in the community if recession damaged the health of the rest of the community and this outweighed the benefit to the unemployed. This distinction is widely ignored and yet it is fundamental to understanding this literature.

Eyer (1977) carried the work of Thomas forward to 1977 with a graphical presentation purporting to show that the Thomas anomaly was still present and that recession still improved health. He also showed that flu epidemics occurred at the peak of economic booms. Later that year he published a paper (Eyer 1977) which attempted to estimate the contribution of a number of factors to the Thomas effect. He suggested that housing and nutrition accounted for about 10%, drug consumption about one sixth, alcohol about 11%, smoking about 6% and social relationships about 72%. "Social relationships" included marriage (2%), migration (9%), strikes, seen as good for health because of the social solidarity induced (17%), overwork (34%), divorces and separation (8%) and unemployment (1%).

At first sight Eyer's work is convincing, not least because it is easier to understand than the complicated statistical techniques of Brenner. But on closer examination the argument doesn't hold. The graphical presentation is convincing mainly because it is such a good fit in the late 19th and early 20th century that the eye fits the rest of the graph to that pattern. But if the period before 1950 is covered up the graph looks totally unconvincing.

An analysis of consecutive five year periods suggests that the Thomas effect dominated the effects of recession on health until the second quarter of this century, but sometime in the second quarter of the century it disappeared.

This is also borne out by the data Eyer presents on flu epidemics.

Postwar they are as follows:

Peak of boom: 1948 1953 1956 1959 1966 1969 1973

Flu epidemic: 1951-53 1957 1960 1963 1966 1968 1972-73

Prewar they are:

Peak of boom: 1902-03 1906 1909 1913 1918-19 1923 1926 1929 1937 1943

Flu epidemic: 1904 1907 1910 1913 1918 1923 1926 1929 1936 1943

The prewar series is convincing. The postwar series is not.

Figure 1: Total Death Rate and Unemployment Rate in the United States 1870-1975

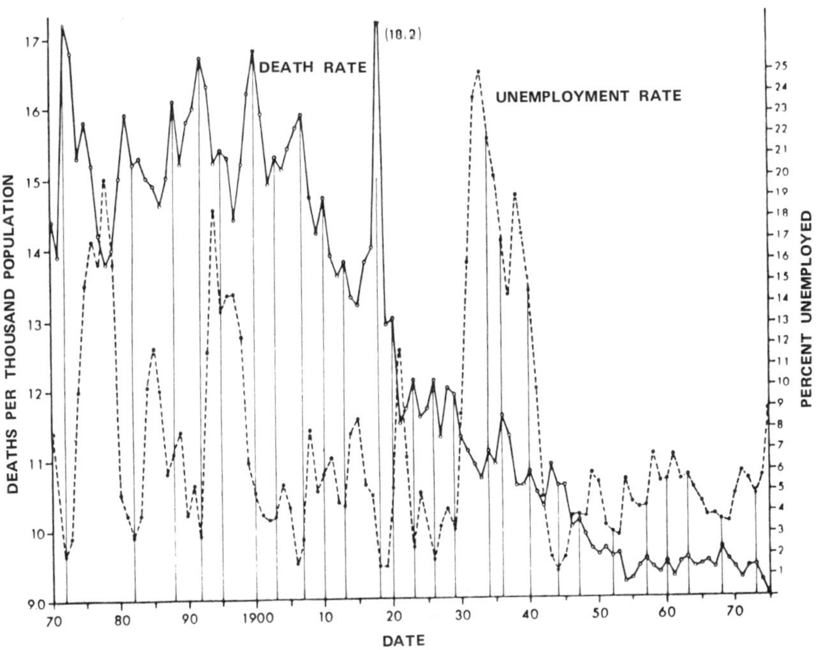

Reprinted from International Journal of Health Services, (1977), vol. 7 no. 1, p. 126

The paradigm which I previously used to explain the Thomas effect can also be used to explain its disappearance. The process of increasing trade union power and increasing social control of industry would continue until the point was reached at which industry was compatible with human health, and became, on balance, no longer harmful. The phrase "on balance" must be stressed because industry undoubtedly has both beneficial and harmful effects.

For industrialists, this is a reassuring explanation, suggesting that, however much harm their predecessors did, industry today is no longer, on balance, health damaging.

However, there is an alternative explanation for the disappearance of the Thomas effect. Since the war, we have seen a decline in the importance of the industrial sector and a growth in the service sector. The majority of the working population are now employed outside the industrial sector. Between 1921 and 1971, the proportion of males employed in non-manual occupations increased from 21 to 31% (Rimmer and Popay 1982).

It should perhaps be stated that the paradigm whih I have used to explain the Thomas effect and its disappearance is an idealised, theoretical and absurd paradigm. In fact, the increased population could not have been housed without expansion of the construction industry and its suppliers, clothed without expansion of the textile industry, supplied with food without expansion of the transport industry, kept warm without expansion of the mining industry, provided with sewers, water and essential domestic supplies without an engineering industry, and brought to full realisation of these health benefits without the manufacture of scientific or medical equipment. It is almost certain that industry, directed to meeting social needs, and with controlled working conditions and environmental effects is beneficial to health. Equally it is almost certain that unrestrained industrial growth in poor working conditions, without environmental control is bad for health. It is highly probable that industry has done more good than harm to health, but <u>at the margin</u> it is highly probable that up to and including the first quarter of this century industrial growth had an adverse effect on health. It is plausible that this is no longer the case due to improved working conditions and greater social control, but it is equally plausible that it is still the case but no longer affects aggregate statistics because industry has ceased to dominate the economy.

These conclusions are of considerable importance to Third World countries who may be considered repeating Western models of unrestrained industrialisation. They may be of importance to Western countries who are considering solving economic problems by relaxing social controls on industry or weakening trade unions.

If the Thomas effect no longer governs the relationship of recession to health, has another relationship taken its place?

This question brings us to the work of Brenner. Brenner's earlier work consisted of an attempt to relate recession to various health problems, including heart disease (Brenner 1971), mental illness (Brenner 1973), aggression and criminality (Brenner 1976), infant and foetal mortality (Brenner 1973b) and overall mortality (Brenner 1976 and Brenner 1977). The unemployment and mortality data were detrended as described in Chapter 1.

In case of mental illness, hospital admissions were used instead of mortality.

In each case Brenner found that the detrended mortality data correlated with the detrended unemployment data so that recession seemed to be associated with deteriorations in health.

In the case of mental illness, this occurred even with unlagged data. In the case of heart disese, however, unemployment rate correlated with the health data of a later year. The optimum lag was determined by a process called Fourier analysis which chooses the lag period that produces the best correlation.

In the case of infant mortality, a lag of one year was used for infant mortality under one day, but a lag of five years was used for postneonatal mortality. This implies that postneonatal mortality is affected by economic conditions before the child was even conceived, presumably through delayed effects on parental health or family stress or family economic conditions.

Winter (1983) attempted to replicate Brenner's work on infant mortality. He concluded that unemployment was not the major factor affecting infant mortality. He did in fact find the Brenner effect for perinatal mortality, but not for infant mortality. He argued unconvincingly that infant mortality ought to have been affected more than perinatal mortality so that his results really refuted Brenner. However, there is another explanation for his findings. Over the period concerned infant mortality fell sharply. It is unlikely that this would have consisted of a steady fall, so that detrended data would have consisted partly of variation around the trend, and partly of variation of the trend from its own regression line. If the latter outweighed the former, then the Brenner effect would be drowned. Perinatal mortality declined much less, and this effect would be much less obvious. It is not surprising therefore that Winter found the Brenner Effect only for perinatal mortality. Probably that is all Brenner actually found as well the 5 year lag on postneonatal mortality seems artificial and odd and was probably a statistical artefact. Winter is undoubtedly right that recession was not the main factor in infant and perinatal mortality. However, when the main factors are peeled away the Brenner effect can be found underneath.

Stokes reported a replication of Brenner's work on mental hospital admissions using data for England and Wales between 1950 and 1978. Using similar techniques he regressed the rate of first admissions to mental hospitals for England and Wales on the long term trend of economic growth, as the annual change in the rate of growth in real per capita income, the residual from the long term economic growth rate, the rate of unemployment, government expenditure on welfare as a percentage of all current expenditure (UK), and dummy variables to control for changes in recording mental hospital admissions. Using UK unemployment data he found a significantlypositive relationship for both sexes, for all age groups combined between 20 and 64, and for most age groups separately at zero lag. Few correlations reached statistical significance when unemployment data for England and Wales were used (Stokes, 1981, and Stokes and Cochrane 1982).

The work on heart disease was reproduced with Australian data by Bunn (1979), who also used GP prescriptions as a measure of national morbidity. Drug prescribing increased 18 months after a change in unemployment. This compares with a 2 year lag found by Brenner in New York.

Brenner also applied the same methodology to alcohol consumption and alcohol related diseases (Brenner 1979). The long term trend was to an increase in alcohol consumption per capita with rises in personal income. The short term fluctuations showed a rise in alcohol consumption and death rates from cirrhosis of the liver within months of an economic downturn. The long term trends affected wine, beer and spirits. The short term trends affected only spirits.

This whole methodology was heavily criticised by Kasl (1979) and polemically attacked by Lew (1979). Kasl criticised the failure to account for changes in diagnostic criteria (at first sight an obvious criticism, but surely they are accounted for by detrending), the arbitrary nature of the lag structure, the possibility of intervening variables (eg a new treatment affecting case fatality) and the fact that if we do not understand secular trends we don't know what the residual variable actually represents. He supports his criticisms by citing previous work by other researchers using similar methodology which had produced ridiculous results, such as a negative correlation of ischaemic heart disease with flour consumption, and another study which correlated IHD mortality negatively with milk consumption at one year and positively at nine years lag. Eyer (1977) also criticised the lag structure, saying that the correct approach was to select the lag before the study from knowledge of the natural history of the disease. He argued that for ischaemic heart disease the lag should be zero, since the study by Kasl, Cobb and Gore (1972) and Kasl, Cobb and Brooks (1968) had shown risk factors to respond immediately to stress. The argument is valid, but the application is ridiculous since risk factors and clinical occurrence are quite different. Moreover Brenner's lags seem on the whole to be compatible with what is known of the natural history of the diseases concerned, and it would be unusual for the natural history to be so precise as to permit preselection of the lag.

John (1983) attempted to reproduce Brenner's work in Germany, but failed to do so. He ascribed this failure to the position of immigrant workers who return home in recession, thereby exporting the health damage to Turkey and also making unemployment rate a poor indicator of recession.

Having demonstrated the correlation between recession and health, Brenner moved on to an attempt to model it econometrically. His first step in that direction was an attempt to estimate the health costs of a 1% rise in American unemployment sustained for 5 years(Brenner 1977).

In 1979 he produced a model of the effect of economic variables on the health of England and Wales from 1936 to 1976 (Brenner 1979).

This model had four main components which contributed to mortality as follows:

a) the smooth exponential trend of long term economic growth measured by real per capita income was associated with a decline in mortality.

b) recession, measured by unemployment rate, was positively associated with mortality.

c) certain indicators of rapid economic growth had a weak association with mortality.

d) government expenditure on welfare as a percentage of total government expenditure was associated with a decline in mortality for infants and young children.

Gravelle, Hutchinson and Stern (1981) criticised the selection of some of these indicators. For example, they thought that GDP per capita was a better measure than personal disposable income. They also criticised the unemployment series which he had used since it excluded the uninsured population.

Much more seriously they demonstrated that the model which he had devised for the period 1936-76 failed to predict satisfactorily for the periods 1922-76, 1922-51 or 1952-76. Using the Chow test, which is a test of the structural stability of models, the principle of which is that the period is divided into two and the model's performance is compared over the two periods, they found that the hypothesis of structural stability was rejected. Re-estimating the model for the period 1936-70, they found that it failed to predict for the period 1970-78.

Finally, they discovered that if certain arbitrary restrictions on the lag structure were removed the model produced quite different results.

Brenner's reply was to argue that his model was not intended to be applicable to periods that include the Great Depression or start after the war. This is a weak response to well substantiated evidence of structural instbility. He did however, point out that the relationship could be found in any four year period between 1922-76 (Brenner 1981).

Brenner's latest model (1983), produced in 1981, is confined to the post war period. The trends found in his earlier models are confirmed, and there are also some new findings about the effects of random changes, such as severe winters or the oil crisis, and about the effects of changes in consumption habits. A separate analysis has been produced for cardiovascular mortality (See Chapter 6)

The latest model also uses age/sex specific unemployment rates, the importance of which have been highlighted by Forbes (1981).

Sogaard (1983) produced a model to explore the hypothesis that changes in patterns of consumption mediated the health damage caused by recession. His model showed that for respiratory diseases in Denmark most, but not all, of the change was statistically explicable by changes in cigarette consumption. This was also true of infant mortality. The changes in cigarette consumption were associated with changes in unemployment. Accident mortality was negatively associated with unemployment, growth and alcohol consumption. Suicide mortality was positively associated with growth, unemployment and divorce rates.

With heart disease mortality there was a direct positive association of growth with mortality, statistically explicable by changes in cigarette and alcohol consumption. Unemployment had a positive effect in short term cycles, but a negative long term effect statistically explicable by its associations with alcohol consumption.

Brenner has more recently (1982) shown that the insertion into his model of certain indices of urbanisation strengthen the model. Although he argues that this can help us decide the precise factors which contribute to the health effects of recession, I do not accept this argument.

The indices which Brenner is using are conventional indices of recession, like unemployment rate, but with a different time relationship. Brenner is therefore inserting lagging and leading indices of the same phenomena into his model. The extra index can therefore be seen as composed of the original index plus a function which represents the difference between the two. It is only this "difference" function which is new.

Assuming that the underlying phenomenon was cyclic and that the lagging and leading indices both perfect, this additional function would be shown by the following diagram:

Figure 2: Effect of including leading and lagging indices

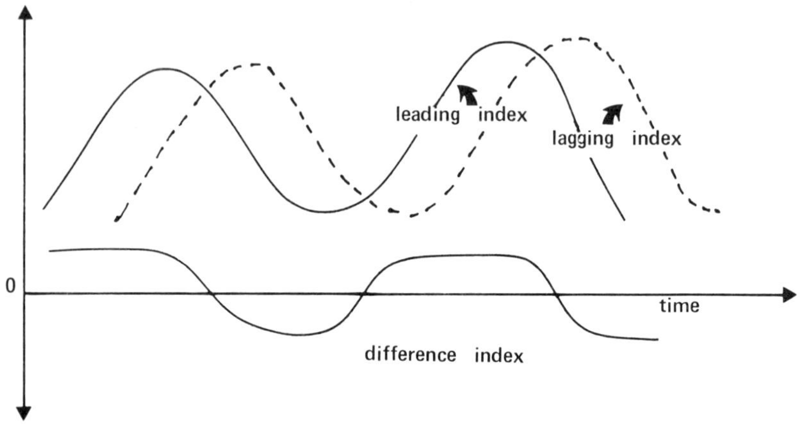

What is therefore being inserted into the model is a function which is positive and constant in terms of boom, negative and constant in terms of recession, and which falls or rises sharply at the points inflection.

If such a function strengthens the model it implies only that there is a correlation with the trend of economic activity rather than with its actual state.

This is perhaps the place at which to discuss the role of econometric analysis in epidemiology. Epidemiological analysis has three stages.

At the first stage significant associations are noted between health indices in the population and factors which may influence health. Such associations cannot be inferred to be causal. If A is associated with B it may be because A causes B, or because B causes A, or because there is a mutual causal link between A and B, or because A and B are both caused by a third factor. When an association is demonstrated it is therefore necessary to devise and test hypotheses to explain the association. Some hypotheses can be excluded at this stage because other associations predictable from them do not prove to be present (for example, the hypothesis that cigarette smoking mediates the relationship between recession and respiratory disease could have been rejected if Sogaard's model had not shown it to explain the relationship statistically). However, no hypothesis can be proved at this stage because associations can never be used to imply causality.

The second stage is to test the hypotheses with epidemiological studies of the retrospective, prospective and intervention types. It is at this stage that causality can be inferred.

The third stage is to measure the risk. Traditionally, this is done either by relative risk (rate in those exposed divided by rate in those unexposed), the former measuring the strength of the contribution to the cause of the disease and the latter measuring the health burden to the community.

Econometric analysis has its place at the first and third stages. There are, however, serious dangers in using econometric analysis before causal relationships have been worked out, except as a way of generating hypotheses. The danger is that considerable reliance may come to be placed on a variable which is a proxy for some other variable (not included in the model) to which it is associated. If there is subsequently a change in the nature of the association between the proxy variable and the real variable, the model will cease to be predictive. Such a change may occur without any intervention. However, the real danger is that it will occur when policy interventions are based on the proxy. A clinical example would be that blood urea ceases to be a measure of renal function when uraemia is treated by a low protein diet. An economic example would be that any measure of money supply ceases to be valid when it is used as an instrument of monetary policy, because there is an artificial constraint on the forms of money included in the measure and a compensatory growth in the forms which are not.

So what are we left with? We are left with the associations between recession and health convincingly demonstrated by Brenner's early work. We are also left with a number of unsatisfactory econometric models, which demonstrate only the difficulty of modelling when it is not known what the variables actually represent in terms of causal relationships. It would be a mistake to believe that the defects of Brenner's more complex models discredit his simpler and earlier work. That work stands undisturbed and it is highly probable that recession causes ill health.

Why does recession cause ill health?

The following hypotheses would explain the relationship:

1. Unemployment causes ill health. I will review the evidence for this hypothesis in the next section and will conclude that unemployment almost certainly causes mental ill health and highly probably causes physical ill health.

2. Fear of unemployment causes ill health. Studies of factory closures, which I will review in the next section, show that health starts to suffer in the run up to closure. We also know that fear of unemployment is widespread. Rimmer and Popay point out (Rimmer and Popay 1982), that between June and September 1980, Gallup recorded an increase from 27% to 38% in the proportion of people who thought their own jobs were under threat. Combining these two findings, it is highly plausible that this factor contributes to the health damage of recession.

3. Recession causes stress which causes ill health. Anecdotally it can be seen that many areas of life become more difficult in recession. Does this cause enough stress to account for a significant part of the health damage of recession? Catalano and Dooley (1983), showed that the chance of suffering an "economic life event" increased in recession, and that, controlling for socio economic and demographic characteristics and for non-economic non-illness events, respondents who experience economic life events will be at greater risk of illness or injury than those who do not. It is plausible that this factor contributes to the health damage of recession.

4. Recession causes deteriorating working conditions which cause ill health. This is highly plausible, but I have been unable to trace any research.

5. Recession causes poverty. So far as the poverty of unemployment is conerned this is one explanation of the health damage caused by unemployment. I will review that question with the literature on unemployment. So far as poverty in the general population is concerned, Stern (1981), points out that living standards only suffer at the depth of recession and may indeed rise, for people in work, for much of the recession. It is therefore unlikely that this factor is important, although it is possible that there may be effects for people who are dependent on deteriorating public services.

6. Recession causes changes in consumption patterns which cause ill health. This is plausible, especially in view of Sogaard's work.

7. Recession causes changes in personal lives which damage health. We know that social support is important to health (Boman 1979; Berkman and Syme 1979; Nuckolls, Cassel and Kaplan 1972; Brown and Harris 1978) and we know that recession causes changes in personal lives (Rimmer and Popay 1982; Hakim 1982) so this is plausible.

Does unemployment damage health?

We have already seen that there is an association of unemployment rate with ill health in time series data, but that unemployment rate is such a good indicator of recession that this association merely demonstrates a relationship between recession and ill health.

There are also associations of ill health with unemployment in geographical studies. Morris and Titmuss (1944) selected 83 county boroughs in England and Wales and grouped them into ten categories based on their 1927-29 level of unemployment and subsequent experiences of unemployment from 1930 to 1938. The twelve years from 1927 to 1938 were then divided into four triennial parts. There was a high correlation between unemployment and rheumatic heart disease rates and there was also a correlation between changes in unemployment rates and changes in mortality due to rheumatic heart disease. The association was strengthened when a mortality lag of three years was introduced.

Gardner, Crawford and Morris (1963) found a strong correlation between unemployment and deaths from cardiovascular disease, bronchitis, lung cancer and cancer of the stomach in middle aged men in sixty one county boroughs in England and Wales. However, similar correlations were found with other socio economic indices such as proportion of the population in low social class and income groups and low rates of car ownership. Indeed these indices were so highly intercorrelated that they were combined into a single index.

Dean and James (1980) showed that the distribution of male first admissions and readmissions for depression in the wards of Plymouth correlated with unemployment rates in the wards. However, there was again a strong inter-correlation with other socioeconomic indices.

Brennan and Lancashire (1978) showed an association between childhood mortality up to the age of four and unemployment rate in another study of county boroughs. The relationship was not found for older children and again there were similar relationships for other socioeconomic factors.

Colledge and Kingham (1983) showed an association between unemployment rates and ill health in the wards of North Tyneside.

All of these studies are open to the alternative explanation that they are demonstrating not the effects of unemployment but the effects of multiple deprivation.

Another approach is to ask what we know about unemployment and what we can infer by combining that knowledge with our knowledge of the health consequences of particular components of this status.

As I have said elsewhere (Watkins 1982) "We know that poverty is damaging to health and that the unemployed are poor. We know that life changes damage health until the individual readjusts and we know that losing your job is a life change and that you are not supposed to adjust to worklessness. We know that social networks are important to health and that the unemployed lose the social network of work and also that they withdraw from other social actions because of stigma and lack of money.

'In order to arrange that unemployment does not damage health, one would have to postulate some beneficial effects of unemployment to outweigh these damaging aspects. The postulated benefit would presumably be absence from the damaging health effects of work. Thus, if it were found that unemployment did not damage health that would be an even greater challenge to our social organisation, suggesting that work damages health even more than being poor, stigmatised and lonely. The Ecology Party could have a field day."

Hakim (1982), points out that 2% of unemployed men had been evicted, threatened with eviction or forced to sell their homes. She cites Smith (1981) as showing that 9% of white unemployed men and 5% of ethnic minority unemployed men had had gas or electricity supplies cut off or goods on hire purchase repossessed or court action over debts, 42% of West Indian, 36% of Asian, and 25% of whites had failed to make payments on rent, mortgages or rates. Rimmer and Popay (1982), review the effects of income loss on the unemployed and conclude that it falls particularly harshly on large families. The Child Poverty Action Group have pointed out the inadequacy of unemployment benefit for the upbringing of children. Sinfield (1970), found significant levels of poverty in his sample. Unemployment seems therefore, to produce genuine poverty and it is highly probable that this will cause the usual health problems associated with poverty.

Hakim (1982) cites Thomas and Collard (1970) and Colledge and Bartholomew (1980), as showing unemployment causes divorce. Stokes (1981) has shown that unemployment is a cause of family tension and Rimmer and Popay (1982) point out that there is also anecdotal evidence to that effect from organisations working in the field. We know of the importance of social support to health (Boman 1979; Berkman & Syme 1979; Nuckolls, Cassell & Kaplan 1972; Brown & Harris 1978), (the standardised mortality ratio (SMR) was 138 for males divorced and 94 for married men, 103 for divorced women and 92 for married women). It is reasonable to infer that unemployment will damage health through this mechanism.

Jahoda (1979) infers the health damage of unemployment from the health benefits of work, pointing out that work provides a sense of identity, a sense of purpose to life, time structuring of the day and the week and social interaction.

Shepherd (1981) draws conclusions about the benefits of work from the literature of psychotherapy. He cites Garfield (1978) as showing that being out of work is widely accepted as indicating a poor prognosis for treatment and cites Wing and Brown (1970) and Vaughan and Leff (1976) as showing the danger of inactivity for chronic psychotic patients, a finding which he suggests can be extrapolated to the rest of the population, although this may, of course, not be a valid inference. Gurney (1980), showed that finding a job led to significant psychosocial development in school leavers.

Clearly there is value in such indirect evidence but it is no substitute for direct evidence. The largest source of such evidence is the literature of the 1930s. Eisenberg and Lazarsfeld in 1938 reviewed 112 references (Eisenberg and Lazarsfeld 1938). This included the classical Marienthal study (Jahoda, Lazarsfeld & Zeisel 1933). This literature cleary documents the psychological and physical impact of unemployment on health.

However, the relevance of this literature to the modern day situation has been questioned by Gurney and Taylor (1981), and more significantly perhaps, by Jahoda (1979), herself one of the Marienthal researchers. The argument is that unemployment today is different in a number of ways. On the one hand the degree of poverty and stigma are both reduced. On the other hand expectations are greater and social solidarity in working class communities has declined. Before leaving the literature of this period, however, we must not overlook the comment by Lane (1978), reminiscing on a lifetime of occupational medicine, that the greatest problem faced by the newly established employment rehabilitation services of the 1940s was to correct the psychological damage to those who had suffered long term unemployment in the 1930s. Amidst all the other pressures of that time (the rehabilitation of TB victims and war casualties for example) this problem of the damaged unemployed registered with him sufficiently to mention in a valedictory address over 30 years later.

The modern literature may perhaps best be looked at in the classical epidemiological categories of retrospective studies, prospective studies, and clinical case studies.

Retrospective studies

In addition to studies on suicide and para suicide (see chapter 3), Hakim (1982) cites White as showing a greater incidence of truancy, reading problems, missing school due to health problems and referral to educational psychologists in the children of unemployed parents.

Cochrane and Stopes Roe (1981) studied a number of sociodemographic variables for their influence on psychological symptom levels in a sample of 232 people living in English cities. Sex, employment, education and social class related to symptom levels, but, age, marital status, social mobility and household crowding were not.

Carr Saunders, in a case/control study in the 1950s found an association between unemployment and delinquency (1959).

Birt (1983), has described a case/control study of the effect of unemployment on physical health, measured by hospital admissions, which is currently under way in Stockport, but for which no results are yet available.

Prospective studies

One of the most obvious ideas for studying the health effects of unemployment is to follow up a cohort of people made unemployed by the closure of a factory and compare them with a control cohort. A number of such studies have been done, of which the best known are the Kasl and Cobb studies (Cobb et al 1968; Kasl and Cobb 1969; Kasl, Cobb and Gore 1972; Kasl, Cobb and Brooks 1968).

In these studies workers from two plants which were closing were compared with a control group drawn from plants which were not closing. The subjects were interviewed before closure, shortly after closure, and 4, 8, 12 and 24 months later. Data was collected partly by structured interview, partly by a health diary maintained by the subject and partly by blood and urine specimens collected by a nurse.

Anticipation of the shutdown was associated with elevated uric acid levels, but normal cholesterol levels, and an increased rate of symptom reporting. After the closure the uric acid remained high, the cholesterol rose also, but there was a drop in symptom reporting. Uric acid and cholesterol remained high until the subject found alternative employment. Those who were still unemployed at the third, fourth and fifth visits showed high levels of symptom reporting again. A similar cycle of changes in blood pressure was observed.

A number of other such studies have been reported (Westin & Norun 1977; Iversen & Glausen 1981; Dept of Employment 1970; Ziegler 1979; Bungener & Horellou Lafarge 1979) all of which show health damage following the closure and poor health in those who remain chronically unemployed. The study of the Nordhaven shipyard (Iversen & Glausen 1981), found worse psychological health. However, it also found improvements in bronchitis, heart trouble and tiredness.

Olsen and Sabroe (1979), found the health of retired members of the Danish carpenter/cabinet makers' trade union to be better than that of non retired members (SMR 82 for non retired members and 70 for retired members).

Stokes (1981) followed up a cohort of unemployed workers in Bradford and found increases in family quarrels and in levels of distress and a decline in social activity.

Owens (1966) found that absence and certified sickness was higher and of longer duration amongst a group of British Rail workers about to be made redundant compared to a group of secure workers.

Parnes and King (1977), followed a cohort of middle aged men for seven years during which time, some of them lost their jobs and others didn't. Those who lost their jobs showed some deterioration in health.

Schlozman and Verba (1978), followed a group of unemployed men to ask the question "Does the new unemployment hurt?". The answer was yes.

The most important prospective studies have been those of Stafford, Jackson & Banks (1980), Cook et al (1982), and Fox & Goldblatt (1982), to which I shall return specifically later.

A retrospective prospective design is implicit in the study by Kitagawa and Hauser (1973) in the United States which showed the SMR of the unemployed to be 291.

Only one prospective study (Ramsden & Smee 1981) shows no difference between the health of the employed and unemployed. This is a study which was carried out incidentally to another study of a different kind and it used a subjective health indicator which has never been validated. Subjects were asked whether their health had improved, deteriorated, or stayed the same in the last year. No other health question was asked.

Clinical case studies

A number of studies have used a clinical case study method, which is really a form of prospective study or cross sectional study which sacrifices the precision of statistical analysis for the greater flexibility of reporting individual experiences. Studies in this category include those of Fagin (1981), Israeli (1934), Hill et al (1973), Jones (1972), Harrison (1976), Swinburne (1981) and Sinfield (1970). All of them show that, whilst some individuals may benefit from unemployment in health terms, the majority found it a psychologically damaging experience.

Some of the clinical studies, such as Hill et al (1973), Harrison (1976), Colledge and Bartholomew (1980), Fagin and Little (1984) and Swinburne (1981), show that the unemployed go through a three phase reaction of denial/optimism, pessimism/distress and fatalism. Swinburne's sample of managers went through this process more slowly than other groups.

A further source of data is the literature on the effect of employment on the health of women. This is an extensive literature. Waldron (1980), reviewed 107 references. Nathanson (1977), has also reviewed this literature. Women demonstrate higher morbidity than men even though they demonstrate lower mortality. The higher morbidity appears to be entirely concentrated at lower levels of morbidity, such as GP consultations or self reported illness. It can be demonstrated that the entire excess morbidity occurs in women without jobs. This could be because work protects women's health, or it could be because women find it easier to quit the workforce when ill, or it could be because the entire excess morbidity of women is a statistical artefact due to the greater availablity to men of health care at the place of work (Watkins 1982), Warr & Parry (1982) have reviewed the literature more critically and suggest that it is only in certain circumstances that work improved the health of women and Arber et al (1982) suggest that part time work is more beneficial than full time work.

Finally it is necessary to look at a small literature which suggests that poverty in childhood may contribute to heart disease in middle age. This is of obvious significance for the long term health of the children of the unemployed.

This literature was initiated by Forsdahl (1977) who showed that geographical variation in the mortality from ischaemic heart disease in Norway followed regional variations in economic circumstances in the 1930s which had since disappeared. Later (Forsdahl 1977) he confirmed this finding for Finland also. Williams et al (1979) showed that it was true for the UK also, but could not be distinguished from the effect of current inequalities because the regional inequalities in the UK were still present. Burr & Sweetnam (1980) used a case control study and showed that a greater number of cases of ischaemic heart disease had come from large families in childhood, or had had an unemployed father.

From this literature we are left with a clear picture that the unemployed have worse health than those in employment. However, there are still difficulties in attributing this to health damage caused by unemployment. Firstly, as Stern (1981), points out, unemployment falls disproportionately on those sections of the population who suffer other multiple deprivations and we may be seeing the end point of those multiple deprivations and attributing it to the wrong one. Secondly, the unemployed are drawn disproportionately from declining industries, in which working conditions are likely to have been worse than average for some time before closure, and we may be seeing the damage from those poor working conditions and attributing it to unemployment. Brinkmann (1983) showed that many of his sample of German unemployed had difficulty finding reemployment because of ill health and this group had a record of working in worse than average working conditions before they became unemployed. Thirdly, it may be that people are selected for unemployment because of ill health, or have difficulty finding reemployment because of ill health. Brinkmann's work supports this hypothesis. In the Kasl & Cobb studies the chronically unemployed tended to have been sick before losing their jobs, because this study was carried out in a time of boom when the majority found work again quickly. Colledge & Bartholomew (1980), Nickell (1979) and Daniell (1974) also present evidence that the sick have greater difficulty finding reemployment.

However, this problem has been elegantly overcome by Stafford, Jackson & Banks (1980) who followed up a group of unemployed school leavers. Using a mental health indicator, which they had previously validated (1980), they measured the health of a group of school leavers before they left school, ie before they knew whether they would find a job or not. There was no difference between those who, as it turned out, subsequenty found work and those who did not, but the mental health of those in work at follow up was significantly better than of those out of work. Moreover, health improved when people found jobs and worsened when they lost them.

This study impressively resolves the doubts whether causality can be inferred for the poor mental health of the unemployed. It is almost certain that unemployment damaged mental health. It could perhaps be argued that school leavers are untypical, but that would be carrying academic scepticism beyond any reasonable doubts.

Regarding physical health, Fox & Goldblatt (1982), draw on the OPCS longitudinal survey to show that those unemployed for reasons other than illness have higher mortality than those in work. The division into those unemployed because of illness and those unemployed for other reasons takes account of the problem of health selection for redundancy, although not necessarily of health selection for reemployment, although it is likely that those who have health difficulties at the time of redundancy and then have difficulty finding work will classify their unemployment as due to illness.

The most elegant study is that of Cook et al (1982). They used the cohort of men enrolled in the British Regional Heart Study. They subdivided the unemployed into those who were unemployed because of illness and those who were unemployed for other reasons and standardised their data for age, social class, town of residence and smoking habits. Table 1 shows the results.

TABLE 1

Percentage prevalance standardised for age, social class, town of residence and smoking habit

	Bronchitis	Obstructive Lung Disease	Ischaemic Heart Disease	Hypertension
Employed	16	10	10	10
Not ill unemployed	18	20	16*	11*
Ill unemployed	24*	22*	26*	9*

*significant at 1% level in comparison with the employed men.

The standardisation for social class <u>and</u> town of residence goes a long way towards meeting the argument about multiple deprivation which Stern raises and the division into ill and not ill unemployed meets the argument about health selection for unemployment. The study does not exclude these arguments perfectly (it is doubtful if any study ever could) but it certainly shifts the ground of debate very considerably.

I conclude that it is highly probable that unemployment damages physical health.

Why does unemployment damage health?

The most important question under this heading is whether unemployment causes ill health because of poverty or because of psychological factors, or both. There is very little evidence on the subject. There must be a psychological component because a number of studies show the effect of psychological factors in moderating the effect. It is not clear to what extent there is also a component of health damage caused by poverty. A further problem is that while it is plausible that the damage to psychological health is due to psychological factors, it is equally plausible that this is not the case, physical health is affected by psychological factors and mental health by problems of poverty. Most of the studies on the effect of psychological factors have looked only at mental health.

One study, that of Little (1973) suggested that unemployed technical professionals were able to cope with the material deprivation but not with the psychological problems. However, I would be reluctant to rule out a poverty effect on the basis of a single study of an atypical group. Indeed, in view of what we know about the poverty of the unemployed and the effects of poverty on health, it seems safer, in the virtual absence of any evidence, to assume that part of the health damage of unemployment is due to a poverty effect than to assume that it is not. In West Germany, Frohlich (1983) found that the degree of economic deprivation affected the likelihood of health damage, but to a much less extent than psychological factors. The effect in Britain, however, is likely to be greater.

I conclude that it is probable that poverty contributes to the health damage of unemployment, although the extent of this contribution is unclear and more research is needed.

Turning now to psychological factors, the following have been shown to be important:

SOCIAL SUPPORT Cobb (1976); Gore (1978); Beckmann & Hahn (1983); Frohlich (1983); and Warr (1981) have all demonstrated that the experience of unemployment is considerably eased by strong social support.

WORK ETHIC Stafford, Jackson & Banks (1980) showed that in their sample of school leavers those who had a high commitment to work experienced a greater damage to their mental health than those who had a lower commitment. Even the lower commitment was still a high one (they found insufficient people in their sample whose work commitment was genuinely low and so could not analyse that theoretical group). Spruit (1983) reviews four Dutch studies (Wezel 1974; Koopmans 1977; Boucher et al 1976; Gravelotte et al 1975) which show the same.

Warr (1981), points out that methods of counselling the unemployed which stress the search for work as of over riding importance, may deepen the work ethic and hence the health damage.

SELF IMAGE Spruit (1983) reviews seven studies which look at the effect that blaming oneself for the loss of a job has on the subsequent health experience. She comments that the results are conflicting.

Brinkmann (1983) points out that the stigma of unemployment is clearly important because health improves when worklessness is redefined as something else eg retirement. Walsworth Bell (1982), has suggested that pregnancy can fulfil this role.

TIME STRUCTURING Hepworth (1980) found that ability to occupy one's spare time was an important factor in diminishing the psychological damage of unemployment. Hartley (1980) found that to have been employed in a job where one was responsible for structuring one's own work subsequently diminished the psychological consequences of unemployment.

Can worklessness be good for health?

Amidst the evidence that unemployment is bad for health, there is a subsidiary theme which we must not lose. The Thomas effect showed that industry is a double edged sword. Deteriorating working conditions in recession may account for part of the Brenner effect. The Nordhaven shipyard study showed some improvements in health in some aspects in those made redundant. Olsen & Sabroe found the retired members of their union to be healthier than those still in work.

Brinkmann found that poor working conditions accounted for much of the ill health which rendered some of his sample unemployable. All the clinical case studies have shown that a minority of the unemployed actually gain more in health terms by leaving health damaging jobs than they lose by unemployment. Arber et al found that it was part time work which was most beneficial to the health of women. Haynes & Feinleib (1980) found that women, with children married to blue collar workers in clerical occupations with a non supportive boss had high levels of coronary heart disease. We must not forget that some work can be more harmful than unemployment.

SCIENTIFIC CONCLUSIONS

From the preceding literature review and having regard to the principles outlined in my opening section and the definitions set out therein, I have reached the following conclusions, upon which my discussions of policy can be based.

1. It is almost certain that recession causes ill health.

2. It is almost certain that unemployment damages mental health and probable that it damages physical health. However, there are some jobs which damage health to a greater extent than unemployment, which accounts for the health benefit observed in a minority of the unemployed.

3. It is probable that poverty accounts for part of the health damage caused by unemployment.

4. It is almost certain that psychological factors, account for some of the health damage caused by unemployment. It is highly probable that these factors include social support and the strength of the work ethic, and probable that they include self esteem and ability to structure time.

5. It is highly plausible that fear of unemployment accounts for part of the health damage caused by recession.

6. It is plausible that a generalised stress in recession causes part of the health damage caused by recession.

7. It is plausible that part of the health damage caused by recession is due to changes in patterns of consumption.

8. It is plausible that part of the health damage caused by recession is due to changes in personal lives.

9. It is highly plausible that part of the health damage caused by recession is due to deteriorating working conditions in the changed state of the labour market.

10. It seems that up until the second quarter of this century recession was associated wth reduced mortality, and in view of our knowledge about occupational and environmental health it is highly probable that this was due to reduction in industrial activity.

It is almost certain that industry, directed to meeting social needs and with controlled working conditions and environmental effects is beneficial to health. It is almost certain that unrestrained industrial growth in poor working conditions without environmental control is bad for health. It is highly probable that industry does more good than harm for health, but *at the margin* it is highly probable that up to and including the first quarter of this century, industrial growth had an adverse effect on health but went hand in hand with increasing social control and trade union power over working conditions which had a beneficial effect. It is plausible that due to improved working conditions and greater social control, industrial growth is now no longer harmful at the margin, but it is equally plausible that it remains harmful, but no longer affects aggregate statistics because industry has ceased to dominate the economy.

REFERENCES

Adelstein & Fox (1978), "Occupational Mortality: Work or Way of Life?", J.Epid.&Comm.Hlth., 32, 74.

Arber, S., Dale, A., & Gilbert, N. G. (1982), "Paid Employment and Women's Health: Enrichment or Role Strain?", paper presented at the BSA Medical Sociology conference.

Banks, M. H., Clegg, C. W., Jackson, P. R., Kemp, N. J., Stafford, E.M., & Wall, T. D. (1980), 'The Use of the General Health Questionnaire as an Indicator of Mental Health in Occupational Studies", J.Occ.Psychol.

Barclay Report (1982), "The Role of Social Workers", National Institute of Social Work, London.

Beckmann, N. & Hahn, K-D. (1981), 'Unemployment and life-style changes' presented at WHO/MEDIS Conferences on Economic Instability and Health, Munich 1981, published in John, J., Schwefel, D., and Zollner, H. (eds) 'Influence of Economic Instability on Health', Springer-Verlag.

Berkman & Syme (1979), "Social Networks, Host Resistance and Mortality - A Nine Year Follow Up of Alameda County Residents", Amer.J.Epidem., 109, 186.

Birt, C. (1983), 'Prevalence of Unemployment Amongst Those Becoming Ill', in John, J. et al (eds), op. cit.

Black Report (1980), "Inequalities in Health", DHSS, London.

Boman (1979), "Behavioural Observations on the Granville Train Disaster and the Significance of Stress for Psychiatry", Soc.Sci.&Med., 13A, 463.

Boucher, Ph. W. G., Robertus, T., Sytstra, H., Wiersum, T. M. K., Wijn, M. A. M. (1976), "Onderzoek Langdurige Werkloosheid; Evaluatie van een Project in Overijssel en een Beeld van de Problematiek 1976", Groningse Stichting voor Personeelbeleid, Groningen, 1976.

Brennan, M. E., & Lancashire, R. (1978), "Association of Childhood Mortality with Housing Status and Unemployment", J.Epidem.&Comm.Hlth., 32, 28-33.

Brenner, M. H. (1971), "Economic Changes and Heart Disease Mortality", Amer.J.Pub.Hlth., 61(3), 606-611.

Brenner, M. H. (1973), "Mental Illness and the Economy", Harvard University Press.

Brenner, M. H. (1973b), 'Foetal, Infant and Maternal Mortality During Periods of Economic Instability', Int. J. Hlth. Svcs., 3(2), 145-149.

Brenner, M. H. (1975), 'Trends in Alcohol Consumption and Associated Diseases', Amer. J. Pub. Hlth., 65(12), 1279-1292.

Brenner, M. H. (1976), "Estimating the Social Costs of National Economic Policy: Implications for Mental and Physical Health and Criminal Aggression", Joint Economic Committee of the Congress of the United States, US Government Printing Office, Washington DC.

Brenner, M. H. (1977), "Health Costs and Benefits of Economic Policy", Int.J.Hlth.Svcs., 7(4), 581-623.

Brenner, M. H. (1979), "Mortality and the National Economy", The Lancet, 15th September 1979, 568-573.

Brenner, M. H. (1981), "Unemployment and Health", The Lancet, 17th October 1981, 874-875.

Brenner, M. H. (1983), 'Mortality and Economic Instability; Detailed Analysis for Britain', in John, J., Schwefel, D. and Zollner, H. 'Influence of Economic Instability on Health', Springer-Verlag.

Brinkmann, C. (1983), 'Health Problems and Psycho-Social Strains of Unemployed. A Summary of Recent Empirical Research in the Federal Republic of Germany', in J. John, D. Schwefel, and H. Zollner, 'Influence of Economic Instability on Health', Springer Verlag.

Brown, G. W., & Harris, T. (1978), "Social Origins of Depression - A Study of Psychiatric Disorder in Women", Tavistock, London.

Bungener, M., Horellou-Lafarge, C. (1979), "Influence des Chomage sur la Sante", Prevenir 1(1), op.cit.

Bunn, A.R. (1979), "Ischaemic Heart Disease Mortality and the Business Cycle in Australia", Amer.J.Pub.Hlth., 69(8), 772-781.

Burr & Sweetnam (1980), "Family Size and Paternal Unemployment in Relation to Myocardial Infarction", J.Epidem.Comm.Hlth., 34, 93-95.

Carr Saunders (1959), cited by Jahoda as "as quoted in Barbara Wooton, 'Social Sciences and Social Pathology', Allen & Unwin, London".

Catalano & Dooley (1983), 'The Health Effects of Economic Instability: A Test of the Economic Stress Hypothesis', in J. John et al (eds) op cit.

Cobb, S. (1976), "Social Support as a Moderator of Life Stress", Psychosomatic Medicine, 38, 5.

Cobb, S., Brooks, G. W., Kasl, S. V., & Connelly, W. E. (1966), "The Health of People Changing Jobs: A Description of a Longitudinal Study", Amer.J.Pub.Hlth., 56(9), 1476.

Cochrane, R., & Stopes Roe, M. (1981), Women, Marriage, Employment and Mental Health, British Journal of Psychiatry, 139, 373-381.

Colledge, M., and Bartholomew (1980), 'The Long Term Unemployed: Some New Evidence', Employment Gazette, 88, 9-12.

Colledge, M., & Kingham, A. (1983), 'Involuntary Unemployment and Health Status. A Sociological and Micro-Epidemiological Perspective', in J. John et al (eds) op cit.

Cook, D. G., Cummins, R. O., Bartley, M. J., & Shaper, A. G. (1982), "Health of Unemployed Middle Aged Men in Great Britain", The Lancet, 5th June 1982, 1290-1294.

Cross, M. (1981), "Redeployment of Managerial and Professional Manpower: A Case Study", paper presented at the KAI Workshop, Hatfield Polytechnic, May 1981.

Daniell, W. W. (1974) "A National Study of the Unemployed", PEP, London.

Dauncy, G. (1981), "The Unemployment Handbook", National Extension College, Cambridge.

Dean, K. G., & James, H. D. (1980), "The Spatial Distribution of Depressive Illness in Plymouth", Brit.J.Psychiat., 136, 167-180.

Department of Employment (1970), "Ryhope: A Pit Closes - A Study in Redeployment", HMSO, London.

Draper, P., Dennis, J., Griffiths, J., Partridge, Popay, J. (1979), "Micro-processors, Macroeconomic Policy, and Public Health", The Lancet, 17th February 1979, 373-375.

Eisenberg, P., & Lazarsfeld, P. F. (1938), "The Psychological Effects of Unemployment", Psychol.Bull., 35.

Eyer, J. (1977), "Prosperity as a Cause of Death", Int.J.Hlth.Sycs., 7(1), 125-150.

Eyer, J. (1977), "Does Unemployment Cause the Death Rate Peak in Each Business Cycle? A Multifactor Model of Death Rate Change", Int.J.Hlth.Svcs., 7(4), 625-662.

Fagin, L. (1981), 'Unemployment and Health in Families', DHSS, London.

Fagin, L., & Little, M. (1984), 'The Forsaken Families', Pelican.

Forbes, J. (1981), "Unemployment and Health", The Lancet, 17th October 1981, 875.

Forsdahl, A. (1977), "Are Poor Living Conditions in Childhood and Adolescence an Important Risk Factor for Arteriosclerotic Heart Disease?", Brit.J.Soc.Prev.Med., 31, 91-95.

Forsdahl, A. (1978), "Living Conditions in Childhood and Subsequent Development of Risk Factors for Arteriosclerotic Heart Disease", J.Epidem.Comm.Hlth., 32, 34-37.

Fox, A. J., & Goldblatt, F. O. (1982), "Longitudinal Study: Socio-Demographic Mortality Differentials 1971-75", Series LS No. 1, HMSO, 1982.

Frohlich, D. (1983) 'Econimic deprivtion, work orientation and health conceptual ideas, and some empirical findings', in J. John et al (eds) op cit.

Gardner, M. J., Crawford, M. D., & Morris, J. N. (1963), "Patterns of Mortality in Middle and Early Old Age in the County Boroughs of England and Wales", Brit.J.Soc.Prev.Med., 23, 133-140.

Garfield, S. L. (1978), "Research on Client Variables in Psychotherapy", in Bergin, A. E., & Garfield, S. L. (eds.), "Handbook of Psychotherapy and Behaviour Change", 2nd Edition, Wiley, New York.

Gore, S. (1978), "The Effect of Social Support in Moderating the Health Consequences of Unemployment", J.Hlth.Soc.Behav., 19(2), 157-165.

Gravelle, Hutchinson & Stern (1981), "Mortality and Unemployment: A Critique of Brenner's Time Series Analysis", The Lancet, 26th September 1981, 675-679.

Gravelotte, R., Hatenboer, A., Koster, A. (1975), "Jeugdwerkloosheid in Leiden II De Belevingsaspecten Nader Onderzocht", Vakgroep Klinische Psychologie, R.U. Leiden, 1975.

Greenblatt, M., Becerra, R. M., Sterafetivides, E. A. (1982), "Social Networks and Mental Health: An Overview", Amer.J.Psychia., 139(8), 977-984.

Gurney, R. M. (1980), "The Effects of Unemployment on the Psychosocial Development of School Leavers", J.Occ.Psychol., 53, 205-213.

Gurney, R., & Taylor, K. (1981), "Research on Unemployment: Defects, Neglects and Prospects", Bull.Brit.Psych.Soc., 34, 349-352.

Hakim, C. (1982), "The Social Consequences of High Unemployment", J.Soc.Pol., 11(4), 433-468.

Harrison, R. (1976), "The Demoralising Experience of Prolonged Unemployment", Department of Employment Gazette, April 1976.

Hartley, J. F. (1980), "The Impact of Unemployment upon the Self-Esteem of Managers", J.Occ.Psych., 53, 147-155.

Hawton, O'Grady, Osborn & Cole (1982), "Adolescents Who Take Overdoses: Their Characteristic Problems and Contacts with Helping Agencies", Brit.J.Psychiat., 140, 118-123.

Haynes, S. G., & Feinleib, M. (1980), "Women, Work and Coronary Heart Disease: Prospective Findings from the Framingham Heart Study", Amer.J.Pub.Hlth., 70(2), 133-141.

Hepworth, S. J. (1980), "Moderating Factors of the Psychological Impact of Unemployment", J.Occ.Psych., 53, 147-155.

Hill, M. J., Harrison, R. M., Sargeant, A. V., & Talbot, V. (1973), "Men Out of Work: A Study of Unemployment in Three English Towns", Cambridge University Press. (According to Newells a summary of this book appears as Hill, J. (1978), "Psychological Impact of Unemployment", New Society, 19th January 1978.)

Israeli, N., "Distress in the Outlook of Lancashire and Scottish Unemployed", J.App.Psych., 19(1), 67-69.

Iversen, L., & Klausen, H. (1981), "Lukringen af Nordavn - Vaerflet", Institute for Social Medicine, University of Copenhagen, Publication 13.

Jahoda, M. (1979), "The Impact of Unemployment in the 1930s and the 1970s", Bull.Brit.Psych.Soc., 32, 309-314.

Jahoda, M., Lazarsfeld, P. F., & Zeisel, H. (1953), "Marienthal - the Sociography of an Unemployed Community, English translation, Tavistock, 1972.

John, J. (1983), 'Economic Instability and Mortality in the Federal Republic of Germany. Problems of Macro-analytical Approach, with Special Reference to Migration', in J. John, D. Schwefel, and H. Zollner (eds), 'Influence of Economic Instability on Health', Springer-Verlag.

Jones, M. (1972), "Life on the Dole", Davis Poynter Ltd., London.

Kasl, S. V. (1979), "Mortality and the Business Cycle: Some Questions about Research Strategies when Utilising Macrosocial and Ecological Data", Amer.J.Pub.Hlth., 69(8), 784-788.

Kasl, S. V., Cobb, S., & Gore, S. (1972), "Changes in Reported Illness and Illness Behaviour Related to Termination of Employment: A Preliminary Report", Int.J.Epidem., 1(2), 111-118.

Kasl, S. V., Cobb, S., & Brooks, G. W. (1968), "Changes in Serum Uric Acid and Cholesterol Levels in Men Undergoing Job Loss", JAMA, 206(7), 1500-1507.

Kasl, S. V., & Cobb, S. (1970), "Blood Pressure Change in Men Undergoing Job Loss - A Preliminary Report", Psychosomatic Medicine, 32(1), 19-38.

Kinnersley, P. (1973), "The Hazards of Work and How to Fight Them", Pluto Press, London.

Kitagawa, E. M., & Hauser, P. M. (1973), "Differential Mortality in the United States", (tables 3.1 and 3.2), Harvard University Press, Cambridge, Mass.

Koopmans, E. (1977), "Onderzoek Onder Worklozen I en II", IVA, Tilburg, 1977.

Lane (1978), "My Fifty Years in Industrial Medicine", J.Soc.Occ.Med., 28, 115.

Lew, E. A. (1979), "Mortality and the Business Cycle: How Far Can we Push an Association?", Amer.J.Pub.Hlth., 69(8), 782-783.

Little, C. B. (1973), "Stressful Response Among Unemployed Technical Professionals", PhD Thesis (Sociology), 1973, University of New Hampshire, op.cit.

Martin, A. R. (1960), "Mental Health and the Rediscovery of Leisure", paper presented at the 13th Annual Meeting of the World Federation for Mental Health, Edinburgh, 1960.

Morris, J. N., & Titmuss, R. N. (1944), "Health and Social Change: The Recent History of Rheumatic Heart Disease", Medical Officer, 1944, 69-87.

Mukherjee, S. (1976), "Unemployment Costs", PEP, Vol. XLIII, Broadsheet 561.

Mullen & Illsley (1981), "Literature Review on Unemployment and Health", Institute of Medical Sociology, Aberdeen.

Munich (1981) refers to papers presented at the WHO/MEDIS Conference in Munich 1981.

Nathanson, C. (1977), "Sex, Illness and Medical Care - A Review of Data, Theory and Method", Soc.Sci.&Med., 11, 13.

Newells, S. (1981), "A Bibliography with Abstracts on the Psychological Impact of Unemployment on the Individual and the Family", Welsh National School of Medicine, Cardiff.

Nickell, S. J. (1979), "Estimating the Probability of Leaving Unemployment", Econometrica, 47(5).

Nuckolls, Cassel & Kaplan (1972), "Psychosocial Assets, Life Crisis and the Prognosis of Pregnancy", Amer.J.Epidem., 95, 431.

Olsen, J., & Sabroe, S. (1979), "A Follow Up Study of Non Retired and Retired Members of the Danish Carpenter/Cabinet Makers' Trade Union", Int.J.Epidem., 8(4), 375-382.

Owens, A. C. (1966), "Sick Leave Amongst Railway Men Threatened by Redundancy", Occup.Psych., 40, 43-52.

Pallis, D. J., Barraclough, B. M., Levey, A. B., Jenkins, J. S., & Sainsbury, P. (1982), "Estimating Suicide Risk Amongst Attempted Suicides", Brit.J.Psychiat., 141, 37-44.

Parnes, H. S., & King, R. (1977), "Middle Age Job Losses", Industrial Gerontology (Washington), 4(2), 77-95, op.cit.

Popay, J. (1981), "Unemployment Centres - The North American Experience", Unemployment Alliance, London.

Ramsden, S., & Smee, C. (1981), "The Health of Unemployed Men", Employment Gazette, September 1981, 397-401.

Rimmer, L., & Popay, J. (1982), "Employment Trends and the Family", Study Commission on the Family, London.

Ross, E. (1982), Exchange of Correspondence Between Ernie Ross, MP (Dundee, East) and Margaret Thatcher, MP (Prime Minister of the United Kingdom), released to the press by Ross.

Schlozman, K. L., & Verba, S. (1978), "The New Unemployment: Does It Hurt?", Pub.Pol., 26(3), 333-358.

Shearman, B., & Jenkins, C. (1979), "The Collapse of Work", Eyre Methuen, London, 1979.

Shepherd & Barraclough (1980), "Work and Suicide - An Empirical Investigation", Brit.J.Psychiat., 136, 469-478.

Shepherd, G. (1981), "Psychological Disorder and Unemployment", Bull.Brit. Psych.Soc., 34, 345-348.

Sinfield, A. (1970), "Poor and Out of Work in Shields", in Townsend, P. (ed.), "The Concept of Poverty".

Smith, "Unemployment and Racial Minority Groups", cited by Hakim as from the Policy Studies Institute, London.

Sogaard, J. (1983), 'Socioeconomic change and mortality - a multivar iate coherency analysis of Danish Time Series', in J. John et al (eds), op cit.

Spruit, I. (1983), 'Unemployment, the Unemployed and Health: An Analysis of the Dutch Situation', in J. John et al (eds), op cit.

Stafford, E. M., Jackson, P. R., & Banks, M. H. (1980), "Employment, Work Involvement and Mental Health in Less Qualified Young People", J.Occ.Psychol., 53, 291-304.

Stellman & Daum (1971), "Work is Dangerous to your Health", Pantheon Books, 1971, Vintage Books, 1973.

Stern, J. (1981), "Unemployment and Its Impact on Morbidity and Mortality", Centre for Labour Economics Discussion Paper No. 93, LSE, London.

Stokes, G. (1981), "The Psychological and Social Consequences of Economically Precipitated Stress", PhD Thesis, University of Birmingham.

Swinburne (1981), "The Psychological Impact of Unemployment on Managers and Professional Staff", J.Occ.Psych., 54, 47-64.

Thomas & Collard (1979), "Who Divorces?", Routledge & Kegan Paul, London.

Thomas, D. S. (1925), "Social Aspects of the Business Cycle", Routledge.

Vaughan, C. E., & Leff, J. (1976), "The Influence of Family and Social Factors in the Course of Psychiatric Illness: A Comparison of Schizophrenic and Depressed Patients", Brit.J.Psychiat., 129, 125-137.

Waldron, I. (1980), "Employment and Women's Health: An Analysis of Causal Relationships", Int.J.Hlth.Svcs., 10(3), 435-454.

Walsworth Bell, J. (1982), personal communication from Dr. Jo Walsworth Bell, North West Regional Health Authority, Manchester.

Warr, P. (1981), "Some Studies of Psychological Well Being and Unemployment", SAPU Memo No. 431, University of Sheffield.

Warr, P. B. (1981), "Psychological Aspects of Employment and Unemployment", Psych.Med., 11, Editorial, also SAPU memo 443, University of Sheffield.

Warr, P. B. (1978), "A Study of Psychological Well Being", Brit.J.Psychiat., 69, 111.

Warr, P., & Parry, G. (1982), "Paid Employment and Women's Psychological Well Being", Psych.Bull., 91(3), 498-516.

Watkins, S. J. (1982), "Unemployment Stress", New Society, 1st July 1982, 30.

Watkins, S. J. (1982), "Occupational Health Services - Part of the Health Care System?", MSc Thesis, Department of Community Medicine, University of Manchester.

Westin, S., & Norun, D. (1977), "NarSardinfabrikken Nedlegges", Institut fur Hygiene oj Sozialmedizin, University of Bergen.

Wezel, J. van (1974), "Beleving van Werkloosheid", Gedrag.T.v.Psych., 2, 63-79.

White, "Long Term Unemployed", cited by Hakim as forthcoming from the Policy Studies Institute.

Whiting, E. (1980), "Unemployment Costs", Financial Times, 24th November 1980 (letter).

Williams, D. R. R., Roberts, S. J., & Davies, T. W. (1979), "Deaths From Ischaemic Heart Disease and Infant Mortality in England and Wales", J.Epidem.Comm.Hlth., 33, 199-202.

Winfield, G. (1981), "Psychology and Centres for the Unemployed: Challenge or Chimera?", Bull.Brit.Psych.Soc., 34, 353-355.

Wing, J. K., & Brown, G. W. (1970), "Institutionalisation and Schizophrenia: A Comparative Study of Three Mental Hospitals 1960-68", Cambridge University Press, Cambridge, England.

Winter, J. (1983), 'Unemployment Nutritian and Infant Mortality in Britain', in J. John et al (Eds) op cit.

Wlodarczyk, W., Szubert. Z., & Bryla, M. (1983), 'An Attempt to Analyse some Dependencies between Economic and Health Status in Poland in the Years 1959-1979', in J. John et al (eds) op cit.

Ziegler, H. (1979), "Sante et Licenciement Collectif: la Sante des Ouvriers d'une Grosse Enterprise de Matallurgie Avant, Pendant et Apres un Licenciement Collectif", Prevenir 1(1), op.cit.

DOES ECONOMIC CHANGE INCREASE MENTAL DISORDER?

A SYNTHESIS OF RECENT RESEARCH

David Dooley and Ralph Catalano

Introduction

Conventional wisdom holds that economic downturns provoke increases in psychological disorder. This view is shared not only by lay people but also by mental health workers (Dooley and Catalano, 1977). The belief that economic contraction causes human suffering appears to be the political foundation for unemployment compensation, full employment policies (see for example the late Senator Hubert Humphrey's preface in Brenner, 1976), and legislation intended to maintain the economic viability of communities threatened by plant closures.

On the other hand, an important tenet of the free enterprise system is that capital must be free to seek the most profitable enterprises and locations. Closing less profitable enterprises may disemploy workers in some regions, but the gains in productivity are assumed to benefit consumers and spur development of new jobs in new technologies at higher wages than the lost jobs. Implicit in this free enterprise perspective is the assumption that workers are adaptable and mobile and that the human costs of their adaptation are compensated by long term improvements in living standards.

These apparently incompatible views about the adaptability of populations to economic change raise a question of considerable importance for policy and for theory: What is the relationship of mental disorder to changing economic conditions? The policy implications of this question obviously reach to the heart of the ongoing debate over balancing the needs to protect human welfare and to maintain productivity. Attempts to answer this question should also advance theory by providing insights into the relationship of the larger social ecology (in this case aggregate economic processes) to individual-level stress, coping and pathology.

There is a long tradition of research on the question of the impact of the economy on mental well being (e.g. Durkheim, 1897)[1]. Historically, research on this topic has increased during major economic depressions (e.g. see the review of the outpouring of work on the Great Depression by Eisenberg and Lazarsfeld, 1938). Recent reviews have covered the literature up to the 1982 recession (Dooley and Catalano, 1980; Jahoda, 1979; Warr and Parry, 1982). The new research stimulated by the most recent recession and the contradictions in the earlier research now invite another appraisal of this body of work.

The first goal was to assemble and organize those English language studies that permitted an inference of causality from economic change to disorder, thereby screening out large numbers of cross-sectional and descriptive reports. The next goal was to explain the persistent conflict in conclusions generated by this literature and to identify the multiple economy-to-pathology pathways assessed by different methods.

Efforts to reduce this literature to a single conclusion have been frustrated by differences in results and methods in the field. These varying types of research approaches do not ask the same question. For example, the strongly positive results found by Brenner (1973) and the mixed results found by Cobb and Kasl (1977), to take the two best known examples of the contradiction, become understandable when these different approaches are understood as addressing different questions.

In the next four sections, the research on economics and psychopathology will be mapped on a matrix of two 3-level dimensions (indicator of psychopathology and level of analysis) and then characterized cell by cell. A more quantitative or meta-analytic approach to reviewing this literature was considered (e.g. Glass et al, 1981) but the small numbers of studies in most cells prohibited application of this approach. The focus is on the specification of an approach that can answer the title question rather than the comparison of results from non-comparable and inadequate approaches. In the final section, we will consider the implications of this analysis for the theoretical guidance of future research and for social policy.

Indicators of Psychopathology

This section explores the meaning of and relationships among the three indicators of psychopathology most commonly employed to measure the mental health impact of economic change: self-reported symptom level, help seeking (usually, but not always, indexed by admissions to specialized mental health care), and suicide. The unstated assumption implicit in comparisons of studies using these different indicators is that they all reflect the same underlying construct of 'true' psychopathology. The possibility that these indicators may not be highly intercorrelated has seldom been raised in the economics and mental health literature and rarely been tested.

Surveyed symptoms

The total amount of behavioral disorder is not known, either over time or at one point in time. At best the amount of behavioral disorder could be estimated from survey samples of 'true' prevalence or incidence. Unfortunately, there are problems with such estimates. First "the major epidemiological population surveys are now almost 25 years old and thus fail to reflect advances in diagnostic and case identification technology" (Regier et al, 1978, p. 685). Second, the questionnaire techniques employed in such large-scale surveys (e.g. the Midtown Manhattan Scale of Langner, 1962) are subject to serious criticism as indicators of treatable disorder (e.g. Seiler, 1973). The prevailing view is that such short symptom checklists do not discriminate types of disorder and, at best, measure generalized distress (Dohrenwend and Crandell, 1970; Seiler, 1973). For example, it is estimated that half of those with severe 'demoralization' as measured by self-report symptom check lists do not have diagnosable mental disorder (Dohrenwend and Dohrenwend, 1982). Third, there has not been a time series survey of true disorder on the scale of such cross sectional studies as the Midtown Manhattan Survey. Given the costs of in-person interviewing, such a large-scale survey with 50 or more repeated panel or cross sectional data points would be prohibitively expensive. Symptom measures are therefore used most commonly in cross sectional or small panel or trend survey studies analyzed at the individual level.

Help seeking and psychiatric admissions

It is well known that symptom level, or the presence of 'true' disorder, is only one of several determinants in the pathway of psychiatric treatment. 'Under-utilization' or 'over-utilization' appear in different demographic subgroups (age, sex, status, ethnicity) compared to expected utilization patterns based on surveyed 'true' prevalence (Tischler et al, 1975). For example, females in treatment, were more likely than males to label their problems as psychiatric, discuss problems with others, enter treatment voluntarily, and have a favorable attitude toward psychiatric treatment (Horwitz, 1977).

In addition to such patient factors, other researchers have identified factors external to the person as determinants of psychiatric admission. The decision to admit or not to admit patients appearing at a psychiatric facility varied with the clinician's discipline and experience and with the patient's resources (Mendel and Rapport, 1969; Streiner et al, 1975). Involuntary admissions to psychiatric care depended not only on symptoms but on the availability of a responsible party who can maintain the patient's equilibrium in the community (Warner, 1961). The existence of social involvements (employment, marriage) tended to prevent admission of former applicants for psychiatric treatment (Richart and Millner, 1968).

The recidivism of mental patients also appears to be a complex matter in that it depends on more factors than the symptomatology of the readmitted (Solomon and Doll, 1979). Greenley (1979) reported that rehospitalizations varied with family expectations but not with symptoms. This is a significant issue because the majority of all mental patients admitted to state and county hospitals in the United States have previously been hospitalized (Rosenblatt and Mayer, 1974).

The effect of the various personal, institutional, and social environmental factors that bear on admission is to reduce treated disorder to a small proportion of survey-estimated true disorder. Regier et al (1978) summarized their estimates of the distribution of persons with mental disorder by treatment seeking in the following way: Specialty mental health sector (including overlap with outpatient medical sector), 21.0%; general hospital inpatient/nursing home sector, 3.4%; outpatient medical sector, 54.1%; not in treatment, 21.5%.

These estimates are consistent with the work by Helgason (1978) who compared cases of mental disorder identified by survey with a case register for the population aged 20 to 49 in Iceland. About 25 to 30% of cases identified by questionnaire could be retrieved by comprehensive case register. Interestingly, there were proportionately more registered psychiatric cases among nonrespondents than among respondents on the survey that had the relatively good completion rate of 80%.

In sum, archival records of admissions for specialty mental health care badly underestimate not only true disorder but also total help seeking, since much care is provided by nonspecialty, formal sources (i.e. general medical practitioners) and by informal sources (such as friends and family). Even worse, many studies fail to measure specialty mental health admissions comprehensively - often omitting the private sector and focusing on either public inpatients or public outpatients. Udell and Hornstra (1975), for example, reported a cross sectional study of specialty mental health care in the late 1960s that found that 40% of the demand for service in the studied community was in the private sector. A severe methodological limitation is posed by the fact that psychiatric admissions are relatively rare. Prospective, individual-level studies of the general population must have large samples in order to find more than a few new psychiatric admissions.

Covariation in true and treated disorder

As can be seen, counts of specialty mental health cases badly underestimate total "true" disorder. Unfortunately it is generally not practical to supplement specialty mental health case counts by counting the psychiatric cases in general hospitals or in outpatient medical care or by surveying large samples of the population. As a consequence, time series studies of treated disorder can be generalized to true disorder only on the assumption that specialty mental health incidence and prevalence are proportional to true incidence and prevalence longitudinally. Only two published studies have attempted to test the assumption of proportionality of treated and true incidence over time (Catalano and Dooley, 1979a; Catalano et al, 1981)[2]. They estimated monthly changes in community mental distress using monthly sample averages of symptom checklist scores. They estimated treated disorder with monthly patient counts provided by the mental health agencies in the two communities. These two series were found, contrary to the assumption of proportionality, to be uncorrelated over time.

One artifactual explanation of this counterhypothetical finding is that the symptom checklist captured relatively narrow variation in symptoms in a sub-clinical set of the population, i.e. it failed to estimate "true" disorder. Another possible problem is that the observed variation in mean symptoms was in part a function of temporal variation in monthly completion rates. A third artifactual explanation of the failure to find an association between treated and untreated disorder arises from the quality of the admissions data. The admissions for specialty mental health units in the studied communities represent an unknown, but probably small proportion of total treated disorder.

The nonartifactual explanation of this finding is that symptom levels may be relatively constant and due to some stochastic process (e.g. genetic basis for disorder with the trait occurring randomly). Variation in treated disorder could then be due to variation in several other variables: personal, clinical, or social environmental factors affecting pathways into treatment as described above, or the supply of mental health service.

Assuming relatively slow shifts in the demographic structure of a community, changes in the age, sex, or social status factors in willingness to enter treatment should not account for much monthly variation in treatment series. Diagnostic policy and staff makeup (e.g. with respect to discipline and experience of admitting clinicians) are also unlikely to account for predictable change on a monthly basis in admission counts. However, changes in the tolerance for disorder and the supply of responsible caretakers could vary over time. Unfortunately, such variables as tolerance or social dislocation are as difficult to measure longitudinally as true incidence.

The variation in capacity of mental health service providers is the other major contender for the cause of variation in treated disorder not accounted for by variation in "true" incidence. Marshall and Funch (1979) partially replicated Brenner's (1973) study Mental Illness and the Economy and found that hospital capacity is a better predictor of the first admission rate for the young and the aged than the state of the economy. It follows that variation in any supply-sensitive measure of treated disorder must be interpreted carefully with respect to at least three plausible causes: true incidence, social dislocation processes, and supply.

Suicide

One possible solution to the problem posed by the supply-sensitivity of treated disorder indicators is to obtain an indicator of disorder that is as objective and archivally available as are admissions data but that is not positively correlated with the supply of care providers. The most frequently studied variable of this type is suicide. (The hypothesis of a negative relationship between supply of mental health services and suicide is generally not supported by evaluations showing little impact of suicide prevention centers on suicide rates.) Several researchers have assessed temporal variability in both suicides and admissions data (Cerbus, 1970; Sanborn et al, 1970; Zung and Green, 1974). Cerbus studied Ohio data from 1962 to 1967. Both suicides and admissions to mental hospitals declined linearly from spring through summer and fall to a minimum in the winter. Sanborn et al studied suicides and psychiatric hospitalizations in New Hampshire for the years 1956 to 1968. Like Cerbus, they found that admissions and suicides peaked in the spring and declined steadily through summer and fall to winter. Over 13 years of seasons, suicides and admissions were positively correlated. In contrast to the above findings, Zung and Green (1974) found no significant seasonal pattern in suicides or admissions for depression in North Carolina from 1965 to 1971. Suicides were not significantly correlated with depression admissions. More recently, psychiatric admissions in the only comprehensive case register in the United States (Monroe County, New York) were correlated with suicides (Catalano et al, 1983). Admissions and suicides were positively correlated in their raw form (i.e. not deseasonalized), but after deseasonalizing, this association disappeared. However, the small monthly incidence of suicide in this study may have prevented finding an association.

There is no evidence about the relationship between surveyed symptoms (or "true disorder") and archival suicide over time. The few trend surveys of self-reported symptoms are typically conducted in relatively small geographic (city) and temporal (months) units. Suicide is so infrequent that average monthly suicide counts in most cities are too small for meaningful time-series analysis. This low frequency also tends to prohibit use of suicide as an outcome measure in individual-level prospective studies of economic change. Moreover, while psychiatric disorder is a risk factor for suicide, suicide can also occur in psychiatric "normals" who choose suicide as a reasoned response to difficult life situations (e.g. painful terminal cancer).

In sum, all three measures of psychopathology are shown to be imperfect indicators of the target construct and to have weak or unknown associations with each other. Studies employing these different outcome measures should be separately interpreted. Studies of the effect of economic change on symptoms, admissions, and suicide may raise three different questions and, therefore, yield three different, equally valid, answers.

Levels of Analysis

Research on economics and mental health typically has been conducted at either the individual or the aggregate level. The individual level of analysis uses panel data to measure the relationship of disorder changes (usually individual symptoms) to earlier economic life events such as job loss (e.g. Cobb and Kasl, 1977). The aggregate level of analysis relates economic indicators to aggregate measures of pathology (usually suicide or admissions to mental hospitals) using time-series methods (e.g. Brenner, 1973). These two approaches neither agree in their results nor exhaust the ways of addressing the question posed above. While there are many cross-sectional attempts to explore this causal question at both levels, our attention will focus on the more internally valid longitudinal literature.

Individual-level approach

Individual-level studies address the question: Are personal job and financial changes associated with subsequent increases in personal symptoms? Survey evidence indicates that, compared to the employed and controlling for occupational status, the unemployed are more dissatisfied with their income, their family life, and their accomplishments, and that access to unemployment benefits does not decrease this dissatisfaction (Schlozman and Verba, 1979). Unfortunately, such cross-sectional survey evidence on dissatisfaction may not translate into similar patterns for more clinical indices of psychopathology. In addition, such surveys may select for unemployed respondents with personal characteristics of long unemployment histories or psychological disabilities.

Cobb and Kasl (1977) provided one of the earliest studies that measured psychopathological symptoms in samples of job losers whose job loss could be confidently regarded as unconfounded with underlying psychological disorder or a history of unemployment. The results were complicated but revealed a relatively weak association of job loss with stress outcomes (see Kasl, 1979). Unfortunately, this study was based on a relatively small, socioeconomically and demographically homogeneous sample. The possible impact of the economic environment (e.g. labor market conditions in the community) was, moreover, not assessed.

Aggregate-level approach

Compared to individual-level studies, aggregate-level studies address a different question: Are aggregate economic changes associated with aggregate indicators of pathology? The aggregate finding that suicide, for example, increases after increases in the unemployment rate cannot be translated to the individual-level conclusion that any job loser committed suicide. Such an interpretation risks the ecological fallacy (Robinson, 1950).

The aggregate-level studies considered here all utilize concomitant time-series methodology. An alternative aggregate-only methodology, analogous to individual cross-sectional studies, would be ecological correlational analysis (e.g. Dunham, 1937). However, ecological relationships may reflect spatial "unit effects" rather than longitudinal causal processes (as demonstrated by Firebaugh, 1980). This problem is illustrated by Lester's (1970) finding of a negative relationship of unemployment and suicide in ecological correlation across spatial units, in contrast to the more usual positive relationship found in time series.

Aggregate-level studies have often found a significant association of economic change and archival indices of pathology, usually with rather large proportions of variance explained (e.g. Brenner, 1973, 1976). Such results conflict with the typically weaker associations found in individual-level studies. Before turning to the studies themselves, some of the reasons for this individual- versus aggregated-level conflict will be noted, and an alternative methodology will be proposed.

Differences in the Magnitudes of Individual and Aggregate Findings

The reasons why individual- and aggregate-level analyses of the economic change-disorder relationship yield such different magnitudes of association are worth reviewing because they illuminate the differences in the questions that these two methods address. The typical finding of greater coefficients in aggregate time-series than in individual-based panel studies is likely to be due both to artifactual and to substantive reasons.

Artifactual sources

Artifacts may be due to method of presentation and to the statistical consequences of aggregation. The presentational artifact pertains to the different ways in which the results of time-series analyses can be summarized. Unlike individual-level studies, aggregate time-series analyses commonly employ predictor variables to control for trend or cyclic threats of spuriousness and to include various types and lags of economic change. If the explained variance is greater in the time-series than in the individual-level study, it may be due to the presence of more explanatory variables in the former. If the variation due to trend and cycle is removed before testing for association, the resulting coefficients describe the contribution of economic change to the variance among residuals of the actual suicide or admission series. The detrended and deseasonalized residual may represent a small amount of pathology in comparison to the original variation. In short, the comparison of aggregate time-series and individual-level studies on the basis of variance explained is difficult.

Even if allowance is made for presentational differences and if the aggregate analysis is conducted on groupings of the original individual-level data, the two levels of analysis could yield different coefficients. One effect of grouping individual data (e.g. by averaging symptom counts over a month) is to increase the reliability of the measure. Correlations of the aggregated data (e.g. over months rather than over individuals) should, other things being equal, be larger to the extent that reliability of measurement is increased (Nunnally, 1978, p. 219). Econometricians recognize this tendency of aggregation or grouping to increase the apparent explanatory power of the predictor (Johnston, 1972, pp. 228-238). Unfortunately, the degree and even the direction of this bias are unpredictable (Moorman, 1980, pp. 140-141).

Substantive sources

Of greater theoretical interest than such presentational and statistical bias explanations are the substantive differences in levels of analyses. Aggregate-level time-series analyses of economic and disorder variables typically deal with different phenomena from those studied at the individual level. These differences may be summarized in four categories.

First, an economic predictor in the aggregate analysis such as unemployment rate may reflect an environmental effect beyond (i.e. controlling for) the sum of individual job losses (Firebaugh, 1978). Such an environmental effect as well as possible environmental-by-individual economic condition interactions are lost in individual-only analyses. Possible environmental effects include (a) the demoralization caused by the anticipation of personal economic loss increased by widespread public concern with the economy; (b) the reduction of alternative employment opportunities that may keep dissatisfied workers in their unpleasant jobs; and (c) the reduction of public services due to declining tax revenues during a recession.

Aggregate-only correlations represent the sum of all direct and indirect causal paths from the economic variable (e.g. unemployment rate) to the outcome variable (e.g. suicide rate), including numerous plausible indirect paths at the individual level intervening between the aggregate variables. In contrast, individual-level studies typically address just one such intervening mechanism (e.g. between job loss and increased suicidal ideation). To the extent that different possible pathways linking the aggregate variables have the same sign, their sum will exceed any single individual-level constituent pathway.

Second, the nature of the psychopathology indicator is likely to lead to sampling differences in individual and aggregate studies. In aggregate research, pathology is commonly indexed by catastrophic outcomes such as suicides or hospitalizations, which are rare or nonexistent in individual research based on small, normal samples. Mentally disordered suicides and hospitalized patients typically have some clinical history that may exclude them from inclusion in panels of the general population with orderly work histories who suddenly lose jobs. Aggregate findings using treated disorder and suicide as criterion variables are therefore based on different populations from those of panel studies of untreated symptoms.

Third, aggregate studies are often based on much longer periods than panel studies, thus allowing more variability in the economic indicator. It is plausible that disorder is not linearly related to the economy. Noticeable increases in pathology may appear only after some threshold of economic recession or depression is experienced (Tennant et al, 1981). Short term studies that fail to include substantial variations in the economy may reveal only that the population can adapt to mild economic changes.

Fourth, recent short term panel studies all fall in an era in which public policy and labor union actions are designed to reduce the negative consequences of job loss. To the extent that these policies are successful, the fear and damage of economic downturns may be considerably reduced from previous eras. Workers in cyclic industries may have become adapted to periodic layoffs and be cushioned psychologically and materially. For example, in one panel study, psychological symptoms appeared not after job loss but rather after unemployment compensation ran out and appeared less for workers who had periodically experienced several layoffs and callbacks with the same employer (Alden and Ferman, 1980). Recent panel studies may therefore reflect an economic change-disorder relationship rather different from the one measured by long term, aggregate studies. In short, lawful relations between economics and mental health may appear to vary "because the facts on which they are based do not generally remain stable" (Gergen, 1982, p. 310).

Cross-level approach

Considering the numerous potential substantive and artifactual sources of differences between individual- and aggregate-level analyses, it should not be surprising that these approaches do not converge. A research strategy that combines levels of analysis and permits an assessment of the effects of both individual life experiences and the economic environment is needed to reconcile the existing differences.

By cross-level research is meant the simultaneous use of individual- and aggregate-level measures of economic experience (e.g. residence in a community experiencing some level of unemployment along with the individual respondent's personal employment situation). Cross-level analysis necessarily requires use of an individual-level outcome variable such as symptoms or psychiatric help seeking. This method allows us to disentangle the potentially different effects of personal condition and of environment as well as to measure the possible interaction between them. For example, might not personal job loss be appraised differently in the context of mass community unemployment versus in a low unemployment economy (as found by Cohn in his cross-level study, 1978)?

The distinction of environmental from individual effects is not new (see Leighton et al, 1963, who showed that a community's social disintegration had psychological consequences over and above those of personal poverty). The cross-level approach is difficult to operationalize since it requires subjects who vary not only on personal economic experiences but who also differ in their economic environment. Cross-sectional, one-site designs are, therefore, inadmissible since, by definition, all subjects experience the same economic environment[3]. Only by sampling different communities (with the problem of possible unit effects as in ecological correlations) or by sampling the same community over time can some variation in the aggregate independent variable be obtained.

An Organization of Recent Research

The research usually cited as evidence that the economy has an effect on the incidence of disorder can be categorized by the combination of dependent and independent variables used in the analyses. The dependent variables can be classed roughly as psychiatric symptoms, psychiatric admissions or help seeking, and suicide. The independent, or economic, variables also can be roughly separated into three groups. The first includes aggregate-level economic indicators (e.g. unemployment rates, total employment, inflation rates). The second includes job and financial events experienced by individuals and assumed to be related to the economy (e.g. loss of a job, difficulty paying bills). A third category of independent variables is formed when individual experiences and economic indicators are combined to form a "cross-level" indicator (e.g. losing a job at a time of low unemployment). When arrayed as in Table 1, these characteristics form a conceptual space in which the existing research will be located. The discussion that follows is organized by the independent variables, or rows, in Table 1.

Based on the foregoing sections, each cell of this 3x3 typology is understood to raise a different question. For example, in the first cell (aggregate economic indicators, psychiatric symptoms), the question would be "Does aggregate economic change lead to aggregate symptom change over time?" Similarly, each of the other eight categories addresses its own unique question. A glance at the table reveals (a) that cross-level sutdies are rare regardless of the type of psychopathology measure, (b) that individual-level studies rarely employ admissions or suicide measures, and (c) that aggregate-level studies are most common in these same columns. As will be seen, this correlation between level of analysis and type of dependent variable has serious implications for the kind of conclusions that can be drawn.

Economic indicators

The studies in the first row of Table 1 have in common the use of time-series methods. While there is a long tradition for this strategy (e.g. Durkheim, 1897), only studies appearing after the introduction of econometric procedures to this literature in the late 1960s are included here. With few exceptions (noted in Table 1), these recent time series studies have each checked the threat of serial correlation of errors (which, if present, leads to an increased risk of making a Type I error). The problem of serial correlation is just one example of a host of technical statistical issues that trouble time-series analysis. Because of these issues, striking positive results (e.g. Brenner, 1976, 1979, and 1983) supporting an unemployment effect on disorder have been sternly criticized (respectively Cohen and Felson, 1979; Gravelle et al, 1981; John, 1982, 1983) on technical grounds. Space does not permit a synopsis of

Table 1: Research on Economics and Mental Health

INDEPENDENT VARIABLES	DEPENDENT VARIABLES Psychiatric Symptoms 1)	Psychiatric Admissions and Help Seeking 2)	Suicide 3)
Economic Indicator (Aggregate time series)	Catalano & Dooley, 1977; 1979a;b Catalano, Dooley & Jackson, 1981 Dooley & Catalano, 1979 Dooley et al, 1981	Ahr, Gorodezky & Cho, 1981 Banzinger, Smith & Foos, 1982 Barling & Handal, 1980[1] Brenner, 1973; 1976 Catalano & Dooley, 1979 Catalano, Dooley & Jackson, 1981; forthcoming Dear, Clark & Dear, 1979 Frank, 1981 Marshall & Funch, 1979 Sclar & Hoffman, 1978 Stokes & Cochrane, 1982	Boor, 1980[1] Brenner, 1976; 1979; 1983 Catalano, Dooley & Jackson forthcoming Cook, Dintzer & Marks, 1980 Hammermesh & Soss, 1974 John, 1982 Mark, 1979 Marshall, 1978 Marshall & Hodge, 1981 Pierce, 1967 Schapiro & Ahlburg, 1982-3 Sogaard, 1983 Stack, 1981 Vigderhous & Fishman, 1978
Job & Financial Experiences (Individual perspective)	4) Banks & Jackson, 1982[2] Brenner et al, 1982 Buss & Redburn, 1983 Cobb & Kasl, 1977 Ferman & Gardner, 1979 Gurney, 1980[2] Hartley, 1980 Lehtinen & Vaisanen, 1981 Liem & Rayman, 1982 Liker, 1982[2] Parnes & King, 1977 Pearlin et al, 1981 Stokes, 1981[2] Thoits & Hannan, 1980[2]	5) Lajer, 1982 Theorell, Lind & Floderus, 1975	6) Fox & Goldblatt, 1982 Olsen & Lajer, 1979 Theorell, Lind & Floderus, 197
Cross-Level	7) Cohn, 1978[3] Dooley & Catalano, forthcoming a, b Dooley, Catalano & Brownell, 1982	8) Dooley & Catalano, forthcoming a Korper, 1976[3]	9)

1 No check on serial correlation
2 Job or income gain rather than job loss or unemployment
3 Ecological correlation

this complex debate (see also Catalano, 1981; Kasl, 1979) but the reader is advised to remember that this dispute continues to confuse the interpretation of the time-series segment of the literature.

The first category of research includes just six studies (based on two data sets) that report time-series associations between community economic indicators and survey measures of symptoms of disorder or risk factors (e.g. stressful life events) for such symptoms. The dependent variables used in these analyses were monthly sample means of life event, depression or symptom inventory scores. Depression was positively related to unemployment in a metropolitan area (Catalano and Dooley, 1977) but not in a more rural community (Dooley et al, 1981). Associations were reported between psychophysiological symptom levels and economic indicators in both metropolitan (Catalano and Dooley, 1979a) and non-metropolitan settings (Catalano et al, 1981), but with different signs. The relationship was intuitive for most subgroups in the metropolitan sample (i.e. more symptoms just after economic downturns) but counter intuitive for all subgroups in the nonmetropolitan sample.

The most obvious connection implied and, often explicitly suggested, by the aggregate research in group one is that shifts in the size or structure of an economy increase the incidence of undesirable, stressful life events implicated in the etiology of behavioral disorder (Dohrenwend and Dohrenwend, 1978). Evidence addressing the connection of economic change to life events is mixed. Results from a metropolitan community (Catalano and Dooley, 1977, 1979b; Dooley and Catalano, 1979) suggest that the mean number of stressful life events experienced by population samples varies with the economy, but no relationship was found in nonmetropolitan samples (Dooley et al, 1981).

The second category includes 13 reports of time-series relationships between economic indicators and the use of mental health facilities. This type of study dates to the often replicated cross-sectional work of Dunham (1937) that reported a correlation between economic characteristics of geographic areas in Chicago and the use of mental health facilities by persons living in those areas.

While most studies in this category find a positive association between unemployment rate and admissions, there are numerous contradictions. For example, in the best known study of this type, Brenner (1973) reports positive coefficients for some subgroups and negative coefficients for other subgroups for first inpatient admissions. While this work was partially replicated in Brenner's original New York State data set (Marshall and Funch, 1979), it has been contradicted elsewhere. For example, while Brenner found that, in general, increasing inpatient admissions followed worsening economic conditions, others found this pattern only for outpatient admissions (Sclar and Hoffman, 1978) but just the opposite for inpatients (Dear et al, 1979; Sclar and Hoffman, 1978). Others find the relationship only for readmissions (Ahr et al, 1981) or a mixture of a few significant relationships among numerous non-significant ones (e.g. Barling and Handal, 1980; Frank, 1981). With few exceptions (e.g. Barzinger et al, 1982, who studied hot line calls and inpatient and outpatient admissions) these studies deal with a limited subtype of psychiatric care. In a study of the most comprehensive psychiatric admissions register available in the United States, unemployment was found generally unrelated to admissions with one exception being a positive relationship for admissions for alcohol and drug abuse problems (Catalano et al, forthcoming).

Aside from the uninterpretable complexity of the results in cell two, the principal issue raised by the findings is whether the supposed relationship implies anything for the hypothesis that the economy affects the incidence of new disorder. As noted by Catalano and Dooley (1979a), a positive correlation of unemployment and admissions could be cited as supporting either a 'provocation' or an 'uncovering' theory. The former holds that economic change increases the use of facilities by provoking new disorder while the latter argues that economic conditions affect decisions as to whether a chronically disordered person can be cared for at home. Two time-series tests designed to discriminate between the provocation and uncovering hypothesis (Catalano and Dooley, 1979a; Catalano et al, 1981) have supported the uncovering hypothesis. These tests suggest that while the economy may influence the incidence of disorder, that relationship cannot be inferred from the association between economic change and the use of mental health facilities. Other literature supporting the uncovering hypothesis reports that readmissions tend to be more strongly related to economic indicators than are new admissions (Ahr et al, 1981) and that the supply of facilities significantly affects longitudinal variation in utilization (Dear et al, 1979; Marshall and Funch, 1979).

The 16 studies in group three of Table 1 describe the time-series association between economic indicators and the rate of suicide. Most of this work converges on the finding that bad economic times are associated with increased suicide. One exception to this general finding is Pierce's (1967) report that economic change in either direction increases suicide, although doubts have been raised about the Pierce findings (Marshall and Hodge, 1981). Some recent analyses find on-time (or synchronous) associations as opposed to lagged relationships (Cook et al, 1980), or little association (Catalano et al, 1983; John, 1982). On balance, however, the literature in this category supports the existence of an association of unemployment rate with suicide at least in large, annual time series.

The relatively consistent suicide findings in group three are, unfortunately, not responsive to the question asked at the outset because of the threat of the ecological fallacy. An association between, for example, the unemployment rate and suicide does not demonstrate that the experience of losing a job increases the likelihood of taking one's life. The association between economic indicators and the rate of suicide can not specify which connecting mechanism is at work. Suicide rates, moreover, may not vary over time with either 'true' incidence of disorder or the use of mental health facilities.

In summary, the time-series literature consistently supports an association between a worsening economy and increased suicide rates. This literature is less consistent on the question of psychiatric admissions but tends to support an association between economic downturns and increases in certain admission rates. This literature is too sparse and inconsistent to support a linkage between the economy and aggregate symptoms or stressful life events.

Job and financial experiences

The studies in the second row of Table 1 all measure the association of personal job or financial experiences (e.g. being out of work, job loss, or job gain) with subsequent symptoms, psychiatric admissions or suicide. This approach is well suited to short term prospective panel surveys, hence the relatively large number of studies in cell four. However, catastrophic outcomes such as psychiatric admissions or suicides are so rare that the required sample sizes are impractical for prospective interview studies. Thus, only four different studies are found in cells five and six. These four studies capitalize on health archives which provide little or no information about original psychiatric status.

The most common personal experience in these studies is being out of work or job loss. However, five studies in cell four (indicated in Table 1) employ a desirable economic event as the independent variable such as receiving increased income or getting a job after graduating from school or leaving prison. The effect of the economic life event is demonstrated in all these studies by contrast between those with and those without the critical event. We cannot be sure, however, that the contrast involving the desirable change is comparable to that involving an undesirable change. Is the contrast of continuing to be unemployed versus getting a job psychologically equivalent to the contrast between losing a job and continuing to be employed?

This overview of the literature concentrates on short term (up to five years following the critical event) effects. Much longer latencies could be imagined, but panel studies long enough to measure such latencies are rare. For example, there may be adverse psychological effects in adulthood in children suffering increased abuse during economic downturns (e.g. Steinberg et al, 1981), but no panel studies have followed such children into adulthood. At best there is some evidence of the economic effects on children reared in the Great Depression (Elder, 1974) and of the effect of economic deprivation on long term marital discord and personality in adults (see Liker and Elder, 1983). To the extent that the major impact of economic change is felt in later decades, the present individual-level literature largely misses such effects.

The fourth category of research measures the relationship between job or financial experience and symptoms across individuals. The best known illustration of the work in this category is Cobb and Kasl's (1977) prospective study of the mental and physical health of 100 workers displaced by two plant closures. When compared to stably employed controls, the workers exhibited increased symptoms when the closures were announced and, to a lesser degree, when jobs actually ended. The effects, however, were not as marked as might be intuitively expected. Kasl (1979), in fact, concludes that losing a job appears to be no more likely to elicit symptoms than job stress when employed.

Not included in category four is a host of cross-sectional studies that assess unemployment correlates at one point in time with or without a comparison to a nonequivalent group of employed workers. Some of these cross-sectional studies compare unemployed workers with employed controls (e.g. Kaufman, 1982; Leventman, 1981) or with representative samples of employed workers (e.g. Schlozman and Verba, 1978). Another type of study involves epidemiological surveys in economically distressed communities (e.g. Rayman and Bluestone, 1982) or of especially vulnerable respondents (e.g. Brown and Harris, 1978; in this regard also see Warr and Parry's (1982) reanalysis of Brown and Harris). Most common are descriptive studies which compare the unemployed not with employed workers but among themselves on such dimensions as length of unemployment or psychological job involvement (e.g. Brinkmann, 1981; Feather and Davenport, 1981; Frohlich, 1981; Goodchilds and Smith, 1963; Hepworth, 1980; Shanthamani, 1973; Stafford et al, 1980; Swinburne, 1981; Thomas et al, 1980; and the review by Warr and Parry, 1982). A major subset of such descriptive studies are those of workers losing jobs in plant closings (see Gordus et al, 1981, for a review).

Failing to control for prior symptom levels, these studies provide only weak tests of the causal impact of unemployment on psychological disorder. Sometimes these studies assess not the trauma of involuntary disemployment but rather the prophylactic value of work (e.g. Brown and Harris, 1978; Stafford et al, 1982; Warr and Parry, 1982). That is, some of the unemployed under study are not job losers but are, apparently, not in the labor force. Negative psychological states found in such nonworkers may or may not bear on the question of the effect of economic change on disorder.

This cross-sectional literature is most pertinent to the question "What individual characteristics are associated with maladaptive responses to unemployment?" Given that so many, perhaps most, unemployed workers react without greatly increased symptoms, psychiatric help seeking, or suicide, perhaps more attention should be given the correlates of positive adaptation to job loss. Several studies seem to converge on one major correlate of such adaptation - the relative attractiveness of the lost job vis-a-vis the alternative. Swinburne (1981) found that favorable adaptation varied directly with how well the unemployed were able to fill their time, and Brinkmann (1981) found that job losers with attractive and legitimate alternative social roles were better off. Looking at the attractiveness of the lost job, Frolich (1981) and Stafford et al (1980) found that the more job-involved losers were worse off than those less involved.

The 14 studies cited in the fourth category are relatively strong examples of causal research. In general, these studies support an association between adverse economic experiences (e.g. job loss or continued unemployment) and increased symptoms. Representative examples include Parnes and King (1977) who found an increased sense of powerlessness following involuntary permanent job loss and Pearlin and his colleagues (1981) who found that disruptive job events led to increased depression. Nevertheless, there are some difficulties with this group of studies and some perplexing inconsistencies. For example, Cobb and Kasl (1977), as noted above, found little support for a major adverse psychological reaction to unemployment, and Hartley (1980) found no decrease in self-esteem in unemployed managers over time compared to their counterparts still at work.

One problem inherent in this group of studies is the timing of the measures. Ideally, the initial symptom measure would be taken before the workers are informed of their job loss, but this has rarely been accomplished. At best, initial measures are taken after notification of planned plant closure but before the end of the job. In such a study by Brenner et al (1982), the pyschological state of those who were unemployed for two months was <u>better</u> than initially. This is consistent with some of Cobb and Kasl's (1977) findings and with unemployment stage theories (e.g. Ferman and Gardner, 1979; Powell and Driscoll, 1973) which suggest that initially, job loss may be a relief. It is also consistent with the notion that for many individuals, the anticipation of job loss is more difficult to cope with than the reality of unemployment, at least in the early stages while unemployment compensation and the optimism about finding a better job still exist.

If the initial measurement of symptom level is delayed too long, the chances of observing an unemployment effect may be lost altogether. For example, Buss and Redburn (1983) studied unemployed steel workers one and two years after their layoffs and found them more stressed than their employed counterparts. Unfortunately, without measures of these groups at or before the plant closure, we cannot tell whether the extended unemployment is cause or effect of the symptoms. In any event, the authors concluded that their unemployed sample's stress was relatively mild and had little effect on mental health service utilization.

Another problem which is rarely addressed in this group of studies is the extent to which unemployment affects people other than the job loser. The Liem and Liem Work and Unemployment Project (described by Liem and Rayman, 1982) found a lagged effect of unemployment on unemployed men and their mates. Controlling for symptoms one month after job loss, those still unemployed after 3 months (and their mates) had higher symptoms than their counterparts (and their mates) who had regained employment. Studies which measure outcomes only in the unemployed may thus underestimate the total social costs of economic change.

A third issue is the previously mentioned distinction of undesirable versus desirable economic events. In one study of a desirable event, ex-felons who obtained more employment after being released from prison had better affective well-being scores than those with less employment (Liker, 1982). Controlling for reverse causation, affective well-being was promoted by employment both directly (extra-economic benefit) and indirectly through the positive effects of improved financial adjustment (i.e. increased income). However, the psychological benefits of desirable economic change were not apparent in a study of subjects given a guaranteed annual income (Thoits and Hannan, 1980). The increased financial security apparently led to increased stressful life events such as divorce, relocation, and job change which may, in turn, have raised symptoms. These two studies thus illustrate the importance of a fourth issue, the distinction between employment (with its intangible benefits of time structure, social support, and status) and income.

The scarce literature in the fifth cell reports a relationship between job or financial stressors and the use of mental health facilities. Only two studies test the proposition that economic experiences lead to increased use of mental health services. Lajer (1982) studied 677 bricklayer union members for 6 years. Their risk of admission to a psychiatric facility was much higher for those unemployed more than half of the time in the preceding year controlling for prior hospitalization. In the monitoring of approximately 3,300 Swedish construction workers, Theorell et al (1975) found that those who experienced more than 30 days of unemployment were significantly more likely to take sick leave for "neurosis" (or commit suicide) than those stably employed. The sample was purged of workers with histories of behavioral disorder to reduce the threat of spuriousness (i.e. chronic disorder caused unemployment).

In the sixth research category only three studies (Fox and Goldblatt, 1982; Olson and Lajer, 1979; Theorell et al, 1975) were prospective. Unfortunately, suicide was not separated from "neurosis" in the Theorell et al study, making it impossible to infer that unemployment caused increased suicide. In the Fox and Goldblatt study, men looking for work were not separated from other inactive men (a category including students). Even if the men looking for work accounted for the excess suicides, the design does not rule out spuriousness, since initial unemployment and subsequent suicide could both be due to pre-existing disorder. In the Olsen and Lajer (1979) study, violent death (both suicide and accident) was associated with unemployment, but again, pre-existing disorder was not controlled. Findings of several retrospective studies not included in Table 1 are also subject to the rival explanation that chronic disorder led to both unemployment and suicidal behavior (e.g. Cumming et al, 1975; Lendrum, 1933; Sainsbury, 1956; Shepherd and Barraclough, 1980; Tuckman and Lavell, 1958). For a comprehensive review of the literature on unemployment and suicide (including attempted suicide or "parasuicide") see Platt Chapter 4.

The research in row two of Table 1 sheds more light on the intervening stress mechanisms by which the economy might affect disorder than does the research of row one. The individual level of analysis, although avoiding the threat of the ecological fallacy, does not measure the relationship between the economic environment and individual disorder. The independent variable is almost always the loss of, or the inability to find a job. Job loss occurs in healthy economies as well as in communities with declining economic bases. Bad economic times in a community, moreover, lead to many real and anticipated adaptation demands other than unemployment. These can include reduced income (by reduction in work hours), changes in work routines and leisure activities, disruption of social support networks and concern over adverse economic or job experiences among friends, family or acquaintances. Elevated unemployment levels can inhibit workers' opportunities to exit unsatisfactory jobs (Shikiar and Freudenberg, 1982), or to bargain successfully in union-management conflicts. The individual level research in row two, therefore, does not capture the subtle shifts in the community potentially tapped by the aggregate research listed in row one. This problem is illustrated by the Thoits and Hannan (1980) discovery that the symptom level, in their income maintenance experiment, differed sharply between communities. This difference was attributed to the unemployment rate difference in the local economies.

Interaction of economic indicators and job loss

Unlike the first two types of research, the "cross-level" research in row three in Table 1 comes closer to measuring the effect of aggregate economic experiences on individual disorder. Studies of this type are so rare, that both longitudinal and ecological examples have been included. One variant provides variability in the economic environment by inclusion of different areas. These ecological correlational studies are noted in Table 1. The other approach provides variability by measuring a single community as its economy changes over time. For reasons noted earlier and detailed by Firebaugh (1980) one cannot assume that these two strategies will yield the same results.

This cross-level research has the unique ability to determine if the economic climate mediates the effect of undesirable life events on outcomes assumed to measure disorder. Unemployed persons living in low unemployment areas, for example, have been found to use mental health facilities more frequently (Korper, 1976 in Cell 8) and to have less self-esteem (Cohn, 1978 in Cell 7) than the unemployed living in high unemployment areas. These findings suggest that economic change may affect the etiology of disorder either by disrupting the mechanisms by which persons adapt to undesirable life events or by leading to "inferred inadequacy" (Dooley et al, 1982; Steinberg et al, 1981). Inferred inadequacy implies that persons experiencing undesirable life events are more likely to attribute their misfortune to personal deficiencies during good economic times than during times when a contracting economy can be blamed. This attribution may, in turn, lead to symptoms of disorder (e.g. depression, Feather and Barber, 1983).

The Korper (1976) and Cohn (1978) findings were, however, contradicted by analyses of survey data from both a metropolitan and a nonmetropolitan community that suggest that the experience of undesirable life events was no more likely to lead to depression during good than during bad economic times (Dooley et al, 1982). Another metropolitan trend survey with self-reported measures of both symptoms and help seeking also found no evidence of an interaction of undesirable economic life events and community unemployment level (Dooley and Catalano, forthcoming and Chapter 8). The research using an interaction of individual and aggregate measures of economic change, therefore, does not converge on an answer to the question posed at the outset. As reflected by the empty cell for group nine in Figure 1, moreover, no research has been found that tests the hypothesis that the interaction of individual life events and the community economy affects suicide.

Although the findings on the interaction between personal job events and the economic climate are mixed, the most recent study does shed light on another matter - the multiple pathways that can link the economy to symptoms and help seeking (Dooley and Catalano, forthcoming and Chapter 8). Aggregate unemployment was positively related to undesirable job and financial life events for some persons (the middle status third of the sample), and these events were positively associated with symptoms. In addition, to this indirect "provocation" pathway from aggregate unemployment there was evidence of two direct links (a) between aggregate absolute change and help seeking controlling for events and symptoms (Dooley and Catalano, forthcoming and Chapter 8) between unemployment and symptoms controlling for events (Dooley and Catalano, forthcoming).

Implications

Summary

The literature on economics and mental health identifies no single, simple relationship between these variables. Aggregate time-series studies of symptoms have been limited to just two communities and have given contradictory results. Aggregate studies of admissions have been more numerous, but they have also yielded contradictory findings. It seems likely that the association of economic change with admissions is at least partially a function of "uncovering" existing disorder rather than or in addition to the "provocation" of new disorder. Of the aggregate variables, only suicide rates appear consistently associated with economic change, particularly unemployment. With few exceptions, the aggregate literature has focused on the unemployment rate to the exclusion of other aspects of the economic climate such as change per se, size of the work force, structure of the economy, or inflation. To the extent that these factors correlate with unemployment, they, rather than it, may be the actual cause. To the extent that they are unrelated to unemployment, we have little knowledge about their impact.

The individual-level studies have concentrated on symptoms, since suicide and psychiatric admissions are so rare. The individual symptom literature has found some evidence for adverse impacts from job loss but is perhaps even more notable for its consistent finding that most individuals adapt successfully to job loss and that job and financial experiences account for little variance in symptoms. The correlates and moderators of the adaptation to job loss are being explored in the growing cross-sectional literature.

The realization that aggregate and individual economic experiences may operate independently and in interaction has spawned the new and, as yet, sparse cross-level methodology. While evidence for an interactive effect (between community unemployment and personal undesirable events) is mixed, this new approach suggests that economic climate can affect different outcomes (e.g. symptoms, help seeking) in different ways (both directly and indirectly via life events.)

Theory

The cross-level evidence suggests that the individual-level studies of job loss may be addressing just one intervening link in the black box implicit in the aggregate-level studies. The interpretation of any findings, whether individual or aggregate, must take into account the multiple hypothetical pathways implicit in the relationship being tested (see Figure 1 for a diagram illustrating some of the paths noted above). For example, as indicated in Figure 1, psychiatric admissions may be related to economic climate by both an aggregate pathway (via Supply of Services) and more than one individual pathway (via Life Events which provoke new Symptoms and Help Seeking and via the direct path from the economy to Help Seeking).

Aggregate-level studies cannot disentangle the pathways between economic change and the dependent variable of interest. When aggregate associations are found, they are often interpreted by the media and lay public, if not by the investigators, in individual-level terms (i.e. ecological fallacy). Individual-level studies ignore the role of economic climate and focus on just one individual-level path, usually that between job events and symptoms. The cross-sectional individual literature concentrates on an even more restricted matter, the mediating effect of individual differences (such as job involvement or role alternatives) on symptoms among the unemployed. How or whether these individual relationships account for the overarching relationships of economic climate and aggregate psychopathology is seldom considered. Instead, a kind of reverse ecological fallacy is often made with individual-level research used to draw implications for public policy interventions on economic climate.

The discrepancies between individual and aggregate approaches and the multiple possible pathways in Figure 1 suggest utilization of a cross-level methodology which permits a simultaneous assessment of many more relationships than in either of the single-level methodologies. For example, the connection between aggregate and individual economic change, typically assumed in both single-level approaches, is measured in the cross-level approach. Moreover, the interaction of these two types of economic experience can be studies (forked, dotted path in Figure 1). Similarly, the cross-level approach helps remind us that individual-level symptoms, suicidal ideation or suicide, and help seeking or psychiatric admission are not identical to their aggregate-level counterparts.

Policy

Just as hypothesis tests and theory have been developed at the aggregate and individual levels, so may interventions be addressed to aggregate- and individual-level targets. Space does not permit a thorough exploration of the options (see Catalano and Dooley, 1980, for a discussion of prevention in this area). The emphasis of this treatment of the economics and mental health literature (which by default has been largely one of unemployment and mental health) has been on its discrepancies. The empirical discrepancies that we have highlighted should especially give pause to those who would recommend changes at the macro-economic level. The variation in psychological response to economic change reported to date would seem to require policy responses tailored to subgroup and even individual differences.

Of the three types of dependent variables, aggregate economic policy makers will be most concerned with suicide (saving lives) and psychiatric admissions (saving health service funds by prevention or extending outreach to more clients). The class of measures consisting of self-reported symptoms does not easily translate into life and dealth or dollar and cents terms. It can be argued that the individual-level finding of an increase in average depressed mood or demoralization by a few symptoms on an item-check list is within the adaptive competence of normal adults and is, therefore, not the proper concern of the government. Unfortunately, the most compelling evidence about the economic precursors of suicide and admission rates is found at the aggregate level. At this level, policy makers cannot be assured that the additional suicides or admissions observed after increased unemployment are previously normal people who have just lost their jobs or are normals who are related to unemployed workers or are previously disordered people with some other connection to the economy. Given

Figure 1: Diagram of Multiple Pathways Linking Aggregate- and Individual-Level Variables

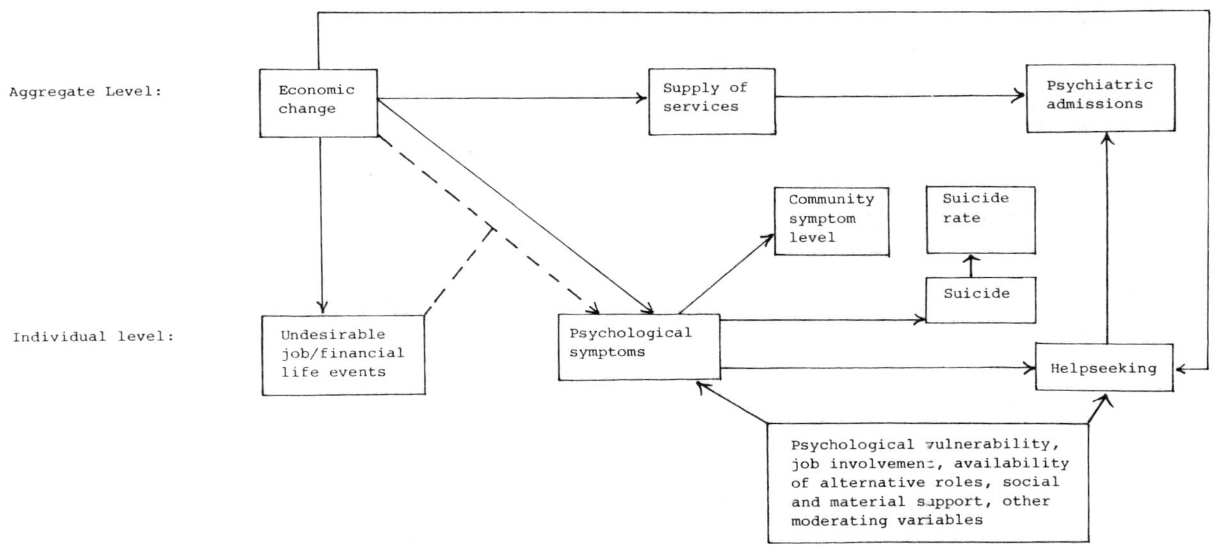

the ongoing dispute about time-series analytic techniques and the perplexing subgroup, lag, and sign differences in the aggregate results, a policy maker will have difficulty knowing when or whether a particular constituency will be benefited by an aggregate-level intervention to reduce unemployment.

While the aggregate-level interventions are typically concerned with changing the source of stress - the economy, individual-level interventions are typically remedial, i.e. involve provision of therapy after the economic dislocation. Individual-level research has provided support for a connection of economic stress to symptoms but is too scarce in the appropriate cells to show a connection to such severe outcomes as suicide or psychiatric admission. Given the evidence that most job losers cope well with their stress, clinical interventions can be justified only if they are mobilized and offered in a timely and focused way to those workers or communities anticipating substantial job dislocation. To date, there is little research on the utilization or cost-effectiveness of such remedial interventions.

It does not follow that we should delay experimental interventions until the theory is completely developed. The positive evidence in cells 2, 3 and 4 seem sufficient to warrant concern for the psychological well being of economically stressed populations. Where possible, interventions in this area should include a research component not only to evaluate the intervention but to shed light on the pertinent theoretical relationships. Thus, differential income maintenance programs for the unemployed, innovative union-based self-help counseling programs, and different state or national plant closure legislative initiatives are all opportunities to clarify experimentally the mechanisms by which economic change affects mental disorder.

Footnotes

[1]Economic change has also been studied in relation to health (e.g. Brenner, 1976; Catalano and Dooley, 1983; Cook et al, 1982, Eyer, 1977), nonpathological psychological characteristics (such as internal-external control, e.g. Andrisani and Nestel, 1976), family disruption (such as divorce, e.g. Hannan et al, 1977; and child abuse, e.g. Steinberg et al, 1981), and crime (e.g. Brenner, 1976). However, consideration of these other potential outcomes of economic change cannot be included here.

[2]There have been three longitudinal surveys (repeated cross sections or trend surveys) of communities using small samples of respondents (500 or fewer respondents per quarter) or short time frames (fewer than 20 monthly or quarterly data points). These three data series were collected in Kansas City, Missouri, Washington County, Maryland (for these two, see Markush and Favero, 1974), and Los Angeles, California (Catalano and Dooley, 1983). None of these sites has a comprehensive longitudinal case register with which to compare the survey estimates of 'true' disorder.

[3]It can be argued that perceived (cognitively appraised) environmental conditions are more important than actual environmental conditions and that the former might vary among subjects within one community at one point in time. This suggests an interesting line of cross-sectional research, but it also raises a possible confound. If different subjects appraise the same environment differently, their appraisal may be correlated with other demographic or personality factors which are linked to the dependent variable. On the other hand, this potential confound might be avoided by manipulation of the appraisal in true experimental designs.

References

Adrisani, P. J., and Nestel, G. (1976), 'Internal-External Control as Contributor to and Outcome of Work Experience', Journal of Applied Psychology, 61, 156-165.

Ahr, P. R., Gorodezky, M. J., and Cho, D. W. (1981), 'Measuring the Relationship of Public Psychiatric Admissions to Rising Unemployment', Hospital and Community Psychiatry, 32, 398-401.

Alden, J., and Ferman, L. A. (1980), 'The Mental Health of Unemployed Workers in Detroit: The Recession of 1975', paper presented at the Meeting of the American Public Health Association, Detroit, October.

Banks, M. H., and Jackson, P. R. (1982), 'Unemployment and Risk of Minor Psychiatric Disorder in Young People: Cross-Sectional and Longitudinal Evidence', Psychological Medicine, 12, 789-798.

Banzinger, G., Smith, R. K., and Foos, D. (1981), 'Economic Indicators of Mental Health Service Utilization in Rural Appalachia', American Journal of Community Psychology, 10, 669-686.

Barling, P., and Handal, P. (1980), 'Incidence of Utilization of Public Mental Health Facilities as a Function of Short Term Economic Decline', American Journal of Community Psychology, 8, 31-39.

Boor, M. (1980), 'Relationships Between Unemployment Rates and Suicide Rates in Eight Countries 1962-1976', Psychological Reports, 47, 1095-1101.

Brenner, M. H. (1973), Mental Health and the Economy, Harvard University Press, Cambridge.

Brenner, M. H. (1976), 'Estimating the Social Costs of Economic Policy: Implications for Mental and Physical Health, and Criminal Aggression', Paper No. 5, Report to the Congressional Research Service of the Library of Congress and Joint Economic Committee of Congress, US Government Printing Office, Washington DC.

Brenner, M. H. (1979), 'Mortality and the National Economy: A Review and the Experience of England and Wales 1936-1976', Lancet, ii, 568-573.

Brenner, M. H. (1983), 'Mortality and Economic Instability: Detailed Analyses for Britain', pp. 27-84 in Jurgen, J., Schwefel, D., and Zollner, H. (eds.), Influence of Economic Instability on Health, Springer-Verlag, Berlin.

Brenner, S.-O., Levi, L., Salovarra, H., Arevstedt, T., Hjelm, R., Sorbom, D., and Tellenbach, S. (1982), 'Job Insecurity and Unemployment: 1) Effects on Health and Well-Being, and 2) Interdisciplinary Evaluation of Coping Measures on Different Levels - Some Preliminary Results', paper in preparation.

Brinkmann, C. (1983), 'Health Problems and Psycho-Social Strains of Unemployed: A Summary of Recent Empirical Research in the Federal Republic of Germany', pp. 263-285 in Jurgen, J., Schwefel, D., and Zollner, H. (eds.), Influence of Economic Instability on Health, Springer-Verlag, Berlin.

Brown, G. W., and Harris, T. (1978), Social Origins of Depression: A Study of Psychiatric Disorder in Women, The Free Press, New York.

Buss, T. F., and Redburn, F. S. (1983), Shutdown at Youngtown: Public Policy for Mass Unemployment, State University of New York Press, Albany NY.

Catalano, R. (1981), 'Contending with Rival Hypotheses in Correlation of Aggregate Time-Series (CATS): An Overview for Community Psychologists', American Journal of Community Psychology, 9, 667-679.

Catalano, R., and Dooley, D. (1977), 'Economic Predictors of Depressed Mood and Stressful Life Events', Journal of Health and Social Behavior, 18, 292-307.

Catalano, R., and Dooley, D. (1979a), 'Does Economic Change Provoke or Uncover Behavioral Disorder: A Preliminary Test', pp. 321-346 in Ferman, L., and Gordus, J. (eds.), Mental Health and the Economy, Upjohn Foundation, Kalamazoo, MI.

Catalano, R., and Dooley, D. (1979b), 'The Economy as Stressor: A Sectoral Analysis', Review of Social Economy, 37, 175-188.

Catalano, R., and Dooley, D. (1980), 'Economic Change in Primary Prevention', pp. 21-40 in Price, R. H., Ketterer, R. F., Bader, B. C., and Monahan, J. (eds.), Prevention in Community Mental Health: Research, Policy and Practice, Sage, Beverly Hills.

Catalano, R., and Dooley, D. (1983), 'The Health Effects of Economic Instability: A Test of the Economic Stress Hypothesis', Journal of Health and Social Behavior, 24, 46-60.

Catalano, R., Dooley, D., and Jackson, R. (1981), 'Economic Predictors of Admissions to Mental Health Facilities in a Nonmetropolitan Community', Journal of Health and Social Behavior, 22, 284-297.

Catalano, R., Dooley, D., and Jackson, R. (1983), 'Selecting a Time-Series Strategy', Psychological Bulletin, 94, 506-523.

Cerbus, G. (1970), 'Seasonal Variation in Some Mental Health Statistics: Suicide Homicides, Psychiatric Admissions and Institutional Placement of the Retarded', Journal of Clinical Psychology, 26, 61-63.

Cobb, S., and Kasl, S. V. (1977), Termination: The Consequences of Job Loss, (Report No. 76-1261), National Institute for Occupational Safety and Health, Behavioral and Motivational Factors Research, Cincinnati, Ohio, June.

Cohen, L. E., and Felson, M. (1979), 'On Estimating the Social Costs of National Economic Policy: A Critical Examination of the Brenner Study', Social Indicators Research, 6, 251-259.

Cohn, R. M. (1978), 'The Effect of Employment Status Change on Self Attitudes', Social Psychology, 41, 81-93.

Cook, D. G., Cummins, R. O., Bartley, M. J., and Shaper, A. G. (1982), 'Health of Unemployed Middle-Aged Men in Great Britain', Lancet, i, 1290-1294.

Cook, T. D., Dintzer, L., and Mark, M. M. (1980), 'The Causal Analysis of Concomitant Time Series', Applied Social Psychology Annual, 1, 93-135.

Cumming, E., Lazer, C., and Chisholm, L. (1975), 'Suicide as an Index of Role Strain among Employed and Not Employed Married Women in British Columbia', *Canadian Review of Sociology and Anthropology*, 12, 462-470.

Dear, M., Clark, G., and Clark, S. (1979), 'Economic Cycles and Mental Health Care Policy: An Examination of the Macro-Context for Social Service Planning', *Social Science and Medicine*, 13, 43-53.

Dohrenwend, B. P., and Crandell, D. L. (1970), 'Psychiatric Symptoms in Community, Clinic, and Mental Hospital Groups', *American Journal of Psychiatry*, 126, 1611-1621.

Dohrenwend, B. S., and Dohrenwend, B. P. (1978), 'Some Issues in Research on Stressful Life Events', *Journal of Nervous and Mental Disease*, 166, 7-15.

Dohrenwend, B. S., and Dohrenwend, B. P. (1982), 'Perspectives on the Past and Future of Psychiatric Epidemiology: The 1981 Rema Lapouse Lecture', *American Journal of Public Health*, 71, 1271-1279.

Dooley, D., and Catalano, R. (1977), 'Money and Mental Disorder: Toward Behavioral Cost Accounting for Primary Prevention', *American Journal of Community Psychology*, 5, 217-227.

Dooley, D., and Catalano, R. (1979), 'Economic, Life, and Disorder Changes: Time-Series Analyses', *American Journal of Community Psychology*, 7, 381-396.

Dooley, D., and Catalano, R. (1980), 'Economic Change as a Cause of Behavioral Disorder', *Psychological Bulletin*, 87, 450-468.

Dooley, D., and Catalano, R. (forthcoming), 'The Epidemiology of Economic Stress'.

Dooley, D., Catalano, R., and Brownell, A. (1982), 'The Relation of Economic Conditions, Satisfaction with Social Environment and Life Events to Depression', submitted for publication.

Dooley, D., Catalano, R., Jackson, R., and Brownell, A. (1981), 'Economic, Life, and Symptom Changes in a Nonmetropolitan Community', *Journal of Health and Social Behavior*, 22, 144-154.

Durham, H. W. (1937), 'The Ecology of the Functional Psychoses in Chicago', *The American Sociological Review*, 2, 467-479.

Durkheim, E. (1897/1966), *Suicide*, (tr. Spaulding, J., and Simpson, G.), Free Press, New York.

Eisenberg, P., and Lazarsfeld, P. F. (1938), 'The Psychological Effects of Unemployment', *Psychological Bulletin*, 35, 358-390.

Eyer, J. (1977), 'Does Unemployment Cause the Death Rate Peak in Each Business Cycle? A Multifactor Model of Death Rate Change', *International Journal of Health Services*, 7, 625-661.

Feather, N. T., and Barber, J. G. (1983), 'Depressive Reactions and Unemployment', Journal of Abnormal Psychology, 92, 185-195.

Feather, N. T., and Davenport, P. R. (1981), 'Unemployment and Depressive Affect: A Motivational and Attributional Analysis', Journal of Personality and Social Psychology, 41, 422-436.

Ferman, L. A., and Gardner, J. (1979), 'Economic Deprivation, Social Mobility, and Mental Health', pp. 193-224 in Ferman, L. A., and Gordus, J. P. (eds.), Mental Health and the Economy, W.E. Upjohn Institute for Employment Research, Kalamazoo, MI.

Firebaugh, G. (1978), 'A Rule for Inferring Individual-Level Relationships from Aggregate Data', American Sociological Review, 43, 557-572.

Firebaugh, G. (1980), 'Cross-National versus Historical Regression Models: Conditions of Equivalence in Comparative Analysis', Comparative Social Research, 3, 333-344.

Fox, A. J., and Goldblatt, P. O. (1982), Longitudinal Study: Socio-Demographic and Mortality Differentials 1971-1975, Her Majesty's Stationery Office, London.

Frank, J. A. (1981), 'Economic Change and Mental Health in an Uncontaminated Setting', American Journal of Community Psychology, 9, 395-410.

Frohlich, D. (1983), 'Economic Deprivation, Work Orientation and Health: Conceptual Ideas and Some Empirical Findings', pp. 293-320 in Jurgen, J., Schwefel, D., and Zollner, H. (eds.), Influence of Economic Instability on Health, Springer-Verlag, Berlin.

Gergen, K. J. (1973), 'Social Psychology as History', Journal of Personality and Social Psychology, 26, 309-320.

Glass, G. V., McGraw, B., and Smith, M. L. (1981), Meta-Analysis in Social Research, Sage, Beverly Hills.

Goodchilds, J. D., and Smith, E. E. (1963), 'The Effects of Unemployment as Mediated by Social Status', Sociometry, 26, 287-293.

Gordus, J. P., Jarley, P., and Ferman, L. A. (1981), Plant Closings and Economic Dislocations, Upjohn, Kalamazoo, MI.

Gravelle, H. S. E., Hutchinson,G., and Stern, J. (1981), 'Mortality and Unemployment: A Critique of Brenner's Time-Series Analyses', Lancet, ii, 675-679.

Greenley, J. R. (1979), 'Family Symptom Tolerance and Rehospitalization Experiences of psychiatric Patients', in Simmons, R. G. (ed.), Research in Community and Mental Health, JAI Press, Greenwich.

Gurney, R. M. (1980), 'The Effects of Unemployment on the Psycho-Social Development of School-Leavers', Journal of Occupational Psychology, 53, 205-213.

Hammermesh, A. S., and Soss, N. M. (1974), 'An Economic Theory of Suicide', Journal of Political Economy, 82, 83-98.

Hannan, M. T., Tuma, N. B., and Groeneveld, L. P. (1977), 'Income and Marital Events: Evidence from an Income-Maintenance Experiment', American Journal of Sociology, 82, 1186-1211.

Hartley, J. F. (1980), 'The Impact of Unemployment upon the Self-Esteem of Managers', Journal of Occupational Psychology, 53, 147-155.

Helgason, T. (1978), 'Prevalence and Incidence of Mental Disorders Estimated by a Health Questionnaire and a Psychiatric Case Register', Acta Psychiatrica Scandinavia, 58, 256-266.

Hepworth, S. J. (1980), 'Moderating Factors of the Psychological Impact of Unemployment', Journal of Occupational Psychology, 53, 139-145.

Horwitz, A. (1977), 'The Pathways into Psychiatric Treatment: Some Differences between Men and Women', Journal of Health and Social Behavior, 18, 169-178.

Jahoda, M. (1979), 'The Impact of Unemployment in the 1930s and the 1970s', Bulletin of the British Psychological Society, 32, 309-314.

John, J. (1982), 'Economic Instability and Health: Infant Mortality and Suicide Reconsidered', paper in preparation.

John, J. (1983), 'Economic Instability and Mortality in the Federal Republic of Germany: Problems of Macro Analytical Approach with Special Reference to Migration', pp. 113-138 in Jurgen, J., Schwefel, D., and Zollner, H. (eds.), Influence of Economic Instability on Health, Springer-Verlag, Berlin.

Johnston, J. (1972), Econometric Methods, (2nd edition), McGraw-Hill, New York.

Kasl, S. V. (1979), 'Changes in Mental Health Status Associated with Job Loss and Retirement', pp. 179-200 in Barrett, J. E. (ed.), Stress and Mental Disorder, Raven Press, New York.

Kaufman, H. G. (1982), Professionals in Search of Work: Coping with the Stress of Job Loss and Unemployment, John Wiley and Sons, New York.

Korper, S. P. (1976), 'Utilization of Community Mental Health Services: Further Consideration of the Implications of Socio-Economic Class and Related Variables', PhD dissertation, Yale University.

Lajer, M. (1982), 'Unemployment and Hospitalization Among Bricklayers', Scandinavian Journal of Social Medicine, 10, 3-10.

Lehtinen, V., and Vaisanen, E. (1981), 'Epidemiology of Psychiatric Disorders in Finland: A Five-Year Follow-Up', Social Psychiatry, 16, 171-180.

Leighton, D. C., Harding, J. S., Macklin, S. B., MacMillan, A. M., and Leighton, A. H. (1963), The Character of Danger, Basic Books, New York.

Lendrum, F. C. (1983), 'A Thousand Cases of Attempted Suicide', American Journal of Psychiatry, 13, 479-500.

Lester, D. (1970), 'Suicide and Unemployment: A Re-Examination', Archives of Environmental Health, 20, 277-278.

Leventman, P. G. (1981), Professionals Out of Work, Free Press, New York.

Liem, R., and Rayman, P. (1982), 'Health and Social Costs of Unemployment: Research and Policy Considerations', American Psychologist, 37, 1116-1123.

Liker, J. K. (1982), 'Wage and Status Effects of Unemployment on Effective Well-Being Among Ex-Felons', American Sociological Review, 47, 264-283.

Mark, M. M. (1979), 'The Causal Analysis of Concomitancies in Time Series', pp. 321-339 in Cook, T. D., and Campbell, D. T. (eds.), Quasi-Experimentation: Design and Analysis Issues for Field Settings, Rand McNally, Chicago.

Markush, R. E., and Favero, R. V. (1974), 'Epidemiologic Assessment of Stressful Life Events, Depressed Mood, and Psychophysiological Symptoms - A Preliminary Report', pp. 171-190 in Dohrenwend, B. S., and Dohrenwend, B. P. (eds.), Stressful Life Events: Their Nature and Effects, Wiley, New York.

Marshall, J. R. (1978), 'Changes in Aged White Male Suicide: 1948-1972', Journal of Gerontology, 33, 763-768.

Marshall, J. R., and Funch, D. P. (1979), 'Mental Illness and the Economy: A Critique and Partial Replication', Journal of Health and Social Behavior, 20, 282-289.

Marshall, J. R., and Hodge, R. W. (1981), 'Durkheim and Pierce on Suicide and Economic Change', Social Science Research, 10, 101-114.

Mendel, W. M., and Rapport, S. (1969), 'Determinants of the Decision for Psychiatric Hospitalization', Archives of General Psychiatry, 20, 321-328.

Moorman, J. E. (1980), 'Aggregation Bias: An Empirical Demonstration', pp. in Borgatta, E. E., and Jackson, D. J. (eds.), Aggregation Data: Analysis and Interpretation, Sage, Beverly Hills.

Nunnally, J. C. (1978), Psychometric Theory, McGraw-Hill, New York.

Olsen, J., and Lajer, M. (1979), 'Violent Death and Unemployment in Two Trade Unions in Denmark', Social Psychiatry, 14, 139-145.

Parnes, H. S., and King, R. (1977), 'Middle-Aged Job Losers', Industrial Gerontology, 4, 77-95.

Pearlin, L. I., Lieberman, M. A., Menaghan, E. G., and Mullan, J. T. (1981), 'The Stress Process', Journal of Health and Social Behavior, 22, 337-356.

Pierce, A. (1967), 'The Economic Cycle and the Social Suicide Rate', American Sociological Review, 32, 457-462.

Rayman, P. M., and Bluestone, B. (1982), Out of Work: The Consequences of Unemployment in the Hartford Aircraft Industry, book manuscript in preparation.

Regier, D. A., Goldberg, I. D., and Taube, C. A. (1978), 'The De Facto U.S. Mental Health System', Archives of General Psychiatry, 35, 685-93.

Richart, R., and Millner, L. M. (1968), 'Factors Influencing Admission to a Community Mental Health Center', Community Mental Health Journal, 4, 27-35.

Robinson, W. S. (1950), 'Ecological Correlations and the Behavior of Individuals', American Sociological Review, 15, 352-357.

Rosenblatt, A., and Mayer, J. E. (1974), 'The Recidivism of Mental Patients: A Review of Past Studies', American Journal of Orthopsychiatry, 44, 697-706.

Sainsbury, P. (1956), Suicide in London: An Ecological Study, Basic Books, New York.

Sanborn, D. E., Casey, T. M., and Niswander, G. D. (1970), 'Suicide: Seasonal Patterns on Related Variables', Diseases of the Nervous System, 31, 702-704.

Schapiro, M. O., and Ahlburg, D. A. (1982-83), 'Suicide: The Ultimate Cost of Unemployment', Journal of Post Keynesian Economics, 5, 276-280.

Sclar, E. D., and Hoffman, V. J. (1978), Planning Mental Health Service for a Declining Economy, (final report to the National Health Services Research), Brandeis University, Waltham MA, January.

Schlozman, K., and Verba, S. (1979), Injury to Insult: Unemployment, Class, and Political Response, Harvard University Press, Cambridge, Mass.

Seiler, L. H. (1973), 'The 22-Item Scale Used in Field Studies of Mental Illness: A Question of Method, A Question of Substance, and A Question of Theory', Journal of Health and Social Behavior, 14, 252-264.

Shanthamani, V. S. (1973), 'Unemployment and Neuroticism', Indian Journal of Social Work, 34, 43-45.

Shepherd, D. M., and Barraclough, B. M. (1980), 'Work and Suicide: An Empirical Investigation', British Journal of Psychiatry, 136, 469-478.

Sherrod, D. R. (1974), 'Crowding, Perceived Control, and Behavioral After Effects', Journal of Applied Social Psychology, 4, 171-186.

Shikiar, R., and Freudenberg, R. (1982), 'Unemployment Rates as a Moderator of the Job Dissatisfaction-Turnover Relation', Human Relations, 35, 845-856.

Sogaard, J. (1983), 'Socio-Economic Change and Mortality: A Multivariate Coherency Analysis of Danish Time Series', pp. 85-112 in Jurgen, J., Schwefel, D., and Zollner, H. (eds.), Influence of Economy Instability on Health, Springer-Verlag, Berlin.

Solomon, P., and Doll, W. (1979), 'The Varieties of Readmission: The Case Against the Case of Recidivism Rates as a Measure of Program Effectiveness', American Journal of Orthopsychiatry, 49, 230-239.

Stack, S. (1981), 'Divorce and Suicide: A Time Series Analysis 1933-1970', Journal of Family Issues, 2, 77-90.

Stafford, E. M., Jackson, P. R., and Banks, M. H. (1980), 'Employment, Work Involvement and Mental Health in Less Qualified Young People', Journal of Occupational Psychology, 53, 291-304.

Steinberg, L., Catalano, R., and Dooley, D. (1981), 'Economic Antecedents of Child Abuse and Neglect', Child Development, 52, 260-267.

Stokes, G. (1981), 'Unemployment Among School-Leavers: A Study of Youth Unemployment in Birmingham', paper in preparation.

Stokes, G., and Cochrane, R. (1982), 'The Relationship Between National Levels of Unemployment and the Rate of Admission to Mental Hospitals in England and Wales 1950-1976', paper in preparation.

Streiner, D. L., Goodman, J. T., and Woodward, C. A. (1975), 'Correlates of the Hospitalization Decision: A Replicative Study', Canadian Journal of Public Health, 66, 411-415.

Swinburne, P. (1981), 'The Psychological Impact of Unemployment on Managers and Professional Staff', Journal of Occupational Psychology, 54, 47-64.

Tennant, C., Bebbington, P., and Hurry, J. (1981), 'The Role of Life Events in Depressive Illness: Is There a Substantial Causal Relationship?', Psychological Medicine, 11, 379-389.

Theorell, T., Lind, E., and Floderus, B. (1975), 'The Relationship of Disturbing Life Changes and Emotions to the Early Development of Myocardial Infarctions and Other Serious Illnesses', International Journal of Epidemiology, 4, 281-293.

Thoits, P., and Hannan, M. T. (1980), 'Income and Psychological Distress', pp. 183-205 in Robins, P. K., Spiegelman, R. G., Weiner, S., and Ben, J. G. (eds.), A Guaranteed Annual Income: Evidence from a Social Experiment, Academic Press, New York.

Thomas, L. E., McCabe, E., and Berry, J. E. (1980), 'Unemployment and Family Stress: A Reassessment', Family Relations, 29, 517-524.

Tischler, G. L., Henisz, J. C., Myers, J. K., and Boswell, P. C. (1975), 'Utilization of Mental Health Services: I. Patienthood and the Prevalence of Symptomatology in the Community', Archives of General Psychiatry, 32, 411-415.

Tuchman, J., and Lavell, M. (1958), 'Study of Suicide in Philadelphia', Public Health Reports 73, 547-553.

Udell, B., and Hornstra, R. K. (1975), 'Good Patients and Bad', Archives of General Psychiatry, 32, 1533-1537.

Vigderhous, G., and Fishman, G. (1978), 'The Impact of Unemployment and Social Integration on Changing Suicide Rates in the USA 1920-1969', Social Psychiatry, 13, 239-248.

Warner, S. L. (1961), 'Criteria for Involuntary Hospitalization of Psychiatric Patients in a Public Psychiatric Hospital', Mental Hygiene, 45, 122-128.

Warr, P., and Parry, G. (1982), 'Paid Unemployment and Women's Psychological Well-Being', *Psychological Bulletin*, 19, 498-516.

Zung, W. W., and Green, R. C. (1974), 'Seasonal Variation of Suicide and Depression', *Archives of General Psychiatry*, 30, 89-91.

SUICIDAL BEHAVIOUR AND UNEMPLOYMENT: A LITERATURE REVIEW

Stephen Platt

Frank Allaun, M.P.: "Has (the Secretary of State for the Home Department, Mr David Mellor) read the recent report of a young worker with a wife and baby who hanged himself, according to the coroner, because he had been out of work for nine months? Does he realise the growing number of tragedies resulting from the spread of unemployment?"

David Mellor, M.P.: "There is no reason to link unemployment with suicide. I should have thought that it would not be seemly to have party disputations on why people commit suicide." [1]

INTRODUCTION

With the inexorable rise of unemployment over the past decade in Europe and the United States to levels unknown since the depression of the 1930's, social scientists have once again turned their attention towards the delineation and measurement of its impact upon society. The negative psychological effects of even short-term unemployment have been clearly identified in studies of redundant steel-workers [2], volunteer male respondents attending an Unemployment Benefit Office [3], unemployed managers [4], and unemployed school-leavers with low academic qualifications [5] [6]. Despite the lack of adequate longitudinal studies of prolonged unemployment [7], there is considerable evidence from case studies and surveys of its effects upon the individual's psychological and social well-being, and upon personal and social relationships within the family [8]. Although some commentators [9] challenge the validity of the temporal sequence of reactions to prolonged unemployment which were first described by Eisenberg and Lazarsfeld [10] - initial shock followed by optimism, then pessimism and finally fatalism [11] - most accounts identify the same core adverse effects. The unemployed person suffers a deterioration in physical and emotional health; experiences reduced levels of morale, self-confidence and self-esteem; complains of boredom, listless depression and idleness; finds the quality and extent of contacts with others outside the family is reduced; loses social status through inability to fulfil the obligations of the work role; suffers a long-term threat to work capacities and enthusiasm for employment; and can sometimes undergo fundamental changes in personality. The rest of the unemployed person's household also pays the price of the breadwinner's unemployment through financial hardship and increased tension, sometimes leading to divorce, violence and family break-up. Children appear to be particularly vulnerable: unemployment may be a contributory factor associated with children going into care and child battering and abuse [12].

Among the most extreme behavioural responses to the experience of unemployment is the act, or even the serious contemplation, of suicide. The existence and nature of any association between the economic climate and suicidal behaviour has been the subject of debate for more than 150 years. Falret [13] contended that suicide rates tend to rise during periods of rapid social change and in times of economic depression. By the time that Durkheim wrote his seminal work on suicide, he believed that Falret's contention had been confirmed to such an extent that he was able to write: "It is a well-known fact that economic crises have an aggravating effect on the suicidal tendency" [14]. However, many contemporary researchers have tended to question Durkheim's assumption. The recent heated exchange between Brenner [15] [16], Gravelle et al [17], and Eyer [18] [19] [20], demonstrates that the issue is far from being resolved.

So what is the evidence on the association between unemployment (nowadays the most commonly used indicator of economic recession) and "the suicidal tendency?" If there is any such association, is it possible to postulate a direct causal link? If unemployment is the new "great plague", then, as a Lancet editorial puts it colourfully, "we need to know the enemy before we choose the weapon - is it the uncertain status of unemployment, the behavioural reaction (more drink, more cigarettes) to being without a job, or the fact of relative poverty, ..., or is it some complex interaction of all three?" [21]. In other words, what is it about unemployment that is suicidogenic? As Gravelle et al. note [17], Brenner's conclusion that fluctuations in mortality are largely explained by current and lagged unemployment rates "is important because it suggests that the social costs of unemployment may be higher than had previously been thought". If Brenner is correct, this may be a rather phlegmatic British understatement. On aggregate, the statistical associations which Brenner derives from a multivariate regression analysis reveal that a single percent increase in the unemployment rate in the United States, if maintained over six years, could be associated with 36 890 additional deaths and a rise in indicators of social morbidity [22].

"THE SUICIDAL TENDENCY": DISTINCTIONS AND DEFINITIONS

In the following review two types of suicidal behaviour (defined as a deliberately self-harmful act) will be distinguished: those with fatal outcome (ie. suicide) and those with non-fatal outcome (once termed "attempted suicide" but nowadays more commonly referred to as "parasuicide" [23] or "deliberate self-harm" (DSH)). Since each study tends to adopt a somewhat idiosyncratic nominal definition of suicide/parasuicide, and it is not unusual to find operational and nominal definitions at variance with each other within the same study, comparisons between different investigators are thereby made more problematic. Nevertheless, a common element in both types of suicidal behaviour is the presence of a deliberate intention to endanger the integrity of the biological organism and influence the potentiality of further conscious experience. Shneidman [24] uses the term "cessation" to refer to the final ending of consiousness, and describes four basic orientations which the individual may adopt towards his own demise: intentioned (where "the individual plays a direct and conscious role in his own demise"), subintentioned ("the individual plays an indirect, covert, partial or unconscious role ..."), unintentioned ("the person psychologically plays no siginificant role ...") and contraintentioned ("an individual who uses the semantic blanket of 'Suicide!' with a conscious absence of any lethal intention"). Although some "suicides" will be unintentioned ("accidents"), most are probably cessation-unintentioned or cessation-contraintentioned. This is not, of course, to deny that some suicides are cessation-(sub)intentioned [25] However, as Stengel and Cook [26] pointed out in their influential monograph twenty-five years ago, the great majority of patients usually described as "attempted suicide" do not have an unequivocal wish to die. While the variety and complexity of motivation for "attempted suicide" has been illustrated by a number of authors [27] most would probably agree with Kessel's view that [25] what is more commonly sought is not the cessation of consciousness but its interruption, defined by Shneidman [24] as "the stopping of consciousness with the actuality, and usually the expectation, of further conscious experience. It is a kind of temporary cessation."

Stengel and Cook [26] were the first to draw a clear distinction between suicide and parasuicide ("attempted suicide"). Decrying the traditional conceptualisation of attempted suicides as merely failed suicides, they not only pointed to the complexity of motivation in non-fatal suicidal behaviour but also identified important epidemiological differences between attempted suicide and completed suicide populations. Subsequent researchers have maintained the distinction between the two types of behaviour [28] ,whilst noting that they are related: "two separate, but overlapping, populations." [29]. There is abundant empirical evidence of epidemiological differences between suicide and parasuicide populations [30] but less widespread consensus on the extent to which the two behaviour types are differentiated on non-e pidemiological variables. However, research evidence is available which suggests characteristic differences in relation to the methods of self-harm which have been used, clinical aspects (eg. psychiatric diagnosis, personality diagnosis, previous psychiatric treatment and physical illness), psychological features and personality patterns [31].

Types of Study Found in the Literature

The numerous quantitative research reports [32] which have been concerned with the association between unemployment and "the suicidal tendency" can be differentiated into four major types. Following Dooley and Catalano [33] we distinguish two orthogonal dimensions: (a) individual versus aggregate measures of unemployment and suicidal behaviour; and (b) cross-sectional versus longitudinal collection of measures. Individual studies measure the relationship between the employment status and suicidal behaviour of individuals, while aggregate studies consider the relationship between the unemployment rate and the (para)suicide rate over time or over geographical areas. The temporal design of the research can either be cross-sectional, measuring the relationship between unemployment and suicide data across individuals or groups at one point in time;or longitudinal, where unemployment in individuals or aggregates is associated with subsequent suicidal behaviour over two or more points in time. The four types of study which result from the intersection of these two dimensions are: individual-cross-sectional (Type 1); aggregate-cross-sectional (Type 2); individual-longitudinal (Type 3); aggregate-longitudinal (Type 4). The methodological limitations of each type will be discussed below and substantive findings presented in the next section.

Type 1: individual-cross-sectional studies

The majority of research projects investigating the association between unemployment (or, more generally, employment status) and suicidal behaviour at the individual level have been based on cross-sectional surveys of parasuicides/suicides. Unfortunately, formidable methodological and conceptual problems arise which tend to make comparisons between studies rather doubtful and perhaps invalid. Wide variations can be found in the definition of both unemployment and parasuicide/suicide. In the case of unemployment, it is rarely made clear whether the non-registered jobless are included in the sample and there is a lack of consistency in the classificaton of married women who are not in paid employment (ie. "housewife" vs. "unemployed"). The definitional problem tends to differ for suicide and parasuicide. In research on completed suicide, the major issue concerns variation between nominal and operational definitions within the same study. While each researcher tends to have a fairly clear idea of what s/he means by suicide, in actual fact the data are almost invariably derived from official records (eg. coroners' courts) or government statistics which use their own operational criteria to decide what consitutes a suicide. In parasuicide research there tends to be a greater correspondence between nominal and operational definitions within the same study, but differences between operational definitions used in the various treatment centres are not uncommon [34]

The major methodological shortcoming of the Type 1 study is that the direction of causality cannot be resolved. While there may be a relationship or association between suicidal behaviour and unemployment, it is not possible,on the basis of a cross-sectional study alone, to claim that unemployment causes suicide or parasuicide. The major alternative model is that individuals with a psychiatric illness or "personality disorder" may be more vulnerable to suicidal impulses and also more likely to behave in such a way that increases their risk of being dismissed from, or impulsively quitting, their job (compared to those who are not psychiatrically ill or personality disordered).

Type 2: aggregate-cross-sectional studies

In Type 2 and Type 4 (aggregate) studies, unemployment and suicide/parasuicide are treated as emergent macro-social variables rather than as properties or characteristics of individuals. In the cross-sectional approach, the investigator calculates relationships (ecological correlations) between unemployment and suicidal behaviour rates across geographical areas (eg. city wards, countries) at one point in time. This type of correlation can point to the presence and strength of association between unemployment and suicidal behaviour, but neither can be used to make any claims about the direction of causality. Furthermore, the relationship between the variables may be spurious. For instance, the variation in suicide/parasuicide rate may be "due to" change in extraneous variables other than the hypothetical causal variable (unemployment rate) [35]. Another major limitation of the ecological approach is that a strong association between two rates cannot be used as evidence of an association at the individual level. Such an eroneous inference would, of course, be an example of the ecological fallacy [36]: even where the suicide and unemployment rates are highly correlated, the suicidal or unemployed populations may consist of the same, overlapping or different individuals. However, sociologists continue to use aggregate data to make inferences about individuals, because appropriate individual-level data are often not available; and, under certain conditions, aggregate level data do provide unbiased estimates of individual-level relationships [37]. Furthermore, it is sometimes possible to investigate empirically whether ecological correlations are accompanied by individual correlations. A relevant example here is provided in the work of Philip and McCulloch [38].

Two further methodological points concerning ecological (geographical) correlations are made by Bagley et al. [39] among others. The first concerns the size of the areas used for the analysis. Although studies have sometimes based their analysis upon boroughs of over 100000 people [40] or on city wards of over 10000 people [38], problems are likely to ensue as a result of the social heterogeneity of such large areas. "In theory the problems of ecological correlations should be decreased if smaller areas are used, since the population of such areas is more homogeneous." [39]. The second problem is that of "spatial autocorrelation". This refers to the fact that while the units of analysis used in calculating correlation coefficients are presumed to be independent of one another, this situation rarely holds with geographical data: contiguous areas tend to be like one another in social and economic characteristics.

> "The practical implication of this problem is that correlation coefficients using ecological data will incorporate two measures in a virtually unquantifiable combination: the covariance of data, and the degree of similarity which contiguous social areas possess. This means that correlation coefficients will be higher than those which measure covariance alone. This also means that the application of significance testing to the correlations obtained is inappropriate." [39].

Type 3: individual-longitudinal studies

Dooley and Catalano note that "few interpretable studies are available to meet the need ... for individual-level analysis of the impact of economic change on disorder." [33]. The most powerful tool in individual longitudinal studies, the prospective cohort design, is in fact almost unknown in research where suicidal behaviour consitutes the dependent variable. This omission is not only due to the technical and practical difficulties associated with quasi-experimentation, but also (and perhaps more importantly) because of the rarity of extreme deviant behaviour such as suicide. According to Dooley and Catalano, the retrospective design suffers from the same major shortcoming as the cross-sectional approach, in that it cannot provide unambiguous evidence in favour of either competing explanation of the economic change - disorder relationship (ie self-selection v causal mechanisms). However, this similarity in methodological deficiency between the approaches may be more apparent than real. Dooley and Catalano apply the label longitudinal to studies by Sainsbury [40], Breed [41] and Tuckman and Lavell [42], among others, which merely report the percentage of suicides who were unemployed at the time of their death. The temporal design of all three studies is cross-sectional, not longitudinal, or else it becomes impossible to differentiate meaningfully between the two types. The distinction between prospective and retrospective approaches depends on whether or not the supposed effects have occurred at the time of investigation. The importance of the distinction lies in certain practical issues and not in any conceptual differences or differences in interpretation of findings [43].

Type 4: aggregate-longitudinal studies

Aggregate-longitudinal studies report the association between unemployment rates and rates [44] of suicidal behaviour in a defined geographical area (city, country) over time (usually measured in calendar years). In early studies it was usual to provide a graph or set of data describing trends in suicide and unemployment without any formal statistical test [45] [46] [47]; regrettably this deficiency continues to be found [48] [49]. However, over the years a number of different analytic strategies have become available for use in assessing more objectively the presence and strength of a relationship over time between two or more aggregate phenomena. Collectively, these methods are usually referred to as concomitant time series (CTS) analysis [50]. The simplest statistical model applied to time series analysis is the ordinary least-squares (OLS) regression model, usually expressed by the Pearson correlation coefficient (r) [51]. OLS regression assesses the synchronous linear relationship between two time-series variables. However, this method of CTS analysis does not probe the temporal precedence of the variables under study; it provides no evidence concerning whether the presumed cause precedes the presumed effect. Another major shortcoming is that autocorrelated error (which occurs when the residuals from an OLS regression are not independent) frequently renders OLS inappropriate. Consequently, various more sophisticated multiple regression techniques (mainly based on cross-sectional analysis) have been applied in order to examine the issue of temporal precedence and overcome the problem of auto-correlated error. The most well-known exponent in this area of research is Harvey Brenner. In his work the unemployment rate has been conceptualised as "a general and sensitive indicator of the extent of the recession phase of the business cycle" [52] and suicide is one of the mortality categories chosen to represent causes of death "reactive to mental stress". A number of other authors interested in exploring the aggregate relationship between unemployment and suicide [53] also use multiple regression methodology; and Mark [50] actually illustrates eight different approaches to the statistical analysis of concomitances in time series by means of data on United States suicide and unemployment rates for the years 1900-1975.

However, a number of technical, methodological and conceptual criticisms have been levelled at time series analysis in general [54] and at Brenner's work, in particular [55]. Thus, Dooley and Catalano question the appropriateness of econometric prediction methods for hypothesis testing in this field:

> "Until the questions of the existence, sign, and lag of the conomic change-disorder relationship are settled, it may be premature to use techniques designed primarily to measure the magnitude of the relationship for forecasting purposes. Econometric techniques, if continued, would be more interpretable and widely convincing if they entailed theoretical specification of detrending techniques, anticipated regression models and distributed polynomial patterns." [33].

Kasl [56] is severely critical of the failure to offer any rationale for the detrending adjustments made in time series analyses, given the likelihood that such adjustments will seriously distort the basic data. He is also sceptical of the manner in which investigators "scan" their data in order to determine the "optimal" lag. Scepticism turns to ridicule when the lag time is extended to minus one year [57]. Kasl follows Eyer [20] in believing that "the selection of a proper lag should be neither an _a priori_ arbitrary decison, nor an _a posteriori_ optimising-of-results decision but should be carried out with reference to relevant data from independent studies" [56].

Gravelle et al [17] have criticised Brenner's work on England and Wales [16] on the grounds that the model is incorrectly specified, it omits relevant variables, that better data could have been used, and Brenner's estimates are artefacts arising from his choice of time period.

On the crucial question of the ability of the aggregate longitudinal strategy to resolve the competing claims of the social causation or selection hypotheses, Dooley and Catalano [33] are doubtful while Kasl [56] is contemptuously dismissive. Brenner himself stresses that:

> "One cannot establish causation with these procedures. At most, one can test specific hypotheses which are ideally grounded on sound theoretical considerations and earlier research findings. In these tests, the hypotheses are either supported or unsupported by the statistical evidence. Even when they are supported on the basis of statistically significant relations, they are not proven since the statistical tests only indicate whether or not the findings may result from "chance" factors at specific levels of probability ...There is also the issue of possible spuriousness even for the relations found to be statistically significant. Regardless of stringent controls, outside infuences may have unobservable effects on the relationships. The possibility remains that we have not taken all relevant factors into account, especially since the state or our knowledge in the fields involved is incomplete. Thus, it is possible that some unknown factor may be influencing both the economic trends and those of the pathological indices." [22].

Cook et al [58] concur with this viewpoint.

Possible candidates for third variables which "account for" the obtained relationship between unemployment and suicide include "confidence in the political system" [59] and "some as-yet not clearly identified societal impulse [which may possibly] influence suicide before it is reflected in the economy".[60]. While these suggestions are insufficiently specific and concrete to be of great heuristic value, the general methodological point remains valid. Unfortunately, a number of CTS analysts are prone to adopt a vulgar Marxist viewpoint which decrees that all changes in the societal superstructure (including health and social customs) are determined solely by changes in the economic infrastructure. Concomitant changes at both levels are assumed to reflect unirectional causation(from the infrastructure to the superstructure). The dangers of this position are well described by Marshall and Hodge:

> "It is also unlikely that the economy is the lumbering, always exogenous *deus ex machina* it is frequently portrayed to be. It is often implicitly assumed that the independent and arbitrary perturbations, trends and cycles of the economy "cause" everything to happen; all social and political life waits for the economy to tell it what to do. It certainly does not require revolutionary insight, however, to suspect that social life influences the "exogenous" economy." [60].

There is a final methodological issue arising out of the use of ecological correlations of (para)suicide and unemployment (Type 2 and Type 4 studies) which does not appear to have been discussed in the literature. This concerns the difference in the type of rates which are characteristically computed for the two variables. The suicide (parasuicide) rate is typically based on the number of individuals committing suicide (parasuicide) over a given period (usually one year) in a specified geographical area, divided by the average number of individuals living in the same area over the same period; the resultant fraction is converted to a rate by multiplying it by a standard figure, conventionally 100000. (Sometimes, age or sex or age-sex specific rates are calculated, eg. a rate for 15-24 year old males would only include males of this age group in both the numerator and denominator. Conventionally, also, the denominator used to calculate the overall suicide (parasuicide) rate excludes the population under 15 or 16 years, suicide in this age group being extremely rare.) Since a person can only commit suicide once, the person and event suicide rates are identical. In the case of parasuicide, however, an individual can be responsible for more than one act in a given period. It is therefore possible to calculate both a person rate (the numerator being the number of *people* committing parasuicide over a given period) and an event rate (where the numerater is the number of parasuicide *events* over a given period). All three types of rates (suicide, parasuicide event and parasuicide person) are measures of *incidence*, ie. they express the frequency with which suicide(parasuicide) occurs during a defined period of time.

The calculation of the unemployment rate, on the other hand, is usually based on a different principle altogether. In Great Britain, for instance, a count of claimants at Unemployment Benefit Offices [61] is made on a certain day each month. This number is divided by the latest available mid-year estimate of all employees in employment, plus unemployed claimants at the same date and the resulting fraction converted into a percentage. A yearly mean unemployment rate is calculated by averaging the numbers of unemployed claimants at each of the twelve censuses; the denominator is the latest mid-year estimate of employees in employment plus this average figure for the unemployed over the year. Separate unemployment rates can be calculated by sex and by age. This type of rate is a measure of *prevalence*. It expresses the amount of unemployment existing in the population at a particular point in time, giving a cross-sectional view of the population (the "stock"). The census count will include all those who happen to be unemployed on the same day, regardless of the duration of their unemployment.

An unemployment incidence rate as such is not published in Great Britain. Nevertheless, it is possible to calculate an approximation to this rate by presenting the total number of unemployment claims or registrations (the "flow") during the calendar year (published as a three monthly average for Great Britain in the Employment Gazette, Table 2.19) as a percentage of the average total economically active workforce during the same period (also available in Employent Gazette) [62]. To my knowledge, no attempt has yet been made in the literature to correlate a (para)suicide rate with an unemployment incidence rate, although such an analysis is feasible (at least in Great Britain). It is difficult to tell whether the sole reliance on an unemployment prevalence rate is the result of oversight or a conscious decision that this type of rate is more appropriate. The latter possibility is rendered less likely by the absence of any discussion on this matter in the suicide and unemployment literature. There is, of course, no reason why two different kinds of rates cannot be compared. If becoming unemployed is held to be crucial to the genesis of suicidal behaviour, then the use of an incidence rate of unemployment appears more appropriate. If, however, there are grounds for believing that prolonged unemployment is of greater aetiological significance, the prevalence measure should be used since it is sensitive to changes in duration of unemployment. Thus, in Great Britain the numbers of unemployed males almost doubled between January 1978 and January1982; during the same period the inflow of male unemployment registrations rose by less than one-third. Therefore the greater part of the rise in the prevalence rate came from changes in duration rather than from changes in the number of entrants to the register [63]. (Median duration of unemployment or males in Great Britan was 21.6 weeks in January 1978 and 30.9 weeks in January 1982.) Evidence presented elsewhere [64] demonstrates that the choice of a prevalence rate for unemployment in aggregate analyses is almost certainly correct. One outstanding feature of unemployed suicidal and parasuicidal populations (compared to the unemployed in the general population) is the over-representation of those undergoing long-term joblessness.

THE RELATIONSHIP BETWEEN SUICIDE AND UNEMPLOYMENT: EMPIRICAL EVIDENCE FROM THE LITERATURE

Type 1 studies (individual-cross-sectional)

Two case control studies report significantly more unemployment among psychiatric patient suicides than their matched psychiatric controls. Robin et al. [65] found that 10 out of 42 male psychiatric patient suicides (in Southend, England, during the period 1952-1965) were unemployed at the time of their death, compared to only one psychiatric control. However, among females, there was only one unemployed suicide (out of 50) but five unemployed controls (also out of 50). Roy [66] reports that 60 (67%) out of 90 psychiatric patient suicides (in Toronto, Canada, during the period 1968 to 1979) were unemployed at the time of their death compared to 44 (49%) of the psychiatric controls ($P<.02$). The difference was extremely pronounced among the men, with 72% of suicides unemployed compared to 43% of the controls, but nonsignificant among the women.

Several other studies have noted the extent of unemployment among a sample of suicides; the main findings are summarised in Table 1. Although none provides information on the extent of unemployment among a suitable control group [67], a few do refer to the level of unemployment prevailing among non-suicides. Thus, Sainsbury contrasts [40] the unemployment rate among the males in his suicide sample (32.5%) with the unemployment rate of 11.1% for the local male population. Tuckman and Lavell note that: "For those below the age of 65, the incidence of unemployment is considerably greater than that found in the general population of Philadelphia, and even this is an underestimation since no information was available on employment for about 30% of cases." [42]. In Yap's sample of male and female suicides, 29% were unemployed at the time of death; the comparable figure for males and females in the general population was 13.2% [68].

Table 1 Uncontrolled studies reporting the proportion of suicides who were unemployed at time of death

Source	Place	Time period covered	N in series*		% unemployed
Stearns (1921) [45]	Massachusetts, U.S.A.	1920-21	167	M & F	69
Sainsbury (1955) [40]	London, England	1936-38	203	M	33
			137	F	
Tuckman and Lavell (1958) [42]	Philadelphia, U.S.A.	1951-55	485	WM	26
			89	BM	25
			69	WF	25
Stengel and Cook (1958)[26]	London England	1953	73	M	7
Yap (1958)[30]	Hong Kong	1953-54	190	M & F	29
Breed (1963) [41]	New Orleans, U.S.A.	1954-59	103	WM	21
Maris (1981) [67]	Illinois, U.S.A.	1966-68	146	M	35
			120	F	32
Sathyavathi (1977)[72]	Bangalore, India	1967-73	919	M	16
			746	F	3
Pallis *et al* (1982) [135]	West Sussex and Portsmouth, England	1968	75	M & F	12
Sanborn *et al* (1974)[78]	New Hampshire, U.S.A.	1968-70	15	M	13**
Ovenstone (1972 (1973)[71][30]	Edinburgh, Scotland	1969-71	56	M	46***
Kraft and Babigian (1976) [70]	Monroe County, New York, U.S.A	1969-71	118	M	21
			61	F	7
Morris *et al.* (1974)[136]	Philadelphia, U.S.A.	1972	103	WM	23
			50	BM	34
			63	WF	10
			20	BF	15

* M = Male F = Female W = White B = Black

** 53% altogether not working

*** Percentage of suicides who were unemployed, or though employed, not working

Four studies compare suicide rates among the unemployed with suicide rates among other groups. Sainsbury [40] reports a suicide rate for the unemployed (73.4 per 100,000) which was over five times that of the local population (14.1 per 100,000). The suicide rate for the unemployed in Yap's sample was 37.2 per 100,000, higher than that of any of the occupational groups [69]. Cumming et al. [69] analyse suicide rates among women in British Columbia, by marital status, age and employment status for the years 1961 and 1971. The 1961 findings reveal that among 25-44 year olds those who are not in the labour force have an excessive rate of suicide compared to those who are in the labour force. While this difference by employment status holds for all marital categories, it is most pronounced for the widowed and the divorced. However, among women aged 15-24 the employed are at greater risk than the not employed. In the 45-64 age group, the not employed have higher rates among the married and single, but the employed have higher rates among the widowed. Overall, the regression analysis shows that the standardised regression coefficient associated with employment status is not significant. By contrast, the 1971 regression analysis points to a clearly beneficial effect of work on the suicide rate. Among married, widowed and divorced of all ages the suicide rate among the not employed is higher than that among the employed. The same finding holds also among the single aged under 45 years, but among those aged over 45 years the suicide rate among the employed is greater. Kraft and Babigian [70] report that the rate of 91.8 suicides per 100,000 among the "chronically unemployed" (not defined) is five times the rate for other groups.

In their discusson of the cross-sectional association between unemployment and suicide a number of authors also comment upon the "reasons for" or "causes of" unemployment in their sample. Thus, Stearns [45] shows that out of 167 suicides "36 were unemployed because they were unable to obtain work, 62 because of sickness or old age and 7 for unknown causes". Tuckman and Lavell [42] claim that in half of the unemployed cases, poor physical or mental health was given as the main reason for unemployment; in 3% of cases, the reasons were lack of seasonal opportunities for work or poor job performance; and the remaining cases the reason was unknown. In Breed's series, 50% were not working full time [41]. The reasons given were as follows: thirteen were "fired" (of whom three were laid off with others in a work force), three quit one to six days prior to suicide, and twelve quit at least seven days prior to suicide. Ovenstone states that the "principal reason" for unemployment (or non-work among those technically employed) was psychiatric morbidity: eighteen out of the twenty-six unemployed/not working were rated as suffering from psychiatric illness or personality disorder [71].

Finally, a number of Type 1 studies attempt to make a retrospective assessment of the extent to which unemployment can be implicated as a likely "cause" of suicide in individual cases. In view of the inherent methodological limitations of this type of exercise, the results should be taken as possibly useful pointers to underlying causal processes rather than accepted uncritically as substantive findings. Stearns [45] claimed that, despite the fact that over 60% of his sample of suicides were unemployed, " ... in no case could [unemployment] be said to be the sole cause [of suicide] ... [N]one of this series show suicide as an immediate reaction to the loss of a job". Likewise, Yap [68] rates only seven out of 136 males and one out of 82 females under the heading "unemployment" in his analysis of suicide by "main precipitating cause". He notes: "A number of cases under [the heading] 'insanity' and 'somatic illness' were in fact unemployed, but they were not classified as such because their unemployment was clearly a consequence of their disease. In some of the other categories too the subjects were unemployed, but unemployment was not considered to be the main precipitating cause of their [suicidal bahaviour]." On the other hand, Sainsbury [40] claims that "lack of occupation was a factor" among 57 out

Table 2 Aggregate cross-sectional studies of suicide and unemployment rates; results from seven* separate studies

Author(s)	Place	Year(s)	Significance of correlation
Sainsbury (1955) [40]	London (29 boroughs)	1929-33	Nonsignificant negative correlations (r=-.14, -.18)
Walbran *et al.* (1965)[74]	Pennsylvania (13 Principal Labour Market Areas)	1954-61	"Little evidence of geographic ... correlation between rates of unemployment and rates of suicide." No formal statistical test.
Lester (1970)[73]	Pennsylvania (13 Principal Labour Market Areas	1954-61	Formal statistical test of Walbran *et al.* data. Negative correlations for 6 of the 8 years (two being significant). Overall, significant *negative* correlation between two variables.
Wallis and Maliphant (1967)[137]	London (28 boroughs)	1960-62	No relationship
Sainsbury *et al.* (1980)[513]	Europe (18 countries)	1961-63	Nonsignificant negative correlation
Bagley *et al.* (1973)[39]	Brighton (19 wards)	1963-69	Suicide rate and percent unemployed correlated r=.55 (p<.01)
Farmer *et al.* (1977)[138]	London (33 boroughs)	1969-73	No relationship
Buglass and Duffy (1978)[76]	Edinburgh (23 city wards)	1968-74	No relationship
Buglass *et al.* (1980)[75]	Edinburgh (23 city wards)	1971-73	No relationship

* Nine references are listed but these cover seven independent analyses (see text.

of the 78 unemployed in his sample who committed suicide: in 24 cases a primary factor, in 33 cases a secondary factor. However, his analysis does not rule out the possibility that the relationship between suicide and unemployment is spurious rather than causal: nine of the unemployed were dismissed from their jobs, 23 were out of work due to illness, and seven suffered from "chronic lack of employment due to mental or physical incapacity". The only study which unequivocally links unemployment with subsequent suicide unfortunately provides no information on reasons for unemployment in the sample. Sathyavathi [72] merely states that 65% of the 171 unemployed suicides took their lives "either due to the sole reason of unemployment or for other reasons in addition to the reason of their unemployment".

Type 2 studies (aggregate-cross-sectional)

Table 2 lists nine publications in which cross-sectional geographical correlations between suicide and unemployment have been reported. It should be noted that the study by Lester [73] is a replication and extension of the previous work by Walbran et al. [74] which uses the same data. Likewise the Scottish Office study of Edinburgh during 1971-73 [75] uses data which are included in the analysis by Buglass and Duffy [76]. Thus, the nine publications cover seven separate and independent tests of the association between suicide and unemployment rates over geographical areas.

Only one conclusion can be drawn from Table 2: there is no such ecological association between suicide and unemployment rates. The findings of Bagley et al. [39] of a significant positive association have to be set againt those of Lester [73] which reveal a significant negative correlation (averaged over eight years). The other studies report no relationship at all between the two variables. Lester [73] puts forward two possible explanations for the negative cross-sectional association between unemployment and suicide: firstly, that in areas of low unemployment, the existence of areas of high unemployment may cause the employed individual to feel threatened with the loss of his job, this threat acting as a precipitant of suicide; and, secondly, that those who are unemployed in areas of high unemployment migrate to areas with low unemployment to look for work.

One relevant non-geographical Type 2 study has been carried out by Rushing [77] who looked at the relationship between suicide rates (and SMRs), median income and unemployment rates among men aged 20-64 in 64 occupations in the U.S.A. during 1950. He found that the effects of unemployment are clearly stronger at the lower income levels. For the high income group of occupations, the unemployment-suicide relationship was non-existent; for the low income group, the corrrelation was highly positive. Rushing's concludes that the results "clearly suggest that unemployment increases the tendency to suicide among low income groups, while employment may do so among high income groups."

Type 3 studies (individual-longitudinal)

I have located eight studies employing a longitudinal design which touch upon the association between unemployment and suicide at the individual level [78]. Three retrospective analyses are reported by Humphrey [79] Olsen and Lajer [80] and Shepherd and Barraclough [81]. Humphrey compared suicide victims (N=98), homicide offenders (N=62) and a control group of (non-suicidal, non-homicidal) psychoneurotic controls (N=76) in respect of their experience of "occupational loss". Occupational loss was measured by allocating points for each permenent loss of job, downward mobility, retirement and being laid off from job for more than two months in the past year. 95% of the total sample with high occupational loss were suicides; only 5% were homicides and none were controls [79]. Olsen and Lajer investigated the associationbetween unemployment and cause of death ("natural" or "violent", ie. "suicide" or "accident") in a re trospective study of bricklayers and carpenters/cabinet-makers in Denmark during the years 1971-5. The bricklayers had significantly more unemployment periods, and a significantly higher suicide rate, than the carpenters/cabinetmakers. For both occupations considered together, it was found that there were significantly more unemployment periods in the group of violent deaths compared with natural deaths [80].

In a case control study, Shepherd and Barraclough [81] looked at the work record of 75 suicides (including 40 males) and 150 controls (80 males) matched by age, sex, location and whether ever married. They found that significantly fewer suicides were in paid employment at the time of their deathand more were off sick or unemployed. Among the men, 10 suicides (25%) were not working although economically active and only four controls(5%). Altogether, nine suicides were unemployed (compared to no controls): two had been dismissed, one for drinking, the other for chronic fault-finding and dissatisfaction; seven had given up their jobs voluntarily and were then unable or unwilling to find another, of whom five gave up work impulsively and two gave up as a result of progressive inability to measure up to the demands of work. There was also evidence that, compared to the controls, the employed suicides had been off sick to a greater extent during the previous year. In the whole group the suicides showed more job instability measured by the number of jobs held in the last three years [82].

The remaining individual-longitudinal studies are prospective in design. Theorell et al [83] found that unemployment lasting over a month or other change at work during the preceding year was significantly associated with subsequent death and 'neurosis' (defined as 'suicide or neurosis, psychoneurosis, anxiety, neurotic depression or asthenia episodes causing sick leave > 30 days'). In order to help ensure independence of the economic change from the dependent variable, all subjects who had been on sick leave for at least 30 days were excluded. The authors do not state how many of the 'neurosis' group (n=32) for 'all death' group (n=42), if any, were in fact suicides.

Cobb and Kasl looked at the frequency of suicidal behaviour in their pioneering longitudinal investigation of the health and behavioural effect of job loss among 100 married male blue-collar workers (aged 35-60) in two factories which were about to close down permanently [84]. There were two completed suicides, giving a rate about 30 times the rate expected of blue-collar men of this age group. One man was also known to have threatened suicide and another "presumably made an attempt". The authors conclude by expressing their belief that "there was an excess of suicide during the period around the closing of the plant though the figures are not statistically significant." [85]

Two prospective longitudinal studies examine the extent of occupational problems among suicides compared to a group of matched controls. In a psychiatric cohort study of 3563 persons (the Lundby study), Hagnell and Rorsman found that 23 men and five women had committed suicide during the 25 year follow up period. Each of these 28 suicides was matched by age, sex and geographical area with two individuals drawn from the cohort and still alive at the end of the observation period. The authors claim that half (50%) of the suicidal group experienced "[major] occupational problems which probably can explain, at least partly, why they took their lives". The comparable figure in the non-suicide group was 18% (10 out of 56). The difference between the two groups was statistically significant at the 1% level. Examples of "major occupational problems" (not formally defined) included dismissal, strain due to excessive responsibility, accident at work, embezzlement and occupational discontent [86]. Borg and Stahl followed up 2 184 psychiatric in and out-patients for one to two years. The 21 males and thirteen females who committed suicide during the period of observation were matched by age, sex, diagnosis and patient status with controls from the original census. In contrast to the findings of the Lundby study, Borg and Stahl discovered more "problems at work" (including unemployment, conflicts with fellow workers, unhappiness at work, high level of stress and bad economy) among the controls (thirteen out of 34) than among the suicides (four out of 34). This difference was not, however, statistically significant [87].

The most impressive evidence of link between suicide and unemployment based on general population data comes from the OPCS Longitudinal Study, a continuous multi-cohort study following random samples of individuals through time. The first report [88] is primarily concerned with relationships between mortality in the five years following the 1971 Census and characteristics of individuals at Census. The sample used is based on those people selected from the 1971 Census (England and Wales) and subsequently traced in the NHS Central Register; these 513 073 persons represent 1.05% of the 1971 Census population. The standardised mortality ratio (SMR) - set at 100 for the whole population - of men of working age (15-64 years) who were seeking work was raised by 30%, whereas for those in work it was 14% less than average. Noting (somewhat surprisingly) that "there are no clear health grounds for expecting this category to record high mortality", the authors recommend that an explanation of the excess deaths among those seeking work should be sought by "looking at the distribution of these men by social class; also at a tendency that men who are less healthy but nevertheless able to work may be unable to hold down a job for a long period and therefore feature disproportionately in their group; and at the possible adverse effects of unemployment." (p.26)

When SMRs are characterised by cause of death, it becomes apparent that factors resulting in excess mortality from accidents and violence (SMR=222) and from malignant neoplasms (SMR=142) have contributed the major part of the excess overall mortality. "Unemployment may have contributed to an excess of deaths from suicide and related causes" (p.27).

Type 4 studies (aggregate-longitudinal)

Table 3 summarises the results of 26 studies which have looked at the temporal association between unemployment (or a related indicator of economic recession) and suicide. The references are listed in approximate chronological order of the time period covered in the analysis.

Seven authors fail to make any statistical test of the data (although it is possible to calculate a correlation coefficient from the information provided by Stearns [45]). The correlational and multiple regression analyses relating to the United States of America are almost unanimous in finding a positive association between undesirable economic change (eg. increased unemployment) and suicide. An exception is Pierce [89] who found a positive association between absolute economic change (ie. change *per se*) and suicide. However, Marshall and Hodge claim that the results of their own analysis of suicide and employment rates provide no support for Pierce's findings:

"... there is little evidence ... to support Pierce's suggestion that the recent history of the United States confirms Durkheim with respect to the importance of change, *per se*, rather than directional change or the state of the economy as an influence upon suicide." [90].

Two studies actually find no relationship between unemployment and suicide rates [91] [92], and Marshal [93], although reporting a significant positive correlation, notes that unemployment's estimated impact on the suicide rate is not significant when multiple regression analysis is employed. However, these findings do not constitute a convincing refutation of the other evidence: in two analyses [91] [93] only restricted age bands are covered, while Catalano et al's attempt to examine trends in suicide and unemployment on a monthly basis is likely to lead to considerable instability in the computed suicide rates [92].

The evidence relating to Great Britain is more conflicting. Swinscow [44] found a significant correlation between suicide and unemployment over the period 1923-47, but his analysis is most unsatisfactory in that it uses actual numbers rather than rates [94]. Brenner [16] states that suicide showed an increase within a year of unemployment increasing in England and Wales over the years 1936-76, but provides no data. When he repeats the analysis for the years 1954/5 - 76, no relationship at all is found; and the positive relationship at two years lag only in Scotland for the same period is shown by Brenner himself to be of doubtful reliability [52]. Brenner's findings were replicated by Boor [51] in his comparative analysis of suicide and unemployment trends in eight countries over the years 1962-76. He found a significant positive relationship between the two rates in the U.S.A., Canada, Japan and France; correlations for Germany, Sweden and Italy, though positive, were not significant. The negative correlation in Great Britain was due to the fact that a consistently decreasing suicide rate was accompanied by a fluctuating but generally increasing unemployment rate. None of the other countries experienced a comparable decline in suicide incidence over the same period [95]. Boor's failure to find a

Table 3. Aggregate longitudinal studies of suicide and unemployment (or associated indicator of economic recession): evidence from the literature

Author(s)	Place	Period	Statistical Procedure*	Findings
Thomas (1927) [139]	England	1853-1913	C	Index of business conditions negatively correlated with suicide rate
Eyer (1977) [20]	U.S.A.	1870-1975	-	Graph of trends in suicide rate by age and unemployment rate. "Suicide typically peak[s] within weeks of the peak of the unemployment rate in the business cycle"
Ogburn and Thomas (1922) [140]	U.S.A. (100 cities)	1900-1920	C	Negative correlation between cycles of suicide rates and cycles of business conditions
Henry and Short (1954) [141]	U.S.A.	1900-1947	C	Suicide rate of males correlated negatively with fluctuations in business (further correlations given for age-sex, race-sex categories)
Cook *et al* (1980) [50]	U.S.A.	1900-1975	C	Suicide and employment rates significantly negatively correlated (zero lag)
Mark (1979) [50]	U.S.A.	1900-1975	C	Suicide and unemployment rates significantly positively correlated (zero lag)
Hurlburt (1932) [47]	U.S.A. (cities of over 100,000 population)	1902-1925	-	Present chart suggesting "a degree of causal relationship between business activity and suicide"
Windschuttle (1979) [49]	Australia	1905-1976	-	Graph of male suicide rate and percent of males unemployed. Claims that "the peaks and troughs in the male suicide rate correlate very closely to the level of unemployment"

Author(s)	Place	Period	Statistical Procedure*	Findings
Stearns (1921) [45]	Massachusetts, U.S.A.	1908-1918	-	Mean annual percentage of unemployment highly correlated with suicide rate**
Dublin and Bunzel (1933) [142]	U.S.A.	1911-31	C	((Inverse correlation between (suicide death rate and index (of business prosperity (((
	Massachusetts, U.S.A.	1910-31	C	
	10 Eastern States, U.S.A.	1910-31	C	
Lendrum (1933) [46]	Detroit, U.S.A.	1912-30	-	Graph of annual suicide rate and stock market averages. Claims "there is little apparent correlation between the two curves", but no statistical test is made
Pierce (1967) [57]	U.S.A	1919-40	C	Percent of labour force unemployed correlated at zero lag and 3 year lag with white male suicide rate, but presence of autocorrelation detected. Public definition of economic situation (index based on common stock prices) and age-standardised white male suicide rate correlated with one year lag - no evidence of autocorrelation
Vigderhous and Fishman (1980)	U.S.A.	1920-69	MR	Zero-order correlation between unemployment and suicide rates (M and F) highly significant. Regression analysis shows that unemployment "had a dramatic impact upon suicide rates of .... males", particularly during period 1920-40
Swinscow (1951) [44]	Great Britain	1023-47	C	Significant correlation between N of male suicides and N of male unemployed

Author(s)	Place	Period	Statistical Procedure*	Findings
MacMahon *et al* (1963) [48]	U.S.A.	1929-59	-	"Suicide rates for males in the 45-54 year age group show a remarkable correlation with total unemployment rates in the same year." Presents graph but no statistical test
Stack (1981) [143]	U.S.A.	1933-70	MR	Significant association between unemployment and suicide rates (M and F combined). Less pronounced in post-war than in pre-war period
Marshall and Hodge (1981) [57]	U.S.A.	1933-76	MR	Adjusted white male suicide rate positively associated with unemployment rate. Absolute change *per se* not a significant influence on suicide rate
Brenner (1979) [16]	England and Wales	1936-76	MR	Short-term changes in unemployment as a measure of economic loss are the most important source of influence on annual fluctuations in mortality. Suicide shows an increase within a year of unemployment increasing (no data provided)
Brenner (1977) [22]	U.S.A.	1940-73	MR	Increases in unemployment are related to higher rates of suicide
Hammermesh and Soss (1974) [53]	U.S.A.	1947-67	MR	Significant association between unemployment and suicide even during relatively mild recessions of postwar period - strongest for older age groups
Marshall (1978) [93]	U.S.A.	1948-72	MR	Significant positive correlation between unemployment and suicide rates among white males aged 65-74. However, using MR analysis, unemployment's estimated impact on suicide rate, though positive, is not significant

Author(s)	Place	Period	Statistical Procedure*	Findings
Brenner (1981)[52]	England and Wales	1955-76	MR	No relationship between unemployment and suicide rates
	Scotland	1955-76	MR	A positive relationship between unemployment and suicide rates at 2 year lag only (but relationship shown to be unreliable by Chow test)
Waldron and Eyer (1975) [91]	U.S.A.	1960-70	-	Doubling of suicide among 15-24 year old males "cannot be attributed to rising unemployment"
Sainsbury *et al.* (1980) [51]	Europe (18 countries)	1961-63 to 1972-74	C	Nonsignificant positive correlation between changes in unemployment and changes in suicide rates
Catalano *et al* (1982) [92]	Monroe County New York, U.S.A	1962-72 (by month)	C	No relationship between *monthly* unemployment rate (M and F) and total, M or F suicide rates
Boor (1980) [51]	West Germany, Sweden, Italy, Japan, U.S.A., Canada, France, Great Britain (England and Wales)	1962-76	C	Significant correlations between suicide and unemployment rates in U.S.A., Canada, Japan and France. Significant *negative* relationship in Great Britain

* Key to statistical procedure used in the study
C Pearson product-moment correlation coefficient
MR Multiple Regression
\- None

** Although no statistical test was made in the original analysis, enough relevant data were given to permit the calculation of a correlation coefficient

significant correlation between unemployment and suicide in the European countries (except France) during the 1960s and 1970s is congruent with the findings of Sainsbury's analysis of the association between changes in unemployment and suicide in Europe over the same period [51]: only a nonsignificant correlation is reported.

THE RELATIONSHIP BETWEEN PARASUICIDE AND UNEMPLOYMENT: EMPIRICAL EVIDENCE FROM THE LITERATURE

Type 1 studies (individual-cross-sectional)

Table 4 presents the available evidence on the relationship between unemployment and parasuicide from cross-sectional surveys of parasuicide samples. Wherever possible, data are given for males only. (If no separate analysis for males has been made, then data refer to both sexes together.) The exclusion of females arises out of the confusion concerning their correct employment status classification, especially among those who are married. In some studies, all married women or women with children (whether married or not) are automatically rate "housewives". In other studies, these groups of women are rated "unemployed" if they are registered as such or even if they merely express an interest in obtaining paid employment. In general, the bulk of studies on parasuicide and unemployment fail to discriminate between groups of women with differing degrees of involvement in the labour market. Warr and Parry [96] have highlighted the same deficiency in studies which examine the relationship between women's psychological well-being and paid employment.

The denominator used in the calculation of the percentage in the final column is usually the total number of male admissions or persons. Ideally, of course, the denominator should be the total number of economically active only. However, although it is possible to obtain these data for Oxford and Edinburgh, they are simply not available in most studies. The use of a rather inflated N in the denominator means that the percentages quoted are somewhat conservative. To give an indication, the percentages for Oxford (1976-82) and Edinburgh (1970-82) would be increased by about 5% and 2% respectively, if the denominator were restricted to the economically active only. Only in rare circumstances would the use of the restricted deonominator make a substantial difference to the figure quoted. The non-economically active include mainly the retired, but also those rated "not known" or "not applicable' (eg. student or in Armed Forces). The only study where the omission of "not applicable" cases makes an appreciable difference to the quoted percentage of unemployed is that of Okaha and Lotaif [97]. Over half of their sample was not economically active (40% were students and 16.5% housewives). Thus while 23% of the total N of male and female parasuicides were unemployed, the figure for economically active parasuicides was 53%.

Most of the data in Table 4 come from British sources. As far as possible the studies are listed in chronological order of the time period covered. The few relevant non-British studies are listed at the end.

Although Table 4 has been set out in rough chronological order to help identify trends over time, the differences in the types of sample used in the surveys makes this a rather difficult exercise. The most valid and generalisable results are undoubtably found in the cohort studies. The first such recent studies with a reasonable sample size (Edinburgh, 1962-63; Newcastle, 1962-64) show identical percentages (34%) of male parasuicides who were unemployed on admission. Thereafter, the tendency is generally towards a higher percentage, although marked fluctuations are evident (eg. Edinburgh, 1970-82). The Newcastle cohort of 1966-69 showed a rate of 47%, which increased to over 50% in Edinburgh and Glasgow in 1971(-72). The Oxford figures are consistently and strikingly lower than those of Edinburgh over the years 1976-82. Both series, however, show marked increases in the percentage of unemployed male parasuicides between 1979 and 1981. The only published study which differentiates the parasuicide group into those with no previous parasuicide history and those with

Table 4. Proportion of parasuicides who were unemployed on admission to hospital

Source	Type of sample	Place/ time period covered	N in series (males (M) or both sexes (MF))*	% of admissions unemployed
Hopkins (1937) [102]	Cohort	Liverpool, 1932-35	50 (M)	52%
Batchelor (1954) [144]	Sample with diagnosis of "psychopathic state"	Edinburgh, 1950-52	25 (M)	60%
Woodside (1958) [106]	Cohort	London, 1956-57	55 (MF)	15%
Patel *et al* (1972) [145]	Retrospective sample obtained from case notes	Glasgow, 1956-60	178 (M)	11%
Bruhn (1962) [99]	Sample from "broken home"	Edinburgh, 1961-62	35 (MF)	43%
Patel *et al* (1972) [145]	Retrospective sample obtained from case notes	Glasgow, 1961-65	307 (M)	19%
Kessel (1965) [23]	Cohort	Edinburgh, 1962-63	165 (M)	34%
Whitlock and Schapira (1967) [102]	Cohort	Newcastle, 1962-64	94 (M)	34%
Jacobson and Tribe (1972) [146]	Referrals to Psychiatric Unit (30% of total N: representativeness uncertain)	Brighton and Hove, 1963, 1967	111 (M)	22%
Patel *et al* (1972) [145]	Retrospective sample obtained from case notes	Glasgow, 1966-70	530 (M)	23%
Smith and Davidson (1971) [108]	Cohort	Newcastle, 1966-69	209 (M)	47%

Source	Type of sample	Place/ time period covered	N in series (males (M) or both sexes (MF))*	% of admissions unemployed
MRC Unit, Edinburgh [147]	Cohort	Edinburgh,		
		1970	344 (M)	42%
		1971	439 (M)	52%
		1972	445 (M)	47%
		1973	428 (M)	49%
		1974	423 (M)	44%
		1975	430 (M)	46%
Patel *et al* (1972) [145]	Cohort	Glasgow, 1971-72	207 (M)	55%
Morgan *et al* (1975) [107]	Non-random sample; representativeness uncertain	Bristol, 1972	121 (M)	36%
Pallis *et al* (1982) [135]	Representative sample	Chichester, 1972-73	146 (MF)	9%
Bancroft *et al* (1975) [34]	Cohort	Oxford, 1972/73	188 (M)	15%
O'Brien (1981) [98]	Cohort of young adults (aged 15-30)	London, 1975	193 (MF)	48%
Hawton [147]	Cohort	Oxford,		
		1976	223 (M)	26%
		1977	252 (M)	26%
		1978	219 (M)	33%
		1979	207 (M)	29%
		1980	205 (M)	33%
		1981	251 (M)	39%
		1982	213 (M)	47%
MRC Unit, Edinburgh [147]	Cohort	Edinburgh,		
		1976	541 (M)	49%
		1977	522 (M)	53%
		1978	465 (M)	47%
		1979	432 (M)	40%
		1980	444 (M)	47%
		1981	571 (M)	57%
		1982	501 (M)	62%
Hawton *et al* (1982) [101]	Cohort 16-18 year olds	Oxford, 1979	25 (MF)	28%

Source	Type of sample	Place/ time period covered	N in series (males (M) or both sexes (MF))*	% of admissions unemployed
Lendrum (1933) [46]	Cohort	Detroit U.S.A., 1927-30	363 (M)	17%**
Yap (1958) [30]	Non-random sample; representativeness uncertain	Hong Kong, 1953-54	127 (MF)	28%
Edwards and Whitlock (1968) [100]	Cohort	Brisbane, 1965-66	197 (M)	18%
Maris (1981) [67]	Cohort	Baltimore, U.S.A. (1970)	64 (MF)	33%
Okasha and Lotaif (1979) [97]	Random sample	Cairo, Egypt, 1975	200 (MF)	23%***

* Data are given for males only, wherever possible (for reasons see text). If no separate analysis for males has been made, then data on both sexes are given.

** 23% of the economically active

*** 53% of the economically active

such a history shows that unemployment among the latter is significantly more prevalent than among the former (32% versus 59%) [98].

Some of the studies listed in Table 4 have drawn attention to the fact that the unemployment rate among parasuicides is far greater than the unemployment rate in the general population. Thus, Lendrum [46] notes that while 22.6% of his cohort of attempted suicides were unemployed, the proportion in the population of which they were a sample was 12.2%. Bruhn [99] contrasts the figure of 43% unemployed in his sample with a figure of 17% among matched controls (psychiatric outpatients with no suicide attempt) and less than 4% for the population of Edinburgh. Edwards and Whitlock [100] found that 18% of their cohort of male parasuicides were unemployed in Brisbane, 1965-6; the rate among general population males was 1.3% in Australia in the same year. Hawton et al [101] show that the proportion of parasuicides who were unemployed was substantially higher than that in the general population in the area at the time of the study while other authors [102] merely state this fact without providing exact information.

I have only been able to locate three published references to parasuicide rates among the unemployed compared to the employed. Yap [68] gives details on a sample (whose representativeness is uncertain) of attempted suicides in Hong Kong, 1953-54. The unemployed constituted 28% of the sample but only 13% of the population (both sexes, 15 years and over). Although no attempted suicide rate is given for the employed as a group, rates are given for individual occupations. The rate for the unemployed (23.9 per 100,000) is second only to the rate for businessmen (36.5); no other rate is above 16 per 100,000. Kessell et al. [103] showed that in a provincial region of Victoria, Australia, the attempted suicide rate of the unemployed over the years 1971-2 was 2 686 per 100 000 unemployed males (1 in 37), more than nineteen times the average area rate of 137 per 100 000 males. The incidence in metropolitan region of Victoria was 1186 per 100,000 males. The rates of attempted suicide among unemployed men and women were very similar. When the employed group was differentiated into different occupational categories, the contrast with the unemployed is even more striking. Thus, the suicide attempt rate per 100 000 males in the provincial region was 21 for professionals/managers; 109 for white-collar workers; 234 for blue-collar workers;and 2 686 for the unemployed. In the metropolitan region the respective rates (males only) were 24, 149, 234 and 1 186. Kreitman [104] gives parasuicide rates for males in Edinburgh over the years 1968-70, by employment status. The rate per 100 000 employed was 92 (1 in 1088); per 100 000 unemployed it was 2 444 (1 in 40), giving a ratio of nearly 27:1. Platt and Kreitman [64] present parasuicide rates among employed and unemployed males in Edinburgh over the years 1968-82. Their analysis shows that although there was a strong temporal association between parasuicide and unemployment rates among males in Edinburgh, the relative risk of parasuicide among the unemployed fell from 29:1 in 1968 to 12:1 in 1982. Whereas the trend in parasuicide rates among the unemployed was generally downwards over this period (from 2824 per 100,000 in 1968 to 1345 per 100 000 in 1982), the rates among the employed fluctuated in a generally upward direction from a low of 97 per 100,000 in 1968 to a high of 173 per 100 000 in 1976, thereafter remaining at around 152 per 100,000 (although the rate for 1982 - 114 per 100,000 - showed a substantial fall over the previous year).

The evidence of the overrepresentation of the unemployed among parasuicides is overwhelming; clearly the relative risk of parasuicide is very much elevated for the unemployed compared to the employed. But is joblessness a significant aetiological factor, and if so, in what way? Cross-sectional surveys of parasuicide populations cannot, as we have seen, provide definitive answers to these questions, but they can give some useful pointers to possible associations between parasuicide and unemployment. For instance, we can examine the extent to which unemployment is given as an immediate cause of parasuicide. A number of studies have examined the events leading up to the parasuicide and Table 5 provides evidence of the frequency with which unemployment or associated socio-economic factors are judged to have been major precipitants. However, before accepting at face value the findings presented in Table 5, a certain number of difficulties should be noted. Firstly, studies differ in the meaning given to "unemployment" and in the range of problems which I have included under the rubric "related socio-economic factors". Secondly, none of the studies listed presents a clear account of the manner in which the rating is made. Is the parasuicide directly asked about the events which precipitated the overdose? If so, how? Is his reply accepted and recorded, or merely used as a guide by the interviewer? If the parasuicide is not asked, how is the information gathered? Thirdly, in some studies only one major precipitant per person is recorded, whereas in others each individual can rate any number of precipitants.

Table 5. Unemployment (or related socio-economic factor) as a "main precipitant cause" leading to parasuicide: a comparison of different studies

Source	Type of sample*	Place/ time period covered	N in series (Males (M) or both sexes (MF))**	Type of event and % or sample with such an event
East (1913) [113]	Cohort	London, 1907-10	1000 (MF)	"Unemployment" 11%
Moore (1937) [105]	Non-random sample; representativeness uncertain	Boston, U.S.A. 1915-36	105 (M)	"Financial embarassment and unemployment 37%
Lendrum (1933) [46]	Cohort	Detroit, U.S.A. 1927-30	363 (M)	"Economic" 33% (including "unemployment" 18%)
Hopkins (1937) [102]	Cohort	Liverpool, 1932-35	50 (M)	"Unemployment" 12%
Robins *et al* (1957) [110]	Non-random sample; representativeness uncertain	St. Louis, U.S.A. 1952-53	86 (MF)	"Trouble at work" 0%
Yap (1958) [30]	Non-random sample; representativeness uncertain	Hong Kong, 1953-54	70 (M)	"Economic" 47% (including "unemployment" 11%)
Woodside (1958) [106]	Cohort	London, 1956-57	55 (M)	"Unemployment" 9%
Harrington & Cross (1959) [112]	Cohort	Birmingham, 1956-68	48 (M)	"Socio-economic stress (occupational difficulties, debts, and housing problems)" 17%

Source	Type of sample*	Place/ time period covered	N in series (Males (M) or both sexes (MR))**	Type of event and % or sample with such an event
Sclare and Hamilton (1963)[148]	Random sample	Glasgow, 1960-62	180 (MF)	"Financial/ employment problem" 9%
Krupinski et al. (1966)[149]	Cohort	Victoria, Australia, 1963	204 (M)	"Finance, work or other environmental troubles" 16%
Whitlock and Schapira (1967)[102]	Cohort	Newcastle, 1962-64	94 (M)	"Worries over money, housing or employment" 11%
Smith and Davidson (1971)[108]	Cohort	Newcastle, 1966-69	209 (M)	"Occupational difficulty" 4% "Financial worries" 3%
Bagadia et al (1976)[111]	Cohort of economically active males	Bombay, India, 1968	255 (M)	"Unemployment" 8% (Among unemployed only 28%)
Morgan et al (1975)[107]	Non-random sample; representativeness uncertain	Bristol, 1972	368 (MF)	"Worries about work or unemployment" 5%
Werry and Pedder (1976) [150]	Cohort	Auckland, New Zealand, 1971-72	194 (MF)	"Financial or job worries" 12%
Lyons and Bindal (1977)[151]	Cohort	Belfast, 1972-75	496 (MF)	"Work problem" 2% "Redundancy" 0%

Bancroft et al. (1977) [109]	Representative sample	Oxford, 1972	130 (MF)	"Work" 7%

* All samples are based on patients admitted to hospital, except East (1913) who describes consecutive admissions to Brixton Prison.

** Data are given for males only, wherever possible. If no separate analysis for males has been made, then data on both sexes are given.

The surprising overall impression generated by Table 5 is of the relative unimportance of unemployment or related socio-economic factors as major precipitants of parasuicide. Although Yap [68], Moore [105] and Lendrum [46] report substantial percentages, only Lendrum's sample is likely to be representative and his figure for unemployment alone as a precipitant (18%) is not strikingly high. Only nine of the 17 studies actually refer to "unemployment" or "redundancy" at all; the average proportion of parasuicides in these samples citing unemployment/redundancy as a causative agent is about 12%. What is of particular interest is a comparison between percent of sample unemployed and unemployment as a major precipitant within the same study. Fortunately, a number of studies present such data. Thus in Hopkins' sample [102], 26 of his 50 males were unemployed but in only six cases was unemployment a precipitating cause; and in none of these was it considered to be a "primary cause". Eight of Woodside's sample [106] were unemployed but in only five cases was unemployment a "precipitating stress". Whitlock and Schapira [102] report that 34% of their sample of males were unemployed but only 11% registered "worries over money, housing or employment" as a "main precipitant cause" of the suicide attempt. Although thirty-six percent of Morgan's sample [107] were unemployed, only 5% claimed that "worries about work or unemployment" triggered that parasuicidal act. Similar discrepancies are found in the studies by Smith and Davidson [108] ,Bancroft et al. [109] and Yap [68]. Robins et al. [110] note that although 41 out of 86 patients admitted to hospital after a suicide attempt had experienced "job difficulties" in the six months prior to the suicide attempt (ie. quitting work, being fired, being demoted, excessive friction with others at work,) "trouble at work" was <u>never</u> given by the patient as a main reason for his behaviour. According to Bagadia et al. [111], "unemployment was the cause for attempted suicide in only 27.8% of the unemployed group". The only exception to this pattern is provided by Lendrum [46], who found that while 63 out of 363 male attempted suicides were unemployed (with a further 76 cases rated "not known" on employment status), 66 mentioned unemployment as a motive for their suicidal behaviour! Otherwise, it would appear that while a significant proportion of parasuicides are unemployed on admission to hospital, only a limited number claim that the state of being unemployed is of significance as an immediate cause or precipitant of their suicidal behaviour. Certainly, unemployment appears to be unimportant as a major precipitant, both absolutely and relative to other precipitants. Virtually all studies reach the conclusion that the most important single type of triggering event in parasuicide is "interpersonal conflict", a broad category which includes marital discord, kin disharmony, broken/unhappy love affair, dispute with parents, infidelity, etc [112]. The relative importance of interpersonal conflict and socio-economic factors (including unemployment) as precipitants of parasuicide are demonstrated in a number of studies. To take only two examples, 65% of a representative sample of suicide attempters in Oxford experienced an event (usually a quarrel) involving a 'key person', whereas only 7% experienced events in the "work" category [34]. Among parasuicide admissions to Bristol Royal Infirmary, 51% described a major precipitating factor involving interpersonal conflict, whereas only 5% referred to worries about work or unemployment [107].

Type 2 studies (aggregate-cross-sectional)

Macro-level analysis of the relationship between unemployment and parasuicide has been extremely limited. Buglass and Duffy [76] demonstrate the existence of a significant association between parasuicide and unemployment (men seeking work, women seeking work and unemployment in young people) across twenty-three city wards in Edinburgh, 1968-73. Significantly ecological correlations for the same town in 1973 alone are also reported, in this case between parasuicide and men and women (separately) seeking work [75]. In both these studies the correlation was higher for men seeking work than for women seeking work. Bagley et al. [39] also report a significant positive correlation between parasuicide rates and percent unemployed across nineteen wards in Brighton, 1966-68. It is noteworthy that the studies in both Edinburgh and Brighton also show high correlations between parasuicide and indicators of poverty (eg. free school meals, non-payment of electricity bills, clothing grants, no inside W.C., no hot tap); and, in Edinburgh alone, parasuicide is linked to juvenile delinquency (eg. truancy, children returned to the Reporter). Buglass and Duffy characterise the areas where parasuicide is common, and suicide relatively rare, as "lower class districts with associated problems of unemployment, poverty and juvenile delinquency" [76 p. 247].

Type 3 studies (individual-longitudinal)

No studies of this type (where parasuicide is the behavioural outcome measure) have been reported in the literature.

Type 4 studies (aggregate-longitudinal)

There is no formal analysis in the literature of the temporal relationship between parasuicide and unemployment. East examined the number of suicides and attempted suicides and the numbers unemployed for the years 1900-1911. He noted that the years 1908-09 showed the highest amount of unemployment for a decade. In 1908 the suicide and attempted suicide rates were also extremely high. "[I]t is clear that the year 1908 is responsible ... for ... unusually high rate[s of suicide and attempted suicide] ... When the reason for this is sought for it appears to be due in some measure, as might be anticipated, to unemployment." However, the following year both rates dropped markedly. Although, therefore, an exact parallel beteen unemployment and suicidal behaviour could not be demonstrated, East concluded that "there would appear to be at least some grounds ... for considering a relation to exist between them" [113]. Writing over 60 years later, Holding et al [114] also noted a peak of parasuicide referrals to the Regional Poisoning Treatment Centre in Edinburgh during 1971: "it was considered possible that this might correspond with the high employment in Edinburgh at about that time." However, unemployment continued to rise in 1972 while unemployment among referrals fell.

In view of the absence of any systematic treatment of this topic, Platt and Kreitman [64] have examined the relevant data for Edinburgh. Table 6 presents a summary of the main findings. It reports the male parasuicide person rate, the male unemployment rate and the percentage of economically active male parasuicides who were unemployed on admission, for the years 1968-82. The rank ordering for each variable across the years is given in parenthesis. A visual inspection of Table 6 appears to reveal a marked tendency for the unemployment and parasuicide rates to co-vary, and this impression is substatiated by formal

Table 6. Male unemployment and parasuicide in Edinburgh: 1968-1982

Year	Male parasuicide (person) rate (per 100,000)*	(rank)	Male unemployment rate (percent)**	(rank)	Percent of economically active male parasuicides who were unemployed on admission	(rank)
1968	157	(15)	2.7	(15)	44.7	(11)
1969	172	(14)	3.3	(14)	40.2	(15)
1970	185	(13)	4.5	(12)	43.1	(12)
1971	218	(9)	5.6	(8.5)	54.2	(3)
1972	223	(6)	5.6	(8.5)	47.1	(6)
1973	207	(11)	4.6	(11)	46.7	(7)
1974	208	(10)	4.4	(13)	42.3	(13)
1975	201	(12)	5.4	(10)	45.2	(10)
1976	247	(2)	6.7	(7)	45.9	(9)
1977	237	(3)	8.0	(3)	50.3	(4)
1978	219	(7.5)	7.2	(5)	46.0	(8)
1979	219	(7.5)	6.8	(6)	41.0	(14)
1980	226	(5)	7.7	(4)	49.2	(5)
1981	269	(1)	10.6	(2)	57.4	(2)
1982	229	(4)	12.8	(1)	63.2	(1)

* Mean rate per 100,000 for hospitalised male parasuicides, Edinburgh residents only, > 15 years old. The boundaries of the city of Edinburgh were enlarged in 1974, resulting in an increase of 5.5% in the total population. The definition of an "Edinburgh resident" was changed accordingly. The Registrar General's mid-year estimate of the male population in Edinburgh aged > 15 years was used as the denominator in the calculation of the rate.

** Males registered with local employment and career services offices covering the Edinburgh, Portobello and Leith employment exchange areas on census day (June) as percentage of all male employees in employment and those registered as unemployed in the same area.

statistical test. Unemployment rate is correlated significantly with both the parasuicide (person) rate (r_s = 0.88, p<.001) and with percent of admissions who were unemployed (r_s= 0.75, p<01). When unemployment is lagged one year, both correlations are reduced but still significant (r_s= 0.71, p<01 and r_s= 0.56, p<.05, respectively).

DISCUSSION

The main findings that emerge from the preceding review of the literature on the relationship between unemployment and suicidal behaviour can be summarised thus. The cross-sectional individual studies revealed that significantly more (para)suicides were unemployed than would be expected among general population samples. Likewise, (para)suicide rates among the unemployed were always considerably higher than among the employed. However, it should be noted that, in the only study of its kind, the relative risk of parasuicide among the unemployed (compared to the employed) was shown to fall during a time of increasing unemployment in the general population [64]. Type 2 (aggregate-cross-sectional) studies provided no evidence of a consistent relationship between unemployment and completed suicide, but a significant geographical association between unemployment and parasuicide rates was found. Results from all but one of the individual longitudinal studies point to significantly more unemployment, job instability and occupational problems among suicides compared to non-suicides. The exception is the investigation by Borg and Stahl [87] which identified (nonsignificantly) more "problems are work" among controls than among suicides (both samples coming from a psychiatric population). The OPCS longitudinal study [88] also found a high suicide rate among the unemployed in the general population. The aggregate longitudinal (Type 4) analyses point to a significant positive association between unemployment and suicide in the United states of America. The negative relationship in Great Britain in recent years has been shown to result from a unique decline in suicide rates in the 1960s due to the unavailability of the most common method of suicide [95].

On the relationship between unemployment and suicide

Despite this plethora of research findings, a definitive choice between the competing self-selection and causal models remains highly probalematic. We can confidently state that there is an association between unemployment and suicide [115] but we cannot specify with the same degree of confidence the nature of this association. It is true that some authors have demonstrated a willingness to make *ex cathedra* pronouncements in support of one or other model, relying more on strongly held personal convictions than on a sound or thorough analysis of available information [116]. The majority of researchers inthis field, however, take a more circumspect position. My own interpretation of the evidence is that empirical support for a *direct* causal link at the individual level between unemployment and suicide is weak. Attempts to abandon completely any element of self-selection in the suicide-unemployment relationship lack credibility because they fail to take cognizance of one crucial fact: namely, that "although mental illness is not a sufffcient cause of suicide, it is for all practical purposes in modern Western culture probably a necessary one" [117]. Retrospective studies by Barraclough et al. [118], and Robins et al. [119] and Dorpat and Ripley [120] show that over 90% of suicide victims are suffering from a major psychiatric illness (most frequently depression but often alcoholism) at the time of death. In his review of the evidence concerning conditions predisposing to suicide, Miles [121] concludes that virtually all the suicides in the United States can be attributed to the following causes: depressive illness, alcoholism, schizophrenia, neurosis and personality disorder, and drug addiction.

Even if this conclusion is considered to be valid [122] it does not ipso facto rule out the possibility that it is the individual's experience of unemployment which increases his/her vulnerability to psychological distress and psychiatric illness, and therefore the risk of suicidal behaviour. Indeed, recently Banks and Jackson [123] have demonstrated a definite causal link between unemployment in young school-leavers and increased psychiatric symptoms (measured by the twelve-item General Health Questionnaire); they also rule out the likelihood of the reverse causation hypothesis, ie. that the psychologically disturbed cannot find jobs. However, this finding cannot necessarily be generalised to other older populations, and the data do not allow a reliable estimate to be made of the extent to which unemployment in the sample was associated with serious psychiatric disorder. About 40% of the unemployed were found to score above the threshold point on the GHQ-12, compared to about 13% of the employed (and up to 20% in other general population surveys) [6].

The results of this type of investigation are therefore of doubtful relevance for our understanding of the association between unemployment and suicide. Close scrutiny of Type 1 studies leads to the conclusion that among those who eventually commit suicide the temporal and causal sequence of events is quite different from the sequence sketched in the model above. Rather than unemployment leading to psychiatric illness and thereafter to suicide, there is more evidence in favour of the alternative model:

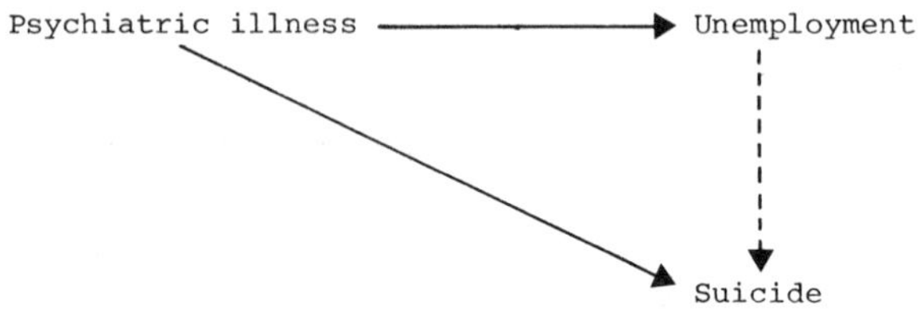

As we have seen, detailed analyses of individual case histories by Tuckman and Lavell [42], Ovenstone [71], Yap [68], Stearns [45], and Breed [41], among others, lend strong support to the proposition that unemployment in suicide victims is to a large extent a consequence or reflection of an underlying psychiatric disorder: rather than unemployment being a cause of psychiatric illness and suicide, it is more likely that the risks of both unemployment and suicide are elevated by the presence of a major psychiatric illness (in particular, depression). This conclusion is in line with Shepherd and Barraclough's speculation that the high prevalence of psychiatric ill-health among their sample of suicides

> "may also have been implicated in the higher rate of unemployment and greater number of job changes ... Rather than their [the suicides'] work loss resulting from broad social and economic trends, it is more likely that their psychiatric morbidity interfered with their capacity for work, resulting in work loss with its attendant disadvantages, so that mental illness at once stimulated in them suicidal thinking and at the same time took away from them an effective protection against suicidal behaviour." [81].

The connection between unemployment and suicide (presented as a dashed line in the diagram above) reminds us of the fact that, while psychiatric illness may be directly implicated in suicidal behaviour, it may also operate via unemployment. In particular, the psychological consequences or correlates of prolonged unemployment would appear to be likely to exacerbate the pre-existing psychiatric condition. The long-term unemployed are not only more vulnerable to, and less protected against, stressful life events and difficulties but also face more of these stressors by virtue of being without work. The effects of the psychiatric condition will be potentiated by the interaction between symptoms, stress and vulnerability.

Thus far we have only considered individual-level (Type 1) studies which necessarily ignore the role of the economic climate. How, then, can we incorporate our conclusions about the relationship between suicide and unemployment at the individual level with the abundant evidence of a temporal association between suicide and the macro-economy, in a more complete model of the pathways to suicide? A simplified version of such a model may be roughly sketched as follows. Macro-economic conditions, although not directly influencing the suicide rate, may nevertheless constitute an important antecedent variable in the causal chain leading to self-harmful behaviour. Consequent upon a deepening economic recession, individuals are subjected to greater levels of psychosocial stress. The experience of severe, undesirable life events and difficulties becomes more widespread leading to an increase in psychological distrubance and acute psychiatric illness in the most vulnerable individuals (some of whom may have previously enjoyed excellent psychological health) [124]. Even if a constant proportion of the psychiatric population becomes suicidal (irrespective of the economic climate), then as the pool of psychiatric cases enlarges the number of suicides (and therefore the suicide rate) will automatically rise. [125]. The additional psychiatric disorder "provoked" by the economic recession may indeed be found disproportionately among the unemployed, causing an increase in the relative risk of psychiatric illness and suicide among the unemployed compared to the employed. (It would be a matter of considerable theoretical and practical significance to discover whether the increased suicide risk was associated with recent job loss or with long-term unemployment.) On the other hand, the health effects of the recession may be more pronounced among the currently employed, inasmuch as they became anxious about job security and anticipate some future negative changes in their lifestyle, standard of living, feelings of "happiness", etc. arising out of the instability of the macro-economy [126]. If this were the case, we would expect to find that the relative risk of psychiatric illness and suicide among the unemployed (compared to the employed) would remain stationary or even decrease, due mainly to a rise in psychopathology among the employed. This trend might well be accentuated by the tendency for some workers made newly unemployed or redundant to experience relief rather than distress at their change in employment status. It is commonly assumed that all employment is "good" and all unemployment "bad". But unemployment may be "good" for individuals who suffer from "bad" employment, ie. jobs that are inherently stressful or psychologically demeaning or subject to insecurity of tenure, or involve continual change of work environment or require some degree of physical separation and isolation from others [127].

On the relationship between unemployment and parasuicide

If the data permitted only the roughest outline of a model describing the pathways between economic climate and suicide, then any attempt to delineate the nature of the relationship between unemployment and parasuicide must be even more tentative. There are no adequate published data based on a longitudinal design, and only two independent aggregate cross-sectional studies. We therefore have to rely almost exclusively on cross-sectional surveys of parasuicidal populations. Despite the inadequacy of this design as a basis for resolving the causal versus self-selection argument, we again find authors arguing vociferously about the meaning of the (universal) finding that there is a higher unemployment rate among parasuicides than among the general population [128]. On the available evidence, can anything be usefully said about this issue?

One point of interest is the discrepancy between the over-representation of the unemployed among the parasuicides, on the one hand, and the infrequent reference to unemployment as a major precipitating cause of parasuicide, at least by those who have committed the act, on the other. This somewhat paradoxical findings does not in fact rule out unemployment as a significant aetiological factor in parasuicide. It has already been pointed out that the rating of "precipitants" of parasuicide is extremely problematic. However the importance of interpersonal conflict as the major precipitant has been demonstrated in so many studies in many different countries, and over at least a quarter of a century, that it appears to be a reliable and valid finding.

Even if unemployment is not a triggering or precipitating event, it could be aetiologically significant as a predisposing factor. That is to say, unemployment may be parasuicidogenic, not in the sense of being a "provoking agent", but as an ongoing situation causing vulnerability which will increase the risk of suicidal behaviour when a provoking agent is present. (Unemployment may, of course, also have more than one aspect of causal importance: it may act as a provoking agent in some cases and a vulnerability factor in others) [129]. Thus, prolonged unemployment may be a significant predisposing factor in suicidal behaviour because it leads to: an increase in family tensions, arguments and violence; more depression and hopelessness; increasing isolation from others; changes in role structure within the family; financial hardship and marital deprevation; loss of self-esteem and self-confidence, and feelings of reduced self-worth; or any combination of these sequelae. A provoking agent (eg. argument with spouse) would be more likely to lead to parasuicide in the presence of unemployment (and its associated behavioural correlates) than in its absence.

This causal model of unemployment as a vulnerability factor, or long-term difficulty, rather than as a crisis event, requires evidence that joblessness among parasuicides is not a recent condition and is of significantly longer duration than would be expected among the unemployed in the general population. The scanty data available on this important issue does indeed show that the long-term unemployed are significantly over-represented in the parasuicide population [130]. However, while this finding supports the vulnerability (causal) model, it is of course also compatible with the possibility that certain individuals are at risk of both long-term unemployment and parasuicide by virtue of certain personal characteristics. Although there is not such a close association between parasuicide and psychiatric illness as was found for suicide, nevertheless surveys of parasuicides have repeatedly claimed that the majority of hospital-based cases are suffering from one or more of the following: a recognised psychiatric illness (usually depression), a personality disorder, alcoholism or alcohol abuse, or habitual drug misuse [131].

Furthermore, comparison between employed and unemployed parasuicides shows that significantly more of the unemployed have a previous history of parasuicide and psychiatric treatment; are classified as personality disordered or alcoholic; report a history of family suicide or parasuicide; have behaved violently towards others in the past five years; disclose a previous criminal record and face police proceedings at the time of admission; have a problem in the use of alcohol; and habitually misuse drugs [132]. These cross-sectional data certainly appear to fit well with the expected pathways of a self-selection model. O'Brien, for instance, concludes that the discovery of a relationship between previous overdose, personal disorganisation and unemployment in her sample of young adult parasuicides

> "suggest[s] that unemployment may be a result of difficulties rather than the main cause. People suffering fom emotional instability, and maybe alcohol or drug problems, will have difficulty in maintaining a job, or seeking employment." [98].

Yet, again, the evidence can be shown to be far from conclusive. For instance, very few parasuicide patients are likely to be suffering from severe psychiatric illnesses [133] and most psychopathology has been shown to be shortlived [134]. Moreover, the significant differences between employed and unemployed parasuicides could equally well rise because long-term unemployment leads to more interpersonal violence, psychiatric treatment, etc.

If, then, we return to the question posed at the beginning of this section ("On the available evidence, can anything be usefully said [about the aetiological significance of unemployment in parasuicide]"), the answer would appear to be: "Not much!". This will remain the case until we have carried out more empirical research based on a longitudinal design, at both the aggregate and individual levels. Admittedly, a prospective cohort study of parasuicide is not a practical or feasible proposition, but retrospective data on reasons for unemployment, duration of unemployment and previous job history should be obtained in order to test out the importance of personality variables in both unemployment and parasuicide. A controlled retrospective longitudinal study similar to that conducted by Shepherd and Barraclough [01] on completed suicides is an urgent requirement in this area of research.

ACKNOWLEDGEMENTS

I received considerable help from a number of individuals in the course of preparing this review. In particular I would like to thank Mr Hugh O'Donnel of the Manpower Services Commission, Edinburgh, Mr. Jim Connel of the Department of Physical Planning, Lothian Regional Council and Mr. A. Spence of the Department of Employment, who all provided me with data on unemployment. Dr. Keith Hawton, Department of Psychiatry, Warneford Hospital, Oxford, kindly supplied me with unpublished data on the employment status of attempted suicides admitted in Oxford. The present revised version has benefitted considerably from the constructive criticism of Dr. Norman Kreitman (Medical Research Council Unit for Epidemiological Studies in Psychiatry, Edinburgh) and Mr. Mike Porter (Department of General Practice, University of Edinburgh). Dr. David Dooley (Public Policy Research Organisation, Program in Social Ecology, University of California, Irvine) brought to my attention a number of relevant references I had originally missed.

REFERENCES

1 House of Commons Parliamentary Debates (Hansard), 37 (67), 366 (3 March 1983).

2 Warr, P.A. A study of psychological well-being. Br. J. Psychol, 69, 111-121, 1978.

3 Hepworth, S.J. Moderating factors of the psychological impact of unemployment. J. Occup. Psychol., 53, 139-145, 1980.

4 Hartley, J.F. The impact of unemployment on the self-esteem of managers. J. Occup. Psychol., 53, 147-155, 1980.

5 Stafford, E.M., Jackson, P.R. and Banks, M.H. Employment, work, involvement and mental health in less qualified young people. J. Occup. Psychol., 53, 291-304, 1980.

6 Warr, P. Some studies of psychological well-being and unemployment. MRC Social and Applied Psychology Unit, Memo No 431, Sheffield, 1981.

7 Warr. P. Psychological aspects of employment and unemployment. Psychol. Med., 12, 7-11, 1982.

8 See e.g., Seabrook, J. Unemployment. Quartet Books, London, 1982; Fagin, L. Unemployment and Health in Families. DHSS, London, 1981; Sinfield, A. What Unemployment Means, Martin Robertson. Oxford, 1981; Colledge, M. and Bartholomew, R. The long-term unemployed: some new evidence. Dept. Employment Gazette, 9-12, January 1980; Hill, J.M.M. The Social and Psychological Impact of Unemployment: A Pilòt Study, Tavistock, London, 1977; Harrison, R. The demoralising experience of prolonged unemployment. Dept. Employment Gazette, 339-348, April 1976; Marsden, D. and Duff. E. Workless - Some Unemployed Men and Their Families, Penguin, Harmondsworth 1975; Jahoda, M., Lazarsfeld, P.F. and Zeisel, H. Marienthal: The Sociography of an Unemployed Community, Tavistock London 1972 (1933); Sinfield, A. The Long-term Unemployed. OECD, Paris 1968; Komarovsky, M. The Unemployed Man and His Family. Dryden, New York 1940; Pilgrim Trust. Men Without Work. Cambridge University Press, London 1938; Eisenberg, P. and Lazarsfeld, P.F. The psychological effects of unemployment. Psychol. Bull., 35, 358-390, 1938; Zawadski, B. and Lazarsfeld, P. The psychological consequences of unemployment. J Soc. Psychol., 6, 224-250, 1935; Baake, E.W. The Unemployed Man. Nisbet, London 1933; Unemployment Unit. A Dossier of Despair: Experiences of Unemployment in the North East. Unemployment Unit, London, N.D. For a selective review of the literature, see Jahoda, M. and Rush, H. Work, Employment and Unemployment: An Overview of Ideas and Research Results in the Social Science Literature. Science Policy Research Unit, Occasional Paper Series, No 12, University of Sussex 1980.

9 E.g. Sinfield, 1981, op. cit.; Warr, 1982, op. cit.; Warr, P. Job loss, unemployment and psychological well-being. In E. van de Vliert and V Allen, eds., Role Transitions. Plenum Press, New York 1983; Fryer, D. 'All the world's a stage': Stages in the psychological response to unemployment. Part One: Phasing: the facts. MRC Social and Applied Psychology Unit, Memo No 523, Sheffield, 1982.

10 Eisenberg and Lazarsfeld, op. cit.

11 For other sequences of response stages see Hill, 1977, op. cit.; Harrison, 1976, op. cit.; Schlossberg, N.K. and Leibowitz, Z. Organisational support

systems as buffers to job loss. J. Vocational Behav., 17, 204-217, 1980; Briar, K.H. The effect of long-term unemployment on workers and their families. Diss. Abst. Int., 37 (9-A), 6062, 1977; Hayes, J. and Nutman, P. Understanding the Unemployed, Tavistock, London 1981.

12 Madge, N. Unemployment and its effects on children. J. Child. Psychol. Psychiatry, 24, 311-319, 1983; Steinberg, L., Catalano, R. and Dooley, D. Economic antecedents of child abuse and neglect. Child Dev., 52, 975-985, 1981; Gil, D. Violence against children, J. Marr. Fam., 33, 637-657, 1971.

13 Falret, J.P. De L'hyponchondrie et du Suicide. Paris, 1822.

14 Durkheim, E. Suicide. Routledge and Kegan Paul, London, 1952 (1897).

15 Brenner, M.H. Estimating the Social Costs of National Policy: Implications for Mental and Physical Health, and Criminal Aggression. Joint Economic Committee of Congess Paper No. 5, US Government Printing Oficer, Washington DC, 1976.

16 Brenner, M.H. Mortality and the national economy: a review and the experience of England and Wales, 1936-76. Lancet, 2, 568-573, 1979.

17 Gravelle, H.S.E., Hutchinson, G. and Stern, J. Mortality and unemployment: a critique of Brenner's time-series analysis. Lancet, 2, 675-679, 1981.

18 Eyer, J. Review of 'Mental Illness and the Economy'. Int. J. Health Serv., 6, 139-148, 1976.

19 Eyer, J. prosperity as a cause of death. Int. J. Health Serv., 7, 125-150, 1977a.

20 Eyer, J. Does unemployment cause the death rate peak in each business cycle? A multifactor model of death rate change. Int. J. Health Serv., 7., 625-662, 1977b.

21 Lancet (editorial) Does unemployment kill? Lancet, 1, 708-709, 1979.

22 Brenner, M.H. Health costs and benefits of economic policy. Int. J. Health Serv., 7, 581-623, 1977.

23 The term 'parasuicide', coined by Kreitman, N., Philip, A.E., Creer, S. and Bagley, C.R. (Parasuicide (letter). Br. J. Psychiatry, 115, 746-747, 1969), refers 'to a behavioural analogue of suicide but without considering a psychological orientation towards death being in any way essential to the definition'. It replaces the term 'attempted suicide' which has been extensively criticised on the grounds that it assumes an intention to die is always present in such behaviour. (see e.g. Kessell, N. Self-poisoning. Br. Med. J, 2, 1265-1270 and 1336-1340, 1965).

24 Shneidman, E.S. Orientation toward death: a vital aspect of the study of lives. Int. J. Psychiatry, 2, 167-200, 1966).

25 Kessel, N. The respectability of self-poisoning and the fashion of survival. J. Psychosom. Res., 10, 29-36, 1966.

26 Stengel, E. and Cook, H.G. Attempted Suicide, its Social Significance and Effects. Chapman and Hall, London, 1958.

27 E.g. Kreitman, N. Social and clinical aspects of suicide and attempted

suicide. In: A. Forrest, ed., A Companion to Psychiatric Studies, Vol. 1. Churchill Livingstone, Edinburgh, pp 38-63, 1973; Birtchnell, J. and Alarcon, J. The motivation and emotional state of 91 cases of attempted suicide. Br. J. Med. Psychol., 44, 45-52, 1971; Bancroft, J., Skrimshire, A. and Simkin, S. The reasons people give for taking overdoses. Brit. J. Psychiatry, 128, 538-548, 1976; Bancroft, J., Hawton, K., Simkin, S., Kingston, B., Cumming, C., and Whitwell, D. The reasons people give for taking overdoses: a further inquiry. Brit. J. Med. Psychol., 52, 353-365, 1979; Stengel, E. The complexity of motivations to suicidal attempts. J. Ment. Sci., 106, 1388-1393, 1960.

28 There are, however, some dissenting views. See e.g. Koller, K.M. and Cotgrove, R.C.M. Social geography and suicidal behaviour in Hobart, Aust. N.Z. J. Psychiatry, 10, 237-242, 1976; Lester, D. Relation between attempted suicide and completed suicide. Psychol. Rep., 27, 719-722, 1970b; Lester, D. Why People Kill Themselves: A Summary of Research Findings on Suicidal Behaviour. Charles C. Thomas, Springfield, Illinois, 1972.

29 Freeman, D.J., Wilson, K., Thigpen, J. and McGee, R.K. Assessing intention to die in self-injury behaviour. In C. Neuringer, ed., Psychological Assessment of Suicidal Risk. Charles Thomas, Springfield, Illinois, pp 18-42 1974 (at p 19).

30 See e.g., Kreitman, N. The epidemiology of suicide and parasuicide. Crisis, 2, 1-13, 1981; Ovenstone, I.M.K. Spectrum of suicidal behaviours in Edinburgh. Brit. J. Prev. Soc. Med., 27, 27-35, 1973; Dorpat, T.L. and Ripley, H.S. The relationship between attempted suicide and committed suicide. Compr. Psychiatry, 8, 74-79, 1967; Wilkins, J. Suicidal behaviour. Am. Sociol. Rev., 32, 286-298, 1967; Kennedy, P., Kreitman, N. and Ovenstone, I.M.K. The prevalence of suicide and parasuicide ('attempted suicide') in Edinburgh, Br. J. Psychiatry, 124, 36-41, 1974; Shneidman, E.S. and Farberow, N.L. Statistical comparisons between attempted and committed suicides. In N.L. Farberow and E.S. Shneidman, eds., The Cry for Help. McGraw Hill, New York, pp 19-47, 1961; Weiss, J.M.A. The gamble with death in attempted suicide. Psychiatry, 20, 17-25, 1957; Gibbs, J.P. ed., Suicide. Harper and Row, New York, 1968; Yap, P.M. Suicide in Hong Kong. J. Ment. Sci., 104, 266-301, 1958; Schmid, C. and van Arsdol, M.D. Completed and attempted suicides: a comparative analysis. Am. Sociol. Rev., 20, 273-283, 1955.

31 For useful summaries of these differences see Kreitman 1973, op. cit., 1981, op. cit.; Kreitman, N. and Dyer, J.A.T. Suicide in relation to parasuicide. Medicine, 36, 1827-1830, 1980.

32 Space precludes consideration of anecdotal, literary or qualitative approaches to this topic. Interested readers might, however, consult Stevenson, J. and Cook, C. The Slump: Society and Politics During the Great Depression. Quartet, London, 1979, for a discussion of the debate in the 1930s on the link between unemployment and suicide; Seabrook (op. cit.), whose moving and sensitive documentary analysis of the experience and impact of unemployment in contemporary Britain includes a number of verbatim accounts of suicidal thoughts among the jobless (e.g. pp. 3, 14, 123); recent newspaper reports of 'death on the dole', e.g. Guardian 30 March 1978 and 28 August 1981; Sunday Sun (Newcastle-upon-Tyne), 13 September 1981; Sunday Mail (Glasgow), 19 September 1982; Scottish Daily

Express, 13 August 182; Glasgow Herald, 12 August 1982; Sunday Times, 30 August 1981; and Fagin's in-depth study of 22 unemployed families in which he includes 'suicidal thoughts' in the list of psychological changes which can be brought about by job loss (Fagin, op. cit.).

33 Dooley, D. and Catalano, R. Economic change as a cause of behavioural disorder. Psychol. Bull, 87, 450-468, 1980.

34 See e.g. difference between Oxford and Edinburgh discussed in Bancroft, J., Skrimshire, A., Reynolds, F., Simkin, S. and Smith, J. Self-poisoning and self-injury in the Oxford area: epidemiological aspects 1969-73. Brit. J. Prev. Soc. Med., 29, 170-177, 1975.

35 See Rosenberg, M. The Logic of Survey Analysis. Basic Books, New York, 1968; and Susser, M. Causal Thinking in the health sciences: concepts and strategies of epidemiology. Oxford University Press, London, 1973, among others, for extended discussions of the methods used to screen causal models for extraneous factors.

36 Goodman, L.A. Ecological regressions and behaviour of individuals. Am. Sociol. Rev., 18, 663-664, 1953; Robinson, W.S. Ecological correlations and the behaviour of individuals. Am. Sociol. Rev., 15, 351-357, 1950; Selvin, H.C. Durkheim's 'Suicide' and problems of empirical research. Am. J. Sociol., 63, 607-619, 1958.

37 Morganstern, H. Uses of ecological analysis in epidemiological research. Am. J. Public Health, 72, 1336-1344, 1982; Firebaugh, G. A rule for inferring individual-level relationships from aggregate data. Am. Sociol. Rev., 43, 557-572, 1978.

38 Philip, A.E. and McCulloch, J.W. Use of social indices in psychiatric epidemiology. Brit. J. Prev. Soc. Med., 20, 122-126, 1966; McCulloch, J.W. and Philip, A.E. Social variables in attempted suicide. Acta Psychiat. Scand., 43, 341-346, 1967.

39 Bagley, C., Jacobson, S. and Palmer, C. Social structure and the ecological distribution of mental illness, suicide and delinquency. Psychol. Med., 3, 177-187, 1973.

40 E.g. Sainsbury, P. Suicide in London. Chapman and Hall, London, 1955.

41 Breed, W. Occupational mobility and suicide among white males. Am. Sociol. Rev., 28, 179-188, 1963.

42 Tuckman, J. and Lavell, M. Study of suicide in Philadelphia. Public Health Rep., 73, 547-553, 1958.

43 MacMahon, B. and Pugh T.F. Epidemiology: Principles and Methods. Little, Brown and Company, Boston, 1970.

44 Exceptionally, the data are presented as raw frequencies rather than rates (e.g. Swinscow, D. Some suicides statistics. Br. Med. J., 1, 1417-1422, 1951).

45 Stearns, A.W. Suicide in Massachusetts. Ment. Hygiene, 5, 752-777, 1921.

46 Lendrum, F.C. A thousand cases of attempted suicide. Am. J. Psychiatry, 90, 479-500, 1933.

47 Hurlburt, W.C. Prosperity, depression and the suicide rate. Am. J. Social., 37, 714-719, 1932.

48 MacMahon, B., Johnson, S., and Pugh, T.F. Relation of suicide rates to sociol conditions. Public Health Rep., 78, 285-293, 1963.

49 Windschuttle, K. Unemployment. Penguin Books, Ringwood, Australia, 1979.

50 For an introduction to time series analysis, see e.g., Cook. T.D., Dintzer, L. and Mark, M.M. The causal analysis of concomitant time series. Appl. Soc. Psychol. Ann., 1, 93-135, 1980; Mark, M. The Causal analysis of concomitancies in time series. In, T.D. Cook and D.T. Campbell, eds., Quasi-experimentaion. Chicago, Houghton-Mifflin, pp 321-339, 1979; Box, G.E.P. and Jenkins, G.M. Time Series Analysis: Forecasting and Control. Holden-Day, San Francisco, 1976.

51 Examples are found in Boor, M. Relationships between unemployment rates and suicide rates in eight countries, 1962-1976. Psychol. Rep., 47 (3 Pt. 2), 1095-1101, 1980; Sainsbury, P., Jenkins, J. and Levey, A. The social correlates of suicide in Europe. In, R. Farmer and S. Hirsch, eds., The Suicide Syndrome. Croom Helm, London, pp 38-53, 1980.

52 Brenner, M.H. Estimating the health costs of national economic policy in Scotland, 1950-1980. Paper presented at Conference on 'Unemployment and Health: The Scottish Perspective', Glasgow, 1981.

53 E.g. Vigderhous, G. and Fishman, G. The impact of unemployment and Familial integration on changing suicide rates in the USA, 1920-1969. Soc. Psychiatry, 13, 239-248, 1978; Hammermesh, A.S. and Soss, N.M. An economic theory of suicide. J. Polit. Econ., 82, 83-98, 1974.

54 See. e.g., Spruit, I.P. Unemployment and health in macro-social analysis. Soc. Sci. Med., 16, 1903-1917, 1982; Kasl, S.V. Mortality and the business cycle. Some questions about research strategies when utilising macro-social and ecological data. Am. J. Public Health, 69, 784-788, 1979; Kasl, S.V. Strategies of research on economic instability and health. Psychol. Med., 12, 637-649, 1982; Eyer, J., 1977a, op. cit, 1977b, op. cit.; Dooley, and Catalano 1980, op. cit.

55 E.g., Stern, J. Unemployment and its impact on morbidity and mortality. Centre for Labour economic, L.S.E. Discussion Paper No 93, London, 1981; Stern, J. Does unemployment really kill? New Soc., 60, 421-422, 1982; Gravelle, et al. 1981, op. cit.; Eyer 1976, op. cit.; Pollack, E.S. Book Review 'Mental Illness and the Economy', Am. J. Public Health, 64, 152-513, 1974; Colledge, M. Economic cycles and health. Towards a sociological understanding of the impact of the recession on health and illness. Soc. Sci. Med., 16, 1919-1927, 1982; and Marshall, J.R. and Junch, D.P. Mental illness and the economy: a critique and partial replication. J. Health Soc. Behav., 20, 282-289, 1979.

56 Kasl, 1979, op. cit.

57 As in Brenner 1973 op. cit. Marshal, J.R. and Hodge, R.W., Durkheim and Pierce on suicide and economic change. Soc. Sci. Res., 10, 101-114, 1981, also refer to the use of Pierce's work (Pierce, A. The economic cycle and the social suicide rate. Am. Sociol. Rev., 32, 457-462, 1967) of 'negative lead' correlations and comment: 'That a hypothesis involving the effect of economic conditions upon suicide could be tested if the dependent variable is lagged one to three years behind the independent variable presents a problem of causation. It is clearly difficult to comprehend

how an event or condition existing in any given year could have an impact on events which occurred between 1 and 3 years earlier

58 Cook et al, op. cit. See also Mark, op. cit.

59 Mark, op. cit.

60 Marshall and Hodge, op. cit.

61 The method of counting the number of unemployed was changed in October 1982. Previously, the unemployed consisted of those persons registered for work with the official employment services - at a Jobcentre, Local Employment Office or Careers Office - on census day and judged by staff to be 'capable of and available for work'.

62 This would, of course, be an incidence event rate, since any individual could have more than one claim/registration during a calendar year. Unfortunately, the manner of collection of unemployment flow data precludes the calculation of an incidence person rate.

63 Huges, I. Flows on and off the unemployment register. Employment Gazette, 527-530, December 1982.

64 Trends in Parasuicide and Unemployment among Edinburgh Men, 1968-1982, Br. Med. J., in press 1984.

65 Robin, A.A., Brooke, E.M. and Freeman-Browne, D.L. Some aspects of suicide in psychiatric patients in Southend. Br. J. Psychiatry, 114, 739-747, 1968.

66 Roy, A. Risk factors for suicide in psychiatric patients. Arch. Gen. Psychiatry, 39, 1089-1095, 1982.

67 Although Breed (op. cit.) interviewed 206 controls (each suicide being matched by sex, race and age with two controls), no information on their employment status is presented in this report; and no comparison with the general population is made. Maris's sample of national deaths is not matched to his sample of suicides. (Maris, R.W. Pathways to Suicide: A Survey of Self-Destructive Behaviours. John Hopkins University Press, Baltimore, Md., 1981).

68 Yap, op. cit.

69 Cumming, E., Lazar, C. and Chisholm, L. Suicide as an index of role strain among employed and not employed married women in British Colombia. Canad. Rev. Sociol. Antropol., 12, 463-469, 1975.

70 Kraft, D.P. and Babigian, H.M. Suicides by persons with and without psychiatric contacts. Arch. Gen. Psychiatry, 33, 209-215, 1976.

71 Ovenstone, I.M.K. An Epidemiological Study of Suicidal Behaviours in Edinburgh. MD thesis, University of Edinburgh, 1972.

72 Sathyavathi, K. Suicide among unemployed persons in Bangalore. Indian J. Soc. Work, 37, 385-392, 1977.

73 Lester, D. Suicide and unemployment. A re-examination. Arch. Environ. Health, 20, 277-278, 1970a.

74 Walbran, B., MacMahon, B., and Bailey, A.E. Suicide and unemployment in Pennsylvania, 1954-61. Arch. Environ. Health, 10, 11-15, 1965.

75 Buglass, D., Duffy, J. and Kreitman, N. A Register of Social and Medical Indices by Local Government Area in Edinburgh and the Lothians (2 parts). Central Research Unit, Scottish Office, Edinburgh, 1980.

76 Buglass, D. and Duffy J.C. The ecological pattern of suicide and parasuicide in Edinburgh. Soc. Sci. Med., 12, 241-253, 1978.

77 Rushing, W.A. Income, unemployment and suicide: an occupational study. Sociol. Quart., 9, 493-503, 1968.

78 Although studies by Ovenstone (1972 op. cit., 1973 op. cit) and Sanborn, D.E., Sanborn, C.J. and Cimbolic, P. Occupation and suicide. Dis. Nerv. Syst. 35, 7-12, 1974, contain some information relating to employment status during the time prior to suicide, they are essentially cross-sectional in design and are included in the section above describing Type 1 studies.

79 Humphrey, J. Social loss: a comparison of suicide victims, homicide offenders and non-violent individuals. Dis. Nerv. Syst., 38, 157-160, 1977.

80 Olsen, J. and Lajer, M. Violent death and unemployment in two trade unions in Denmark. Soc. Psychiatry, 14, 139-145, 1979.

81 Shepherd, D.M. and Barraclough, B.M. Work and suicide: an empirical investigation. Br. J. Psychiatry, 136, 469-478, 1980

82 Sanborn et al (op. cit.) found that 10 out of 15 male suicides experienced some form of job change within the 12 months preceding their deaths, and six exhibited a history of job-hopping or job loss during their occupational lives. Ovenstone (1972 op. cit) reports that about half of 37 male suicides who were unemployed, not working or retired at the time of their death had been in the same situation for at least two years prior to death.

83 Theorell, T., Lind, E. and Floderus, B. The relationship of disturbing life-changes and emotions to the early development of myocardial infarction and other serious illnesses. Int. J. Epidemiol. 4, 281-293, 1975.

84 See e.g., Kasl, S.V., Gore, S. and Cobb, S. The experience of losing a job: reported changes in health, symptoms and illness behaviour. Psychosom. Med., 37, 106-122, 1975; Kasl, S.V. and Cobb, S. Some mental health consequences on plant closing and job loss. In L.A. Ferman and J.P. Gordus, eds., Mental Health and the Economy. W.E. Upjohn Institute for Employment Research, Kalamazoo, pp 255-299, 1979; Cobb, S. and Kasl, S.V. Termination: The Consequences of Job Loss. D.H.E.W. (N.I.O.S.H.) Publication No. 77-224, Cincinatti, 1977.

85 Cobb, S. and Kasl, S.V. Some medical aspects of unemployment. Industr. Geront., 8, 8-15, 1972.

86 Hagnell, O. and Rorsman, B. Suicide in the Lundby Study: a controlled prospective investigation of stressful life events. Neuropsychobiology, 6, 319-332, 1980.

87 Borg, S.E. and Stahl, M. Prediction of suicide: a prospective study of suicides and controls among psychiatric patients. Acta Psychiatr. Scand., 65, 221-232, 1982.

88 Fox, A.J. and Goldblatt, P.O. Longitudinal Study: Socio-demographic and Mortality Differentials, 1971-1975. H.M.S.O., London, 1982.

89 Pierce, op. cit.

90 Marshall and Hodge, op. cit., p 106.

91 Waldron, J. and Eyer, J. Socioeconomic causes of the recent rise in death rates for 15-24 year olds. Soc. Sci Med., 9, 383-396, 1975.

92 Catalano, R.A., Dooley, D. and Jackson, R. Selecting a Time-Series Strategy. Unpublished MS. 1982.

93 Marshall, J.R. Changes in aged white male suicide: 1948-1972. J. Gerontol., 33, 763-768, 1978.

94 The dangers of using numbers rather than rates is nicely illustrated by Cook et al (op. cit.) who show that the Pearson correlation between the N of suicides and the N of employed persons in the USA over the years 1900-1975 was +0.83! Once population growth is 'controlled for' by using detrended data, the relationship becomes significantly negative (r-0.59).

95 Kreitman, N. (The coal gas story: UK suicide rates 1960-1971. Br. J. Prev. Soc. Med., 30, 86-93, 1976) shows that the carbon monoxide (CO) content of domestic gas fell markedly in Great Britain after 1962, and that during the following decade suicides specifically due to CO decreased dramatically (in both sexes and all age-groups). He argues convincingly that there is a direct causal relationship between these two phenomena. At the same time, however, suicide due to other causes increased among women of all ages and among young men, with a decline registered only among men aged 55 years plus. Overall, the decrease in CO suicide was sufficiently large to lower the total suicide rate and accounts for the unique finding of a negative correlation between unemployment and suicide in Great Britain. (An analysis by the present author of the association between unemployment and non-CO suicide over the period investigated by Boor (op. cit.) shows, as expected, that the sign of the correlation changes from negative to positive. For males, r+0.76, p>.01. See Kreitman, N. and Platt, S. Suicide, Unemeployment, and Domestic Gas Detoxification in Great Britain, J. Epidem. Comm. Hlth., 38, 1-6, 1984.

96 Warr, P. and Parry, G. Paid employment and women's psychological well-being. Psychol. Bull., 91, 498-516, 1982.

97 Okasha, A. and Lotaif, F. Attempted suicide. An Egyptian investigation. Acta Psychiatr. Scand., 60, 69-75, 1979.

98 O'Brien, S.E.M. A survey of young adults admitted to hospital for self-poisoning in a central London district, February 1975-August 1976. PhD Thesis, University of London, 1981. In an unpublished analysis of male parasuicide admissions to the Regional Poisoning Treatment Centre in Edinburgh, it was found that 59% of those with a previous parasuicide history were unemployed compared to 31% of those with no previous history. These figures are virtually identical to those given by O'Brien.

99 Bruhn, J.G. Broken homes among attempted suicides and psychiatric outpatients: a comparative study. J. Ment. Sci., 108, 772-779, 1962.

100 Edwards, J.E. and Whitlock, E.A. Suicide and attempted suicide in Brisbane. Med. J. Aust., 1, 932-938, 1968a.

101 Hawton, K., O'Grady, J., Osborn, M. and Cole, D. Adolescents who take overdoses: their characteristics, problems, and contact with helping agencies. Br. J. Psychiatry, 140, 118-123, 1982.

102 E.g., Hopkins, F. Attempted suicide: an investigation. J. Ment. Sci., 83, 71-94, 1937; Whitlock, F.A. and Schapira, K. Attempted suicide in Newcastle-upon-Tyne. Br. J. Psychiatry, 113, 423-434, 1967.

103 Kessell, A., Nicholson, A., Graves, G. and Krupinski, J. Suicidal attempts in an outer region of metropolitan Melbourne and in a provincial region of Victoria. Aust. N.Z. J. Psychiatry, 9, 255-261, 1975.

104 Kreitman 1973, op. cit.

105 Moore, M. Cases of attempted suicide in a general hospital: A problem in social and psychological medicine. N. Eng. J. Med., 217, 291-303, 1937.

106 Woodside, M. Attempted suicide arriving at a general hospital. Br. Med. J., 2, 411-414, 1958.

107 Morgan, H.G., Burns-Cox, C.J., Pocock, H. and Pottle, S. Deliberate self-harm: clinical and socio-economic characteristics of 368 patients. Br. J. Psychiatry, 127, 564-574, 1975.

108 Smith, J.S. and Davidson, K. Changes in the pattern of admissions for attempted suicides in Newcastle-upon-Tyne during the 1960s. Br. Med. J., 4, 412-415, 1971.

109 Bancroft, J., Skrimshire, A., Casson, J., Harvard-Watts, O. and Reynolds, F. People who deliberately poison or injure themselves: their problems and their contacts with helping agencies. Psychol. Med., 7, 289-303, 1977.

110 Robins, E., Schmidt, E.H. and O'Neal, P. Some interrelations of social factors and clinical diagnosis in attempted suicide: a study of 109 patients. Am. J. Psychiatry, 114, 221-231, 1957.

111 Bagadia, V.N., Ghadalia, H.N. and Shah, L.P. Unemployment and attempted suicide. Indian J. Psychiatry, 18, 131-139, 1976.

112 See e.g., Bancroft et al, 1975 (op. cit.) 1977 (op. cit.); Fieldsend, R. and Lowenstein, E. Quarrels, separations and infidelity in the two days preceding self-poisoning episodes. Br. J. Med. Psychol., 54, 349-352, 1981; Whitlock and Schapira (op. cit.); Harrington, J.A. and Cross, K.W. Cases of attempted suicide admitted to a general hospital. Br. Med. J., 2, 463-467, 1959; Kessel 1965 (op. cit.); Adam, K., Bianchi, G., Hawker, F., Nairn, L., Sanford, M. and Scarr, G. Interpersonal factors in suicide attempts: a pilot study in Christchurch. Aust. N.Z. J. Psychiatry, 12, 59-63, 1978; Morgan et al, 1975a (op. cit.).

113 East, W.N. On attempted suicide, with an analysis of 1000 consecutive cases. J. Ment. Sci., 59, 428-478, 1913.

114 Holding, T.A., Buglass, D., Duffy, J.C. and Kreitman, N. Parasuicide in Edinburgh - a seven-year review 1968-1974. Br. J. Psychiatry, 130, 534-543, 1977.

115 <u>Pace</u> Mr David Mellor (see note 1).

116 The most extreme example of an ideological commitment to the self-selection model is found in the general discussion of suicide by MacEarlean, D.A. Some aspects of suicide. Ir. J. Med. Sci., 102, 241-254, 1934, who notes that the rate of suicide is nearly twice as high among unemployed as among employed males. 'This is an instance of the 'weaker going to the wall'', he states. 'The man with a strong healthy inheritance is more likely to be a fighter and to obtain employment, but the reason why his suicide rate is lower is not because he is employed but because his physiological system is the sounder of two, which enables him to retain his employment longer.' Walbran et al, (op. cit.) are more tentative in their expression of the same viewpoint. They tend towards agreement with the statement that 'unemployment is not an etiological influence in any appreciable number of suicides' rather than that 'unemployment is a precipitating factor is suicide'. They suggest that the high proportion of unemployed among suicides may result from a social or occupational 'drift' associated with characteristics of the impending suicide syndrome (quoting evidence in Breed, op. cit.). On the other hand, Windschuttle (op. cit.) rejects out of hand the argument that certain personality characteristics tend to increase the individual's vulnerability to both unemployment and suicide, claiming that longitudinal and cross-sectional analyses establish the causal significance of unemployment in suicidal behaviour.

117 Brown, J.H. Suicide in Britain. More attempts, fewer deaths, lessons for public policy. Arch. Gen. Psychiatry, 36, 1119-1124, 1979.

118 Baraclough, B., Bunch, J., Nelson, B. and Sainsbury, P. A hundred cases of suicide: clinical aspects. Br. J. Psychiatry, 125, 355-373, 1974.

119 Robins, E., Gassner, S., Kayes, J., Wilkinson, R.H. and Murphy, G.E. The communication of suicidal intent. A study of 134 consecutive cases of successful (completed) suicide. Am. J. Psychiatry, 115, 724-733, 1959.

120 Dorpat, T. and Ripley H.S. A study of suicide in the Seattle area. Compr. Psychiatry, 1, 349-359, 1960.

121 Miles, C.P. Conditions predisposing to suicide: a review. J. Nerv. Ment. Dis., 164, 231-246, 1977.

122 It should be noted that many non-psychiatrists are loth to accept the validity of this association between suicide and psychiatric illness. Baechler, J. Suicides. Basil Blackwell, Oxford, 1979, for instance, contends that since suicide is a positive act ('one logical and universal way ... of resolving a problem'), the 'really mentally ill' cannot commit suicide. 'Where consciousness is eclipsed, no suicides are to be found.' (p 45). According to Maris (op. cit.), 'most suicides are not psychotic, nor even necessarily irrational'. He goes on to criticise studies which report a prevalence of mental illness among suicides approaching 100%: 'it is well-known that when invesigators are aware in advance of their

diagnosis that they are evaluating a suicide, their post factum diagnosis of mental illness is higher than when the subject is evaluated without prior knowledge of suicide.' (p 207).

123 Banks, M.H. and Jackson, P.R. Unemployment and risk of minor psychiatric disorder in young people: cross-sectional and longitudinal evidence. Psychol. Med., 12, 789-798, 1982.

124 Evidence of an association at the aggregate level between changes in the economy and changes in the incidence of psychiatric illness, though strong (e.g., Brenner, M.H. Mental illness and the economy. Harvard University Press, Cambridge, Mass, 1973; Brenner 1976, op. cit.; Marshall and Funch op. cit.; Stokes, G. and Cochrane, R., The relationship between national levels of unemployment and the rate of admission to mental hospitals in England and Wales, 1950-1976. Social Psychiatry in press), is not conclusive (see e.g., Catalano, R.A., Dooley, C.D., and Jackson, R.L. Economic predictors of admissions to mental health facilities in a non-metropolitan community. J. Health Soc. Behav., 22, 284-297, 1981; Barling, P. and Handal, P. Incidence of utilisation of public mental health facilities as a function of short term economic decline. Am. J. Community Psychol., 8, 31-39, 1980; Dooley, C.D., Catalano, R.A., Jackson, R.L. and Brownwell, A. Economic, life, and symptom changes in a non-metropolitan Community. J. Health Soc. Behav., 22, 144-154, 1981). Partial support for the hypothosised link between economic contraction, an increase in undesirable stressors and in increase in the incidence of illness and injury has been reported by Catalano, R. and Dooley, D. The health effects of economic instability: a test of the economic stress hypothesis. J. Health Soc. Behav. (in press). Qualified support is also reported for the provocation explanation, whose central tenet is that economic instability somehow causes disorder in previously healthy people which, in turn, increases their likelihood to seek help. However, the same study found evidence in favour of a rival explanation which assumes that economic instability can lead to help seeking without causing disorder in previously healthy people. Dooley, D. and Catalano, R. Why the Economy Predicts Help Seeking: A Test of Competing Explanations. (See Chapter 8)

125 According to an alternative version of this model the impact of economic conditions upon the health of the population would not be reflected in an increase in the number of persons with psychiatric symptoms, but in an increase in the proportion of the psychiatric pool suffering from a major disorder. Given the association between such disorders and suicide, the suicide rate would be likely to rise also.

126 For further discussion on the stressful effects of the recession upon the employed as well as the unemployed, see e.g. Brenner, 1981, op. cit.

127 Warr, 1983 op. cit.; Brodsky, C.M. Suicide attributed to work. Suicide Life Threat. Behav., 7, 216-229, 1977. See also, Karcher, C.J. and Linden, L.L. Is work conducive to self-destruction? Suicide Life Threat. Behav., 12, 151-175, 1982.

128 Thus Hopkins (op. cit.), while acknowledging the fact that 'prolonged unemployment has far reaching influences on outlook, health, domestic relations, etc', reaches the firm conclusion that his finding of a high prevalence of unemployment 'among suicidals [more than half his sample of male attempted suicides were unemployed] is a result of inferiority of personality rather than a cause of suicide.' However, Lendrum (op. cit.), who found a less marked relationship between unemployment and parasuicide than Hopkins, reached a diametrically opposite conclusion:

'The distinctly greater proportion of unemployment in the group of persons who attempted suicide suggests that unemployment is not merely an excuse for suicide, but that it is actually a predisposing factor of considerable importance'. More recent discussions of this issue have been less strident, and it is perhaps signficant that none can be found which wholeheartedly embrace Lendrum's position. For instance, Edwards, J.E. and Whitlock, F.A. Suicide and attempted suicide in Brisbane, Med. J. Aust. 1, 989-995, 1968b note the chacacteristic association between high rates of unemployment and times of economic depression, on the one hand, and high suicide and attempted suicide rates on the other.

> 'Nevertheless, it would be wrong to infer that attempted suicide by unemployed persons necessarily means that unemployment was a factor responsible for the suicidal act. Personality disorders affect employability, leading to a higher incidence of unemployment which has been brough about largely by the make-up of the individual. In 1965, in Brisbane, there was no major employment problem, although in Newcastle in 1962 and 1963 unemployment was heavy. Nevertheless, in both cities, among those making attempts at suicide, there was a higher rate of unemployment in comparison with the general population.' (p 990).

129 I am here following the terminology of Brown, G.W. and Harris, T. Social Origins of Depression. Tavistock, London, 1978, p 47.

130 Smith and Davidson, op. cit.; Morgan et al 1975a, op. cit.; Platt and Kreitman, op. cit.

131 In their study of overdose patients assessed using the present state examination, Newson-Smith, J.G. and Hirsch, S.R. Psychiatric symptoms in self-poisoning patients. Psychol. Med., 9, 493-500, 1979, found that psychiatric symptoms were common during the four weeks preceding the act. 31% of patients had a definite psychiatric disorder and a further 29% were in the borderline or 'threshold' category. All but one patient in these two groups were diagnosed as suffering from depressive disorders. Urwin, P. and Gibbons, J.L. Psychiatric diagnosis in self-poisoning patients. Psychol. Med., 9, 501-507, 1979, found that 30% of their sample of self-poinsoners had definite disorders and 42% were in the borderline group. Most were suffering from depression. A quarter of the men and just over 1 in 10 of the women were classified as having personality disorders. Only one third of male parasuicide admissions to the Regional Poisoning Treatment Centre, Edinburgh, in 1980 were not classified as either psychiatrically ill or personality disordered or alcoholic. This proportion rose to just under a half in 1981. About a third of male admissions in both years had received previous inpatient psychiatric care. Just under one in five males reported habitual drug misuse (unpublished data).

132 Platt, S. and Duffy, J. in preparation.

133 Morgan et al op. cit. report that only 12% of their sample of 337 parasuicides were diagnosed as suffering from a major functional psychotic illness.

134 Newson-Smith and Hirsch, op. cit.

135 Pallis, D.J., Barraclough, B.M., Levey, A.B., Jenkins, J.S. and Sainsbury, P. Estimating suicide risk among attempted suicides: I The development

of new clinical scales, Br. J. Psychiatry, 141, 37-44, 1982.

136 Morris, J.B., Kovacs, M., Beck, A.T. and Wolffe, A. Notes toward an epidemiology of urban suicide. Compr. Psychiatry, 15, 537-547, 1974.

137 Wallis, C.P. and Maliphant, R. Delinquent areas in the county of London: ecological factors. Br. J. Criminology, 7, 250-284, 1967.

138 Farmer, R.D.T., Preston, T.O. and O'Brien, S.E.M. Suicide mortality in Greater London: changes during the past 25 years. Br. J. Prev. Soc. Med., 31, 171-177, 1977.

139 Thomas, D.S. Social Aspects of the Business Cycle. Knopf, New York, 1927.

140 Ogburn, W.F. and Thomas, D.S. The influence of the business cycle on certain social conditions. J. Am. Stat. Assoc. 18, 324-340, 1922.

141 Henry, A.F. and Short, J.F. Suicide and Homicide, Free Press, New York, 1954.

142 Dublin, L.I. and Bunzel, B. To Be or Not To Be, A Study of Suicide. Harrison Smith and Robert Haas, New York, 1933.

143 Stack, S. Divorce and suicide: a time series analysis 1933-1970. J. Fam. Issues, 2, 77-90, 1981.

144 Batchelor, I.R.C. Psychopathic states and attempted suicide. Br. Med. J., 1, 1324-1327, 1954.

145 Patel, A.R., Roy, M. and Wilson, G.M. Self-poisoning and alcohol. Lancet, 2, 1099-1103, 1972.

146 Jacobson, S. and Tribe, P. Deliberate self-injury (attempted suicide) in patients admitted to hospital in mid-Sussex. Br. J. Psychiatry, 121, 379-386, 1972.

147 Unpublished data.

148 Sclare, A.B. and Hamilton, C.M. Attempted suicide in Glasgow, Br. J. Psychiatry, 109, 609-615, 1963.

149 Krupinski, J., Stoller, A. and Polke, P. Attempted suicides admitted to the mental health department, Victoria, Australia: a socio-demiological study. Int. J. Soc. Psychiatry, 13, 5-13, 1966.

150 Werry, J.S. and Pedder, J. Self-poisoning in Auckland, N.Z. Med. J., 83, 183-187, 1976.

151 Lyons, H.A. and Bindal, K.K. Attempted suicide in Belfast. Irish Med. J., 70, 328-332, 1977.

EPIDEMIOLOGICAL STUDIES OF THE PSYCHOLOGICAL RESPONSE TO ECONOMIC INSTABILITY IN ENGLAND: A SUMMARY

Graham Stokes

I intend to concern myself in this paper with a brief and what may inevitably seem a rather superficial review of some research I have carried out over the past 6 years into the psychological and social consequences of economically precipitated stress in general and job deprivation in particular. A time series analysis of mental hospital admission rates in relation to the level of unemployment for England and Wales from 1950 to 1976 is described elsewhere (Stokes and Cochrane 1984a, see also p26). This paper describes three epidemiological studies of unemployed workers and school leavers carried out in Bradford and Birmingham between 1978 and 1982.

The experience of redundancy: a six month study of job loss and unemployment in Yorkshire 1978 - 1979

While the life problems associated with economic recession are varied, it is reasonable to assume that the people who are exposed to the most potentially stressful demands, events and situations at a time of economic contraction, in terms of both frequency and severity, will be those experiencing the primary effects of the economic situation, for example, the unemployed.

However, when reviewing the literature concerned with the psychological effects of unemployment, many of the conclusions drawn are confounded by a serious methodological problem. In addition to the evidence that poor health is associated with unemployment (Metcalf & Nickel, 1977), Baxter (1972) revealed that the unemployed were more likely to come from large families and have disturbed backgrounds, while Metcalf & Nickel established that those people with below average incomes were more likely to become unemployed. It is evident, therefore, that among the unemployed there are many people whose health and social background may place considerable strain on their psychological well being, regardless of their employment status. It may well be that these factors create psychological and social instability, which in turn is responsible for the experience of job loss and any 'subsequent' health or social problems identified during unemployment. A review of the unemployment literature (eg Jahoda 1982; Stokes and Cochrane 1984b) reveals the extent of this methodological difficulty is revealed for the majority of studies have recruited their samples from individual cases of job loss which are possibly 'illness related' events (Brown et al 1973).

Fortunately for researchers, as a consequence of mass redundancy being the most common experience of many who become unemployed today (an event 'independent' of the personal characteristics of the workers), the methodological weakness evident when recruiting a sample of unemployed workers from, for example, Job Centres or Benefit Offices, is no longer of great concern. Yet in the interests of meaningful research the question of whether a study is being made of antecedents or consequences should always be borne in mind.

In the light of these considerations I conducted a research project among the unemployed workforce of a large electronics factory in Bradford, West Yorkshire which in closing down had made 2,000 people redundant.

As a consequence of involved negotiations it was not possible to interview the workers prior to the factory closure and I was therefore unable to identify the nature and effect of the period of anticipation of job loss which Kasl, Gore and Cobb (1975) found to be at least as threatening as the event itself.

However, it was reported by personnel management and trade union officials that there were increasing signs of anxiety, depression, despair and apathy amongst the workforce. Accepting that the aims of social research are invariably not appreciated, and sometimes even misunderstood (eg Hill, 1977), the response rate to a request for participation in the study of 3.1%, which yielded a sample of 48 workers, can be taken as indirect evidence of the sense of apathy, resignation and alienation that prevailed amongst the workforce. As Hill noted in his pilot study of the unemployed in 1977, the state of mind of the unemployed, or as in this case the soon to be unemployed, provides "strong motives for not wishing to expose themselves to an interview". I feel that a possible reason for the finding that unemployment research is predominantly small scale, anecdotal and methodologically unsound revolves around this difficulty of access.

The interviewing of the volunteer subjects commenced on the first day of their unemployment and each of the unemployed respondents were interviewed once every four weeks during a total observation period of 24 weeks. Using standard measures I collected data concerning psychiatric symptomatology, emotional state, level and direction of hostility, social attitudes, self concept, interpersonal and family relationships, and life quality at each interview. In order for comparisons to be made a matched control group of employed workers was also recruited and monitored.

Results and discussion

In brief, significant differences between the unemployed who remained out of work for the entire 24 week observation period and the employed control subjects were found on the measures of symptomatology, hostility, self satisfaction, interpersonal relations and familial role behaviour. In each case the redundant workers manifested greater levels of personal distress and dysfunctional behaviour (Stokes and Cochrane 1984b).

In this brief review I intend to mention in further detail only two of the most salient observations. First, the finding that the unemployed revealed higher levels of mild undifferentiated psychiatric disturbance compared with those workers still in stable employment although living and working in an area of economic instability, indicates that while the effects of economic stress are likely to be felt throughout a locality, distress is more acutely experienced by those undergoing job loss. Hence, it is this group who are more likely to require psychiatric treatment, a finding in accord with the results of previous studies (eg Israeli, 1935; Jaco, 1960). Consistent with this statement the study also revealed that the unemployed showed a greater tendency to hold negative self attitudes and feelings of guilt. This does not support the contention of Cohn (1978) that being unemployed in a period and/or area of high unemployment is less likely to be considered an indicator of personal failure, and would therefore, be unlikely to lead to low self esteem. In my opinion while there was an external locus of responsibility for their joblessness available to the redundant workers, the pervasive feelings of helplessness and hopelessness resulted in an increased dissatisfaction with the self, rather than a maintenance of self esteem. Dissatisfaction with the self was undoubtedly reinforced by the continuing social stigma attached to unemployment, and the regular conservative press coverage at the time of "scroungers" on the "dole", and the number of unfilled vacancies (known as the mismatch phenomenon) with the implication that some people prefer to live, and maybe prosper, on the "dole".

Finally, I would like briefly to discuss the finding that the unemployed women in the sample were as socially and psychologically distressed as a result of experiencing job loss as their male counterparts. It has been stated that women tend to view paid employment as being of secondary importance, rather obtaining gratification and self expression through the traditional female roles. This difference in the importance of employment status has been attributed to either "differential socialization" or the availability of alternative roles such as motherhood and wifehood, which can be meaningful sources of self definition. Unfortunately there is a lack of published work on female unemployment, which places a limitation on any conclusions that are made. Kasl (1979) found that most of the data on job loss in the United States was obtained from male blue collar workers, and in Great Britain, because most studies on unemployment utilize the Department of Employment register of unemployment or gain access to the unemployed through the Department's local offices, there is an absence of non registered unemployed in any such research, and as a result of women having a lower propensity to register, this is undoubtedly a major contributory factor in there being a lack of any substantial work on female unemployment in Great Britain.

However, in the light of my research and other studies which found that employment outside the home has a beneficial effect on the psychological health of women (eg Brown & Harris, 1978; Cochrane & Stopes-Roe, 1981) it is clear that the plight of the female unemployed deserves to be examined. At a time when female unemployment is an increasingly serious problem, the denial of "the increasing need and desire for women to seek paid work" (Bruegel, 1979) cannot be dismissed out of hand.

In conclusion, the results of my study show that unemployment in Bradford in the late 1970s was still a disturbing and threatening experience, giving rise to mild psychiatric disturbance, self doubt, hostility and rejection. The levels of distress identified were detected as a result of direct interviewing in the community using standard measures, and not as a consequence of establishing observable "illness behaviour", such as visits to GPs or drug usage for stress related disorders. Thus, the identification of "untreated" negative responses to unemployment cannot be discounted as being a function of the workless probably having more time to bring their health and welfare problems to the attention of the medical or social services as has been occasionally maintained by politicians of a conservative persuasion.

Unemployment among school leavers: a six month study of youth unemployment in Birmingham 1979 - 1980

While the difficulties which have plagued the British economy during the 1970s and 1980s have resulted in unprecedented levels of unemployment overall, they have had an identifiably disproportionate effect on young people, so that the unemployed family member today is increasingly likely to be a teenage son or daughter. Between 1975 and 1982 overall unemployment quadrupled yet unemployment among under 18 year olds multiplied five times, despite the introduction of special employment measures (most notably the Youth Opportunities Programme). Teenagers attempting to make the transition from school to work have fared particularly badly. The Manpower Services Commission in 1981 forecast that when taking no account of the effects of special measures, 59% of the labour force aged under 18 years would be unemployed by 1984.

My research on the psychological impact of unemployment on school leavers was located in Birmingham in the West Midlands, a region which has experienced a dramatic decline in its economic fortunes. As with the experience of Great Britain as a whole, the adverse economic conditions have led to a widespread increase in unemployment among school leavers something which had not happened in Birmingham since before the 1939-45 war. By June 1982 there were 6 082 registered unemployed under the age of 19; 4 277 young people on special schemes and only 251 job vacancies.

I followed the experiences of a group of school leavers who had left full time education in the Summer of 1979 and had been unable to find employment on leaving school, for a period of six months between November 1979 and May 1980. The unemployed school leavers were seen in their homes on three occasions. A total of 47 youngsters were interviewed within a structured format using standard measures. They were predominantly unqualified, 60% having no qualifications at all. A group of employed school leavers was also recruited as a control group.

Results and discussion

The discussion of the results of my study will be confined to the incidence of personal distress identified among the young unemployed. For a more detailed account see Stokes (1983a).

The finding of greater levels of anxiety among the unemployed school leavers (as indicated by the performance on the Symptom Rating Test) runs counter to the results of Daniel & Stillgoe in 1977 who considered that unemployment among the young was far from a devastating experience. This disparity can be accounted for by the increase in long term involuntary unemployment among young people since the mid 1970s, as distinct from the traditional pattern of relatively short periods of voluntary unemployment. However, in accordance with the view that research on the effects of unemployment among school leavers may be contaminated by the personal qualities of the young people, it is possible that the observed association between employment status and poor psychological health may simply reflect the prevalance of disorder at school which led to unemployment after the termination of full time education.

Feelings of anxiety were accompanied by a strong sense of being undesirable and worthless. It seems that the regular media coverage of the employment problems confronting young people, and the increasing likelihood that unemployment is becoming a part of everyday experience for many teenagers, did not remove feelings of failure and inadequacy.

The unemployed were also significantly less satisfied with their personal identity, for finding a job when leaving school represents a crucial aspect in the general development from dependent adolescence to independent adulthood. Frustration of this development leads to the perpetuation of a status which is inconsistent with the demands of society, expectations of parents and positive regard of peers.

My research also revealed that not only were there significant differences between the unemployed and employed school leavers on the measures of reaction, but that the well being and attitudes of the jobless changed during the six months of observation. Forty three members of the original group of 47 school leavers remained unemployed during the period of study, and I found that they experienced an apparent improvement in their condition as the period without a job progressed. However, the reduction in distress and upset revealed by the research questionnaires cannot be regarded as representing a genuine improvement in psychological health and social well being. The impression gained while interviewing indicated that the unemployed had come to terms with their situation by restricting their potential. As a result of redefining their position, subjecting expectations to a reappraisal and restructuring beliefs, self image improved, anxiety diminished and feelings of frustration and hostility were reduced. They had become resigned to their privation. Hope for the future was restricted, and fatalistic apathy permeated everyday life. The unemployed tended to withdraw from official contact, on average visiting the Careers Service, the specialist agency concerned with the job placement of young people, only twice a month. This phase of fatalistic apathy did not represent an initial lack of interest in work, nor does it mean that the unemployed enjoy being without a job, or would refuse suitable employment if it should become available, it is an understandable, defensive reaction to a situation that gives rise to stress, strain and worry.

A clear deterioration in social and practical skills also accompanied what Anna Freud has labelled, "restriction of the ego". Many of the sample were socially inadequate when compared to their employed counterparts and cannot have presented an attractive picture to prospective employers. Being deficient in social skills only served to compound the plight of the teenage unemployed, for not only were they predominantly unqualified, and many had an inadequate knowledge of the "3 Rs", but their attitudes, manner and appearance were now at variance with the demands and requirements of employers. Thus, nearly a year after leaving school many of the unemployed had accepted their pernicious situation and in the process had become less attractive as potential workers.

The disconcerting conclusion to be drawn from this study is that long term unemployment may well be responsible for a large number of young people becoming resigned and apathetic, withdrawing from meaningful and constructive social contact and having little commitment to a society that seems to be offering no worthwhile future. What was dismissed in the early 1970s as a 'folk theory' namely long term unemployment among the young after leaving school leading to lethargy, apathy and settling down to a "street corner" life style, was an apt description of the young unemployed interviewed in Birmingham. This finding clearly justifies official efforts to provide special assistance for the unemployed youth of this country, although consideration should be given to whether the Youth Opportunities Programme or any other special measure which presents as its raison d'etre the improvement of a young person's chances of getting a job, is appropriate when a large proportion of contemporary unemployment is structural and cannot be regarded as a temporary aberration from a situation of comparatively full employment. If government schemes are designed solely to improve employability they will fail to prepare and equip young people for life in a time of technological change and declining employment opportunities.

An examination of the attitudes, experiences and perceived life skills deficits of two groups of school leavers facing unemployment in Birmingham 1982

As Reubens (1979) has suggested, "the absence of dramatic new approaches to youth unemployment is the most conspicuous feature of the widespread effects in the 1970s" to offer protection to teenagers in the labour market. The Youth Opportunities Programme (YOP), which was introduced in 1978, (now replaced by the Youth Training Scheme) provided a six month placement with an employer in which training should be given. The Trainees were paid an allowance by the State, very slightly in excess of their benefit while unemployed.

The assumption on which the Youth Opportunities Programme operated was that a short period of work experience would improve the readiness of young people for a permanent job, which should eventually be forthcoming. I feel this assumption is inaccurate and inappropriate for it is probable that the high levels of unemployment now being experienced represent as Jenkins & Sherman (1979) have dramatically termed, "a collapse of work", a condition symptomatic of structural changes in the economy. It is therefore necessary for young people to realize that a job is not the only social activity of importance for there is little social value in restoring and developing a motivation and orientation to work through job related schemes if permanent employment is not likely to be achieved. This can only serve to hinder rather than help in coping with a lengthy period without work.

However, with the unwillingness of official, political and governmental institutions either to recognise or publicly acknowledge that future economic growth and affluence will go hand in hand with less available employment opportunities (Jenkins & Sherman, 1981) young people are not formally prepared for unemployment and thus are unaware of the type of problems they will face and the probable timing of their onset, thereby making them vulnerable to the adverse psychological consequences which have been identified (eg Gurney, 1980; Stafford et al 1980; Stokes, 1983a).

I therefore decided to examine the potential for instituting a programme of skills training for unemployed school leavers that focussed on both job seeking and unemployment 'survival' skills, the latter inevitably involving a reappraisal of the meaning of work. The programme was designed to satisfy the desire among young people for greater effectiveness in the job market, yet which gradually introduced the belief that life could be rewarding and enjoyable if alternatives to employment were considered, and practical coping skills could be acquired to deal with the 'hassle' of being unemployed, and help to inhibit or remove the emotional upset of joblessness.

The questionnaire designed to gain opinions on the content and timing of the skills training programme was administered to a group of 20 unemployed unqualified school leavers along with an unemployment questionnaire aimed at assessing their attitudes, activities, experiences and skills. The research project also required the use of a group of school leavers who had left school at the same time (easter, 1982) and had entered onto YOP schemes.

I will briefly detail the results of the project which relate to the attitudes the unemployed young people and YOP trainees held toward the education system, the careers service and the Youth Opportunities Programme, as well as their views regarding the proposed unemployment counselling programme.

Schools were seen as failing to prepare young people adequately for either the prospect of work or possibility of unemployment. When combining the two groups, 60% reported that they were not told about what type of jobs were available locally and 73% could not recall a local employer visiting the school to talk about his industry or business. Overall approximately half of the youngsters felt that school had done either 'little' or 'nothing at all' to prepare them for work. Similarly, the young people's opinions on the role of their schools in helping them to prepare for unemployment were not favourable. The conclusion must be that schools are "not fully succeeding in generating an understanding of the nature of the unemployment situation, nor enabling young people to cope with unemployment" (Whittaker et al, 1981).

Turning to the questions of how the careers service was regarded by the young people, significant differences were revealed between the groups. While the unemployed were overall 'mostly dissatisfied' with the attitude of the staff and job placement procedure, the trainees were 'pleased' with these aspects of the service. I believe this more than likely reflects the fact the YOP participants had obtained something tangible and, to varying degrees, rewarding as a result of their attendance at the careers office. However, neither of the groups attended their local office regularly and this reflects an increasingly negative regard for its relevance in the present economic situation and thus in increasing rates of non usage. The decline in employment opportunities is preventing the careers service from carrying out its function as a vocational guidance and job finding agency, while the introduction of YOP has relegated careers advisers to mere placement officers for increasingly unsatisfactory special employment schemes. They receive no training and possess no formal skills to help them meet the demands of young people who are experiencing the frustration of aspirations and the onset of a crisis of identity, and are thus having to improvise in the face of this new and unwelcome sitation.

It is clear that the employment services need to attract and assist these alienated non users, yet this is unlikely to occur if the service has very little to offer other than temporary schemes of increasingly doubtful quality and outcome. While in my study YOP was favourably regarded by the trainees, firm resistance was revealed by many of the unemployed who dismissed it as a source of cheap labour which provided inadequate training. This view is likely to become increasingly apparent as the number of 'alienated' youngsters increases as deteriorating placement rates make it particularly difficult to persuade young people of the value of a place on YOP or any similar employment measure.

Table 1: Unemployment among school leavers and young workers (under 19) in Birmingham, 1980 - 1982

(June)	1980	1981	1982
School leavers	2452	3577	5072
Young workers	1821	1501	1010
TOTAL REGISTERED UNEMPLOYED	4273	5078	6082
No of young people on special schemes	1635	3704	4277
No of current vacancies	800	257	251

Given the negative response of the school leavers to the existing provision of support services it is not surprising that there was an overwhelmingly favourable reaction to the proposed unemployment counselling and skills training programme which the teenage respondents were quite adamant should be provided before leaving school. Information on job search strategies, interview techniques, how to cope with rejection, family tensions and friendship difficulties, and how to deal with the problems of occupying time and budgeting was considered to be essential if they were to develop ways of confronting difficult or unpleasant situations. Such a programme, in conjunction with the establishment of social institutions wherein purposeful activities could be conducted that would enhance self esteem, reduce boredom, remove loneliness and maintain a sense of time, may create the opportunity for young people to become more versatile and adaptable in what may be a period of fundamental change in the previously accepted pattern of work and leisure (Stokes 1983b).

I hope my studies have contributed to an understanding of the meaning of contemporary redundancy and unemployment, but there still remain many under researched questions that require examination, not by descriptive, anecdotal and methodologically unsound observation, but through a rigorous reseach methodology that enables definitive conclusions to be drawn and policy decisions to be made that reflect the needs of the unemployed.

The complexity of the social world and the idiosyncratic response of different individuals does not facilitate the achievement of these objectives. However, unless many people are to be abandoned to an uncertain and deprived existence to which inadequate and inappropriate measures are administered, there can be few more worthwhile areas of study and research.

References

Baxter, J. L., 'Long Term Unemployment in Great Britain 1953-1971', _Bulletin of the Oxford University Institute of Economics and Statistics_, 34, 4, 1972.

Brown, G. W., Sklair, F., Harris, T. O., & Birley, J. L. T., 'Life Events and Psychiatric Disorders: Part 1 - Some Methodological Issues', _Psychological Medicine_, 3, 1973, 74-87.

Brown, G. W., & Harris, T. O., _Social Origins of Depression_, Tavistock Publications, London, 1978.

Bruegel, I., 'Women as a Reserve Army of Labour: A Note on Recent British Experience', _Feminist Review_, 3, Autumn 1979, 12-23.

Cochrane, R., & Stopes-Roe, M., 'Women, Marriage, Employment and Mental Health', _British Journal of Psychiatry_, 139, 1981, 373-381.

Cohn, R. M., 'The Effect of Employment Status Change on Self-Attitudes', _Social Psychology_, 41, 2, 1978, 81-93.

Daniel, W. W., & Stillgoe, E., 'Where Are They Now? A Follow-Up Study of the Unemployed', _Political and Economic Planning_, London, 1977.

Freud, A., _The Ego and the Mechanisms of Defence_, Hogarth Press, London, 1937.

Gurney, R., 'The Effects of Unemployment on the Psycho-Social Development of School Leavers', _Journal of Occupational Psychology_, 53, 1980, 205-213.

Hill, J. M. M., The Social and Psychological Impact of Unemployment: A Pilot Study, Doc. No. 2T 74, Tavistock Institute of Human Relations, 1977.

Israeli, N., 'Distress in the Outlook of Lancashire and Scottish Unemployed', Journal of Applied Psychology, 19, 1935, 67-69.

Jaco, E. G., The Social Epidemiology of Mental Disorders, Russell Sage Foundation, New York, 1960.

Jahoda, M., Employment and Unemployment, Cambridge University Press, Cambridge, 1982.

Jenkins, C., & Sherman, B., The Collapse of Work, Eyre Methuen, London, 1979.

Jenkins, C., & Sherman, B., The Leisure Shock, Eyre Methuen, London, 1981.

Kasl, S. V., Gore, S., & Cobb, S., 'The Experiencing of Losing a Job: Reported Changes in Health, Symptoms and Illness Behaviour', Psychosomatic Medicine, 37, 2, 1975, 106-122.

Kasl, S. V., 'Changes in Mental Health Status Associated With Job Loss and Retirement', in Barrett, J. E., et al (eds.), Stress and Mental Disorder, Raven Press, New York, 1979.

Metcalf, D., & Nickell, S., 'The Plain Man's Guide to The Out-of-Work: The Nature and Composition of Male Unemployment in Britain', unpublished paper, 1977.

Reubens, B. G., 'Review of Foreign Experience', in Sawhill, I. V., & Anderson, B. E. (eds.), Youth Employment and Public Policy, Prentice Hall, Englewood Cliffs, 1979.

Stafford, E. M., Jackson, P. R., & Banks, M. H., 'Employment, Work Involvement and Mental Health in Less Qualified Young People', Journal of Occupational Psychology, 53, 1980, 291-304.

Stokes, G.J., 'Out of School - Out of Work: The Psychological Impact', Youth and Policy, 2, 1983a, 27-29.

Stokes, G.J., 'Work, Unemployment and Leisure', Leisure Studies, 2, 1983b, 269-286.

Stokes, G. J., & Cochrane, R., 'The Relationship between National Levels of Unemployment and the Rate of Admission to Mental Hospitals in England and Wales 1950-1976', Social Psychiatry 1984a (in press).

Stokes, G.T. & Cochrane, R., 'A Study of the Psychological Effects of Redundancy and Unemployment', Journal of Occupational Psychology, 1984b, (in press).

Whittaker, J., Royle, D., & Smith, D., 'The Stoke-on-Trent Employment Survey', unpublished paper, 1981.

Part II

The health effects of unemployment: new studies

A: Time series studies

ECONOMIC CHANGE AND MORTALITY BY CAUSE IN SELECTED EUROPEAN COUNTRIES: SPECIAL REFERENCE TO BEHAVIOUR HEALTH RISKS, EMPHASISING ALCOHOL CONSUMPTION

M Harvey Brenner

In previous research it has been shown that economic growth is strongly related to declines in mortality rates in industrialized societies (1). It has also been demonstrated that departures from smooth economic growth, or "economic instability", especially as measured by unemployment rates, are related to mortality increases in the United States, Canada, England and Wales, Scotland, France, West Germany, Sweden, Italy, and Spain (2).

These relations between national economic changes and mortality trends and fluctuations have been measured largely utilizing a relatively simple version of the economic change model of pathology. That simple version includes the exponential trend of real per capita income, the residual cyclic fluctuation of economic growth, lagged rates of unemployment and measures of social welfare expenditure. It is only for the United States (3), England and Wales (4), and Scotland (5) that a more complex version of the economic change model of pathology has been shown to be effective in the explanation of mortality rate changes since World War II.

In the present paper it is shown that the basic economic change model of pathology, consisting only of economic indices, is usefully supplemented by a number of variables that reflect currently understood epidemiological risks to health in the post World War II era. These risks to health can be conceptualized as adaptational errors associated with economic growth because they depend on a minimal level of affluence in industrialized societies. These health risks include elements of consumption, production, and social isolation.

The consumption factors include immoderate use of alcoholic beverages, cigarette smoking, and diets heavy in animal fat and overall calories. Production factors include, especially, environmental contamination and exposure to toxic levels of synthetic organic chemicals. Social isolation includes breakdown in social networks (family structures in particular), and it is identified by high divorce rates and the proportion of the population living alone.

In this paper, the structure of control variables has been expanded to cover each of the above health risks. In particular, the alcohol consumption factors have been substantially elaborated to include potential representation of each of the three major beverages - spirits, wine, and beer. The main reason for expanding the alcohol investigation is that in different countries alcohol is differently used according to beverage type, and therefore the effects of the three beverages on health in each country may vary considerably. Specifically, there is reason to believe that a relatively high ethanol beverage such as spirits may be more readily used for its anesthetic and stress-relieving effects. Wine and beer, on the other hand, are more likely to be used as meal-enhancing beverages.

Also, there is now considerable evidence to suggest that moderate alcohol use (as distinguished from very high or very low use) may be beneficial in cardiovascular disease and especially in ischemic heart disease (6 - 8). At the same time, it is possible that alcohol - especially heavy use - may be a risk especially in hypertension-related disease.

The present study examines mortality patterns in nine countries - Australia, the United States, Canada, England and Wales, France, West Germany,

Denmark, Sweden, and Finland. The mortality patterns involve all cause (or total), heart disease, suicide, and infant mortality. The investigative model includes measures of economic growth and instability, adaptational error related to economic growth, and random shocks to the population such as climate change and epidemics.

The measures of economic instability have been expanded to involve not only unemployment rates, but business failure rates, and average weekly hours worked in manufacturing industries. For some countries additional recessional indicators have been examined such as immigration (which increases during economic upturns), and emigration and work stoppages (both of which increase during recessions).

The reader will observe that the data presented in this paper are drawn from a number of different studies, so that some of the control variables will vary by country. Nevertheless, the uniform set of variables that are consistently tested in all countries are: the exponential trend in real per capita income, the unemployment rate, alcohol consumption (total, and by beverage type), and cigarette consumption.

It will be seen that the alcohol beverage variables are measured in three forms: (1) rates of consumption per capita, (2) annual changes in rates of consumption, and (3) ratios of specific beverages consumed to total alcohol consumed. The reason for this three-fold distinction is that any one (or more) of three models of alcohol effects may be operating in a particular cause of death. For example, annual changes in alcohol consumption may affect mortality particularly strongly when the trends in alcohol consumption are relatively benign or are correlated with beneficial trends.

Further, it is often the case that large subpopulations of a single national population are frequent consumers of more than one (or two) beverages. Thus, increases in consumption of one beverage are inevitably linked to that of another even though the effects of each may be quite different - indeed, even contradictory. The consumption ratio of one beverage to total (alcohol) consumption implicitly involves interaction of beverages (i.e., reciprocal relations). Thus, while under certain conditions we may not be able to test the effect of individual beverages by themselves, we can test the health effects of <u>relative shifts</u> toward each of the specific beverages by examining the consumption of each beverage in ratio to that of the others.

In order to include the wide range of control variables in the explanatory equations, it was obviously necessary to substantially expand the framework of the economic change model of pathology. The expanded framework is reported in the next section of this paper. The empirical findings based on the expanded framework are described in the third section of the paper, which also includes an array of statistical tables.

Part II: THE ECONOMIC CHANGE MODEL OF PATHOLOGY

Introduction

A general theoretical model, the economic change model of pathology, was designed to account for the impact of changes in the economy on physical and mental health in industrialized countries during the past 30 years.

Specifically, the model brings together a variety of economic conditions, organizes them in context and shows the relationships among them. Both the major economic stresses of recession and the beneficial and deleterious factors related to economic growth and development are emphasized. Thus, it is a model which can be used in times of economic growth as well as economic contraction so that different periods can be compared statistically and, over time, better understood.

Scope of the Study

There is both ample and historical evidence, and continuing indication, that low socioeconomic status is associated with poor health status (1 - 7). Furthermore, it is argued that economic loss and downward mobility typically associated with economic instability are related to increased morbidity and mortality, particularly for the lower status person.

The economic change model of pathology is designed to contribute to a more accurate picture of the complex relationship between the economic environment and individual well-being by taking into account the impact of changes in the economy on the social areas of physical and mental health. Changes in measures of the aggregate economic status of the population are seen in relation to changes in the pathological indices. Two steps are involved in this process. The first is to associate indicators of health and social pathology with each of the following model elements: economic growth, economic instability, economic inequality, adaptation errors associated with economic growth, and random shocks. The second is to generate and test hypotheses which emerge from the resulting relationships.

Indices of social pathology and mortality are measures of human happiness and well-being. Mortality rates are indications of the changing life span. Mental health indices - mental hospital admission rates and suicide and cirrhosis mortality rates - cover a number of broad mental health problems, which taken together, generally reflect the overall mental health status of the population.

A distinction between long-term trend and cyclical change is crucial to an understanding of this model. Long-term trend refers to the lengthy, relatively even process of growth which is healthy for the economy. The economic cycle is the semi-periodic movement of many aspects of national economic activity (employment, investment, consumption patterns, etc.) in a nearly concurrent sequence. Such cyclic patterns are common in market economies, as well as in planned economies whose economic activity is partially interdependent with that of market economies.

The cyclic movement is one of two aspects of economic instability. The second component involves the problem of obsolescence that is based on increased productivity. Actual increased productivity occurs through the process of invention and replacement: tractors replace horses and automated equipment replaces factory workers. This process pushes some portion of the population out of the work process. In this way, short-term cyclical changes frequently interact with longer term or structural changes.

In market economies, during periods of economic growth, the long-term decline in average weekly hours worked in manufacturing and other industries is a reasonably good indicator of increased leisure time and favourable working conditions. In contrast, the short-term decline in average weekly hours worked which is associated with the recessional activity of the business cycle, is an indicator of economic loss, both for individuals, business organizations and the population as a whole.

A detailed discussion of model elements and related hypotheses follows.

Lag Structure

It is also necessary in the general model to specify the range over time, during which the relationships are expected to take place. In general, we expect increases in mortality rates, mental pathology indices and criminal justice indices to be seen within a six-year period including and following recession (or other economic decline). Based on previous research in the United States and European countries, we expect that there will characteristically be two peaks of the relationships within that six-year lag period. The first of these peaks, occurring during the first year of the recession, usually reflects: (1) sharp psychological reactions to substantial economic loss such as occurs in the suicide rate, in mortality affecting highly vulnerable populations, and in criminal justice indices; (2) decline in nutrition and medical care utilization affecting infant mortality and mortality among the chronically ill.

The second peak typically occurs at 2 - 3 years following recession (or other economic decline) as measured at the highest level of the unemployment or business failure rates. Though chronic disease mortality (especially cardiovascular disease) is especially involved, nearly all sources of ill health and social pathology are implicated. The 2 - 3 year peak reflects a period of continued economic loss for the population that is downwardly mobile in socioeconomic status as a result of recession. This sequence can be observed through the examination of standard economic indicators.

In market economies, recessions usually will occur over a period of less than twelve months which covers the time from the peak to the trough of economic activity. However, specific "lagging" economic indicators, such as the unemployment or labour force participation rates, will usually not return to their pre-recession level for 2 - 3 additional years. Following very deep recessions, 4 - 5 years may pass before employment-related indices return to pre-recession levels. These have been called the "period of depressed employment following recession" by the author. During this entire period of recession and subsequent depressed employment, the downwardly mobile population experiences continuous erosion of economic and social status with attendant damage to social relationships.

It is noteworthy as well that much of the post-recession period of depressed employment occurs at a time when the majority of the population is experiencing sustained economic improvement. This post-recession period, then, represents the time of maximal psychological deprivation for those who are seriously damaged by recession. At this time the downwardly mobile population loses both in absolute terms and in relative terms of economic inequality as compared to the population majority. Adding further to the psychological trauma of the downwardly mobile at this time is that it becomes clear to them, their families, and associates that their situation of status loss is probably permanent.

The 0 - 5 year interval of increased mortality associated with recession (or other economic decline) is understood to partially reflect increases in the incidence or severity, of chronic illnesses which in some instances result in mortality. It is further assumed, however, that the majority whose ill health is aggravated by recession probably do not die within a six year period of recession. Rather, this more seriously ill population now becomes more vulnerable to mortality at least over the subsequent decade. This heightened vulnerability results from three different mechanisms.

The first is simply an acceleration of the natural progression of chronic disease processes that have been stimulated or exacerbated by recession. A second source of subsequent vulnerability arises from the fact that recessions will occur and inflict more serious health consequences on the population whose health has already been put at risk. For this reason among others, the extent of recessional damage on a population's health is in part related to the degree of damage that was associated with previous recessions.

A third source of heightened vulnerability to mortality during the decade following the initial 0 - 5 year period (of recessional damage) reflects the increased probability of economic loss following increased severity of recession-related illness. If, for example, a chronic mental or physical disorder becomes incapacitating as a result of recession, then the incapacitating condition itself will increase the difficulty of maintaining or regaining a job or income. This secondary condition of deterioration in the subject's socioeconomic position is then likely to further increase the longer-term risk of chronic disease or mortality.

To recapitulate, the general model specifies damage to mental, physical and social well-being during the six-year interval which includes the average recessional period and the following five years. It also assumes continued damage over at least the subsequent decade to general physical health especially involving chronic diseases.

The Economic Change Model

Economic Growth

The first element of the economic change model of pathology, long-term economic growth, is taken to be the underpinning of social well-being and increases in the life span. This element is responsible for increased resources of wealth per capita, by which society is better able to manage the natural and human environments. The relation between growth and mortality derives from the basic definition that economic growth produces higher levels of resources within a population. Resources can be allocated to (1) improvements in the standard of living; (2) investment in the development of new knowledge; and (3) investment in the applications of existing knowledge (35, Ch. 9), including medical care and education of the population. Economic growth is also the basis for improved working conditions, including health and safety measures, leisure and social insurance, e.g., unemployment, health, and aid to the disabled, elderly and those in poverty.

Over the long run, the net effects are the result of both beneficial and adverse factors made possible by growth. Beneficial factors include the potential of social investment in the development of new knowledge. The application of that knowledge may result in a higher standard of living:

good nutrition, climate control via housing, clothing and the use of fuel; parasite control; education; comfortable working conditions; and adequate monetary and social remuneration for work. A major beneficial factor that is specifically important to severe morbidity and mortality involves the provision and utilization of primary health services.

A number of risk factors to physical and mental health, made possible by high mass consumption and technological development related to long-term economic growth, have become unusually prominent during the past two decades. Included are the immoderate consumption of alcoholic beverages, tobacco and animal fats; increased reliance on non-human energy sources and the corresponding effects of a sedentary life, such as a decline in cardiovascular fitness and overconsumption of calories; and the improper use of medicine and psychotropic drugs.

Economic growth is also related to a decline in strength and stability of primary relationships, especially nuclear family and extended kinship networks, as indicated by high and increasing divorce rates; high proportions of the population living alone; and the prevalence of female-headed households, career- and recession-related disruptions to family formation and childbearing. Disruption to career and social integration is also seen in the diversion of manpower to military service, especially under conditions of conscription, but even on a volunteer basis in times of war when the threat of injury and loss of life is substantial.

This general theoretical conception on the effects of economic growth on health and social well-being leads to the following specific hypothesis:

> *The overall mortality rate for all ages, both sexes, de-decreases in relation to long-term increases in real per capita income.

Long-term economic growth is defined according to a measure of real per capita disposable income (i.e., accounting for the rate of inflation). The "pure" trend element of economic growth tends to have an exponential form. We therefore fit an exponential trend to the real per capita income, thus eliminating the "cyclical" component, which is measured by the variables discussed in the section on economic instability. The relation between an increase in economic growth and the decrease in the overall and specific mortality rates will continue to hold under statistical controls for trends in detrimental factors historically associated with economic growth, such as cigarette smoking, very heavy consumption of alcoholic beverages and animal fats, and measures of social isolation.

Economic Instability

Economic instability is the generic term for recessional and structural economic changes that are damaging to particular subsections of the society. In market economies, downturn in the business cycle, indicated by a rising unemployment rate, high rates of business failures and declines in labour force participation among other changes, is known as recession. In both planned and market economies, a disturbance to economic activity involves recession in economic growth, which then proceeds at a slower rate, stalls, or actually declines. As a result, the population fails to gain benefits that it would have received had growth continued at a previous rate. The loss, or interruption of gain, in benefits is not evenly distributed.

Persons with little or obsolete skills, workers in declining industries, older workers and persons living in economically declining areas are likely to lose status permanently.

Under these conditions, certain groups in the population experience downward mobility, or the process whereby socioeconomic position is lost or seriously damaged. In the population that is downwardly mobile, the greatest psychological hardships occur when hope of re-establishing their former position is lost. Among the mechanisms involved which lead to psychological harm are fear of loss of social identity; loss of basic economic resources; loss of primary social relationships; forced migration and fear of the inability - and intensive striving - to re-establish socioeconomic position.

It is also assumed that the effect of recession particularly will affect adversely those who work as well as those who lose their jobs. A secondary set of mechanisms affect employees who remain at work. These include a lack of promotion and poor or competitive relations among staff; emphasis on high productivity; and work overload caused by critical shortages of employees and an atmosphere of anxiety and tension. Such conditions may generate for much of the population a series of stresses nearly equivalent to employment loss.

We can derive the following general hypothesis from these theoretical conceptions on the effects of economic instability on morbidity and mortality:

*Economic instability relates to a higher incidence of morbidity and mortality.

Specific hypotheses which flow from the general one stated above are as follows:

Economic decline in specific regions, industries or occupational groups is related to increases in:

*total mortality rates;
*cardiovascular mortality rates;
*cirrhosis mortality rates;
*suicide rates;
*mental hospital admissions rates;
*homicide rates;
*imprisonment rates; and
*infant mortality rates.

In countries with market economic systems, the unemployment rate tends to be the principal indicator of recessional economic loss. At the macro or population level of analysis, increase in the unemployment rate is an indicator of the extent of recession and/or structural economic decline. These forms of economic distress reflect for some part of the population loss of the work role; loss of income; downward social mobility; increased stress; and possible increases in poverty levels. At this level of analysis, we can identify relations between the aggregate unemployment rate - acting as an indicator of several sources of social distress - and measure of health and aggression.

Other hypotheses which use additional indicators of recessional damage as experienced in countries with market economies are as follows:

*The increased failure rate of economic organizations is related to increases in total mortality rate, cardiovascular mortality rate and suicide rate.

The industrial failure rate is a prominent recessional indicator and is important in the age group over 45, and especially over 65, for the service, manufacturing and agricultural worker and manager. As in the case of leaving the labor force, this indicator tends to reflect a period of chronic anxiety and struggle to keep the economic organization from economic destruction prior to failure, as well as a major change in social status and way of life. We therefore anticipate a lag of within two years between an increased industrial failure rate and increased pathology rates.

*Decreases in labor force particpation rates are related to increases in total mortality rates, including infant mortality, cardiovascular mortality, and suicide.

*Short-term declines in production or wage rates are related to increases in total and chronic disease mortality rates.

Economic Inequality

Economic inequality relates to the distribution of the product of economic development. For reasons which usually depend on structural changes in the economy, specific populations may not gain - or may actually experience loss - while the majority of the population takes part in the process of economic growth. For example, youth, the elderly, women and ethnic minorities frequently experience this situation in European countries.

Economic inequality has an even greater adverse impact which is compounded during periods of economic growth, when the majority of society is earning at least moderate incomes and is not experiencing very high unemployment. This is occasionally the condition of a significant proportion of youth of lower socioeconomic status and especially of minority ethnic backgrounds. This description also extends to many of the elderly who may be in chronic economic difficulty and to a significant number of female heads of households. Finally, these problems of structural economic deprivation (as opposed to the short-term losses of recessionary periods) and low income have, in the last decade, been extended to former workers in several of the durable goods industries which have suffered structural declines in employment in Western Europe.

In periods of economic instability, the economic loss and downward mobility typically associated with a recession leads to further expansion of socioeconomic differentials; thus the effects of recession become an even greater burden, proportionally, on the downwardly mobile. Economic inequality becomes even more acute when the general population is moving out of a recession. While some individuals gain, a portion of the population has lost income and never recovers. This group subsequently exhibits lower socioeconomic status and higher mortality rates.

The model allows for the impact of economic inequality on the two preceding relationships by developing hypotheses for specific populations.

*In countries with market economic systems, increases in the unemployment ratio for all ages and all sexes are related to pathological indices.

The reason is that each of the age/sex-specific unemployment rates does not correspond exactly to the fluctuations of the overall unemployment rate, and we would additionally like to identify the relation of each age/sex group's unemployment rate to its pathological pattern. This can be done by using the ratio of age/sex-specific unemployment rates to the total unemployment rate.

The unemployment rate and age/sex-specific ratios indicate much of the effect of recessional losses and anxieties, but they actually measure only the extent to which members of the population are looking for work. Substantial proportions of those who look for work, however, do not find it, are therefore "discouraged workers", and leave the labor force entirely. This is especially true of males over age 45 during the past two decades. Since there is likely to have been a span of one or two years of unemployment prior to leaving the labour force, we expect decreases in labour force participation to lead to increased pathology within two years.

As in the situation where the total unemployment rate does not measure perfectly the unemployment situation of specific age-sex groups, so it is with the total per capita (real) income not precisely measuring the real income gain or loss situation of each of the age/sex groups. The proposed solution is the same; namely, in addition to the total per capita income, the age/sex median income ratios are used.

In countries with either planned or market economies the age/sex income ratio is a reasonable indicator of economic differentials.

Adaptational Error

Adaptational error associated with economic growth refers to the pathological results of specific patterns of consumption and production. Pathological results occur either because of ignorance, difficulty in changing habitual behaviors, or potential damage to economic interests, if changes were to significantly decrease consumption or production of specific items. Examples are immoderate alcohol consumption, abuse of prescription or illicit drugs, cigarette smoking, regular consumption of foods that are overly high in fat content, environmental contamination with chemical toxins, greatly increased numbers of motor vehicles in the population and neglect of protective devices, e.g. seat belts, crash helmets, air bags, in road traffic. Another adaptational problem associated with economic growth pertains to disturbed social relations such as social isolation due to divorce or solitary living arrangements.

Two sets of hypotheses emerge, one to address those adaptational errors resulting from increased mass consumption and the other, to explain the social disorganization that is strongly associated with an increased life span.

The hypotheses involving risks resulting from high mass consumption are as follows*

> *An increase in the heavy consumption of alcoholic beverages is related to high mortality rates, especially for cirrhosis, cardiovascular illness, certain malignancies, accidents, infant mortality, suicide, homicide, and mental disabilities.

Although moderate levels of drinking may be protective with respect to some illnesses (especially ischemic heart disease), prevalence of heavy consumption of alcoholic beverages is expected to show a positive relation to general mortality, including especially cardiovascular illnesses, specified malignancies, abortions, infant mortality, and alcohol dependence syndrome possibly involving aggression or depression with relatively short lags. In the case of relatively short lags (0 - 5 years), we are concentrating on the already chronically morbid populations, as well as on changes in cognitive ability and mood.

> *An increase of cigarette consumption per capita is related to higher motality rates, especially for cardiovascular and respiratory diseases, certain malignancies, infant mortality, and accidents.

The consumption of cigarettes per capita is expected to be positively related to mortality rates, especially for cardiovascular and respiratory disease and specific malignancies, both at relatively short and at long lags, i.e. 10 - 15 years. The shorter-lag relationship is due to a population already morbid for whom the additional smoking is expected to exacerbate serious illness levels within a period of 6 months to 6 or 7 years.

> *A high level of consumption of animal fat is associated with higher mortality rates, especially from cardiovascular disease and malignancy.

A high level of consumption of animal fat is a risk factor in a great many causes of illness - especially in cardiovascular disease and malignancies. The consumption of animal fats per capita is expected to be related to total and ischemic heart disease mortality at relatively short (under 5 years) and long (15 - 20 years) lags. The short lag relationship is particularly pertinent to populations already morbid with cardiovascular disease.

> *Increases in automobile registration rates and miles driven per capita are related to higher mortality rates due to injuries.

Automobile registration rates and miles driven per capita are expected to be positively related to mortality due to injuries - especially involving youth - at lags of under 3 years.

Hypotheses involving risk factors related to a decline in primary relationships include:

> *The divorced population is at considerably greater risk of mortality and mental health problems.

This is one of two prime indicators of potential lack of social integration or social support. It is a standard finding in psychiatric epidemiology and recent studies of morbidity that the divorced population is at considerably greater risk of mortality.

*Persons living alone are at greater risk of mortality and mental health problems.

The number of persons living alone and an increase in the proportion of female heads of households are additional indicators of the potential lack of social support. They are meant to reflect recent findings on the importance of social contact as a negative influence on morbidity as well as the classic sociological literature on the malintegrative aspects of advanced urban living conditions.

*An increase in the proportion of female household heads is related to an increase in the total mortality of persons under age 15.

The proportion of female heads of households is also related to low income, as households headed by females are disproportionately represented in the number of low socioeconomic households. Low socioeconomic status places children at far greater risk of morbidity and mortality.

Ameliorative effects of social welfare aid to families of low socioeconomic status are tested by the following hypothesis:

*Increases in the number of low socioeconomic households receiving social welfare aid are related to decreases in the mortality of the young.

Random Shocks

An additional set of factors, "random shocks" to the population, needs to be taken into account in order to use this elaborated economic change model for detailed explanation or prediction. These factors include (1) extremely disruptive phenomena, e.g. climatic irregularities such as severe winters; (2) minor epidemics; (3) events which damage the economy and the population in ways that go beyond usual economic predictions, e.g. natural disasters, political or international economic crises; (4) important demographic changes such as were brought about by sharp increases in the birth rate, or "baby boom".

An emergent hypothesis would then be that:

*An increased proportion of males aged 15 - 24 in the population is associated with an increase in criminally aggressive activity and accidents.

Involvement in war is a random shock adversely affecting the population's health and life span, particularly of those actually involved in military actions. Size of the military population is correlated with the number of people on active duty for combat. The hypothesis was developed that:

*As the rate of military personnel in the population goes up, indices of pathology and mortality rates increase, especially for the military-age population.

Limitations of the Model

The question of the correct causal specification of a relationship generally involves the possibility that an unobserved external phenomenon is responsible for changes in both the predictor and predicted factors. In that case the observed correlation between "explaining" and "explained" factors does not reflect a causal relation between them and instead results from their joint relation to a third factor.

In the present study, there is no external unspecified factor which is known to regularly influence both the state of the economy and, independently, mortality or mobidity rates, for example. On occasion, unusual conditions such as war, may influence economic conditions and health. However, war and similarly rare factors obviously do not influence either the economy or health on a continuous basis. More generally, there is no known external factor which regularly influences the state of the economy. Indeed, if such a factor were known, we would be able to use it in efforts to forecast economic conditions.

A somewhat different approach to this question of an unknown external factor is to ask whether phenomena that are, for example, influenced by economic conditions also influence health. In this study we ask that question with respect to several factors known to affect health adversely - alcohol, cigarette, and fat consumption per capita, social isolation, etc. The problem then is whether, if one controls for the effects of such additional factors, the relations between economic conditions and health and social well-being still can be observed. In this study such external factors are explicit in the model to be tested, under the general classification "adaptational errors associated with economic growth". In fact, we find that controlling for the adaptational error factors usually strengthens rather than weakens the relations between economic conditions and the populations' health and well-being.

We conclude, therefore, that the findings usually observed do not appear to be influenced by problems of random occurrence or lack of control for factors which should have been taken into account. However, as in all studies based on statistical tests, the findings can only be taken as evidence in favor of, or against, specific hypotheses.

In this case, for example, considerable statistical support is usually found for the statement that economic instability is related to adverse change in national health and well-being. But it cannot be said that such findings prove the existence of causal relationships. Statistical studies only permit statements of probability rather than absolute proof.

Part III: FINDINGS

Exponential Trend in Real Per Capita Income

The trend of economic growth, adjusted for inflation, is found to be significantly inversely related to age-adjusted total mortality and to infant mortality in all nine countries (see Tables 1 and 3). This exponential trend is almost always significantly inversely related to heart disease mortality, except in France, where it does not show statistical significance (see Table 4). For suicide, an inverse relation to economic growth is observed in England and Wales, Australia, Denmark, and Finland; in no country, though, was a positive relation found (see Table 2).

The Rate of Unemployment

For total mortality, the relation to unemployment is positive and significant in all nine countries. In all countries except Australia, there is positive relation at under five years' lag (see Table 1).

In all countries examined, recessional factors are found to influence mortality. Thus even where the total age-adjusted mortality rate is not significantly correlated with unemployment rates, it is correlated with business failure rates. The potential long-lagged effects of unemployment rates on total mortality were examined in the United States, England and Wales, Canada, Denmark, and Australia. In all five cases, positive relations were found to peak within the 7 - 15 year lag period.

For age-adjusted heart disease, mortality relations to the unemployment rate are found within a five-year lag, except for Finland. As in total mortality, in the case of Finland the relation is not seen over age 65, but is measured at under that age.

In eight of the nine countries examined, the principal relation of unemployment to heart disease mortality is found at a three-year lag. In France, the peak relation is at a one-year lag, while in England and Wales a one-year lagged relation is found in addition to the principal three-year lag (see Table 4).

Of the five countries in which long unemployment lags (7 - 15 years) were examined for relations to age-adjusted heart disease mortality, three countries showed positive relations (Australia, Denmark, and the United States; see Table 4).

The infant mortality rate shows a deleterious influence of the unemployment rate in eight of the nine countries (see Table 3). Even in Australia, where the unemployment rate did not show a significant relation, another recessional variable - business failure rates - did.

For suicide, the unemployment rate is again virtually always positive and significant, except for Australia, where nevertheless the business failure rate is positive and significant (see Table 2).

Average Weekly Hours of Work in Manufacturing Industries

This variable, tested in England and Wales, Canada, France and West Germany, is an indicator of recession in its short-term pattern of variation.

In Canada, average hours worked was inversely related to total mortality; in England and Wales, however, it was inversely related to both heart disease and total mortality. In France, it was inversely related to infant mortality (see Table 3). In West Germany, it was inversely related to suicide (see Table 2). In none of the four countries were positive relations observed.

Immigration and Emigration

In- and out-migration to and from a country are classic indices of recessions. During recessions, emigration increases and immigration decreases. These indices were tested in Denmark, Sweden, and France in connection with suicide and infant mortality. In Denmark and France, immigration was inversely related to suicide, while emigration was positively related to suicide in Denmark (see Table 2). For infant mortality, immigration showed inverse relations in Sweden and France.

For West Germany, immigration and emigration are tested with a different objective. Here the issue was whether the process of immigration had contributed to mortality, either through the potentially stressful adaptation process or because in-migrants were of typically lower socio-economic status who might have contributed to a higher national mortality rate. The data indeed indicate that for West German total mortality increased immigration is associated with higher mortality within three years, while emigration is related to decreased mortality within one year.

Business Failure Rates

The business failure rate was tested in seven of the nine countries (i.e. except for Denmark and France, where data were not then available).

For total mortality, all seven countries showed a positive significant relation; in six of the seven countries, at a two- or three-year lag. In Finland, the peak lag is a one-year, and in England and Wales there is a peak at zero lag in addition to a two-year lag.

For heart disease, significant and positive relations are found in six of the seven countries. In the six countries involved, the principal lag is at two or three years, but an additional zero lag is found for Australia, West Germany, and the United States, and an additional one-year lag is found for Finland.

For infant mortality, positive relations are found for Australia, Canada, and Finland.

For suicide, positive relations are found in Australia, Canada, England and Wales, the United States, and West Germany.

Alcohol Consumption Per Capita

For age-adjusted heart disease mortality, all nine countries except Denmark show a damaging effect due to either spirits or wine consumption within a three-year lag period; spirits show a damaging effect in six countries, while wine does so in four. Beer consumption, on the other hand, typically shows a beneficial effect on heart disease within a six-year lag period. In three of the nine countries, an inverse relation of beer consumption to overall heart disease mortality was observed that was not immediate; Sweden and Canada show no significant relation and West Germany actually shows a positive relation.

However, when we examine ischemic heart disease mortality, rather than the overall heart disease category, the inverse relation of beer consumption to mortality can be observed even in these three countries. This inverse relation regarding beer consumption is measured either in rates of consumption per capita, or annual changes in consumption rates, or in the ratio of beer consumption to total alcohol consumption. (See Table 5).

In the last case, it is important to recognize that the inverse relation for the beer consumption ratio is not due to a positive relation for spirits or wine consumption. Spirits and wine consumption (and overall beer consumption as well) are either controlled by already being in the equation or, if not present, were found not to affect heart disease mortality in a statistically significant manner.

In comparison with the extensive influence of alcohol consumption (deleterious as well as beneficial) on heart disease mortality, its influence on total mortality is rather minimal. Total alcohol consumption shows a positive relation to total mortality in one country (Australia), spirits consumption in three countries (Canada, Sweden, and West Germany), and wine consumption in two (France and West Germany). Beer consumption, on the other hand, shows no positive relation to total mortality and two inverse relations (Finland and France).

Suicide, by contrast, shows a deleterious influence of alcohol consumption in all countries except West Germany. Most of this deleterious influence is via spirits (six countries), but some clearly occurs in the combination of at least two beverages as measured by total alcohol consumption (four countries; see Table 2). However, no deleterious effects on suicide are found specifically for wine or beer; indeed, in two countries beer consumption is inversely related to suicide rates (England and Wales, and Sweden).

The relation of per capita alcohol consumption to infant mortality is again extensive. Six of the nine countries show deleterious effects of spirits consumption, three of total alcohol consumption, three of wine consumption, and one of beer consumption. There is in fact some indication, though, that the beer consumption ratio is actually beneficial in France. This is plausible for France, where wine is used regularly at meals. If pregnant women shift their consumption toward beer (i.e. increase beer consumption at the same time that they decrease wine consumption), the result is that they would consume overall fluid levels of lower ethanol content. The decreased ethanol would then represent a lower risk to fetal developmental abnormalities.

Cigarette Consumption

Mortality rates appear to be harmfully affected by the influence of cigarette smoking over a period of 0 - 20 years. This reflects (a) cohort effects in the 10 - 20 year range; (b) medium-term effects on chronic illness incidence of 5 - 9 years' lag; (c) short-term effects - usually of stopping smoking - of 0 - 2 years' lag.

For total mortality in three of the nine countries, a peak lag is found at zero, in four countries at 3 - 6 years, and in four countries at

10 - 20 years (see Table 1). Similar but not identical lags can be seen in heart disease. In both total and heart disease mortality, all nine countries show the effects of smoking. For infant mortality, eight of the nine countries show the effect; the peak lag is always within two years.

SUMMARY OF RESULTS AND CONCLUSION

Overall, the statistical viability of the economic change model of pathology is affirmed in nine countries. Data from these countries consistently show the fundamental beneficial effects of economic growth and the harmful effects of economic instability* and recession. The data also show the considerable harm to health of cigarette smoking. The effects of alcohol consumption are highly varied. Substantial harm is measured in high-level ethanol beverages (especially spirits and occasionally wine) in several causes of death. Beer, though, is the least damaging (and lowest-ethanol) alcoholic beverage. Moreover, beer consumption per capita appears to show beneficial effects in heart disease for nearly all countries studied.

* A previous analysis of economic instability in Denmark failed to show these relationships due to (a) lack of use of the entire economic change model of pathology and (b) incorporation of pre-World War II years as well as post-World War II years in the same analysis. Besides the analytical tables for Denmark, See Figures 1 - 3.

References to Part I

1. Cochrane, A., A. S. St. Leger, and F. Moore. "Health Services 'Input' and mortality 'Output' in Developed Countries". Journal of Epidemiology and Community Health 32:200-205, 1978.

2. Brenner, M. H. "Mortality and Economic Instability: Detailed Analyses for Britain and Comparative Analyses for Selected Industrialized Countries". International Journal of Health Services 13:563-620, 1983 (forthcoming).

3. Brenner, M. H. Estimating the Effects of Economic Change on National Health and Social Well-Being. U.S. Congress, Joint Economic Committee. U.S. Government Printing Office, 1983 (forthcoming).

4. Brenner, M. H. "Mortality and Economic Instability: Detailed Analyses for Britain and Comparative Analyses for Selected Industrialized Countries". International Journal of Health Services 13:563-620, 1983 (forthcoming).

5. Brenner, M. H. "Mortality and Economic Instability: Detailed Analyses for Britain and Comparative Analyses for Selected Industrialized Countries". International Journal of Health Services 13:563-620, 1983 (forthcoming).

6. Gordon, T. and W. B. Kannel. "Drinking Habits and Cardiovascular Disease: The Framingham Study". American Heart Journal 105:666-673, 1983.

7. Gordon, T. et al. "Diet and its Relation to Coronary Heart Disease and Death in Three Populations". Circulation 63:500-515, 1981.

8. Klatsky, A. L. et al. "Alcohol Use and Cardiovascular Disease: The Kaiser-Permanente Experience". Circulation 64 (Suppl III): 32 - 41, 1981.

References to Part II

1. U.S. Department of Health, Education, and Welfare. Health Status of Minorities and Low-Income Groups. DHEW Publication No. (HRA) 79-627.

2. U. S. Department of Health and Human Services. Health Resources Administration. Health of the Disadvantaged: Chart Book-II. DHSS Publication No. (HRA) 80-633. September 1980.

3. Parron, D. L., F. Solomon, and C. D. Jenkins, eds. Behaviour, Health Risks, and Social Disadvantage. Health and Behavior: A Research Agenda, Interim Report No. 6. Washington: National Academy Press, 1982.

4. Hamburg, D. S., G. R. Elliott, and D. E. Parron, eds. Health and Behavior. Washington: National Academy Press, 1982.

5. Egbuonu, L. and B. Starfield. "Child Health and Social Status". Pediatrics 69, 550, 5 May 1982.

6. Great Britain. Department of Health and Social Services. Inequalities in Health. Report of a Research Working Group. August 1980.

7. Morris, J. N. "Social Inequalities Undiminished". The Lancet 1:87-90, 1979.

8. Brenner, M. H. "Importance of the Economy to the Nation's Health". In The Relevance of Social Science for Medicine (ed. by L. Eisenberg and A. Kleinman), p. 371. Dordrecht, Holland: D. Reidel Publishing Company, 1981.

9. Townsend, P. "Inequality and the Health Service". The Lancet 1:1179-1184, 1974.

10. Bolger, G. B. "Social Class and Access to Health Care Systems". McGill Medical Journal, 19 - 24.

11. Aday, L., R. Andersen, and G. V. Fleming. Health Care in the U.S.: Equitable for Whom? Beverly Hills: Sage Publications, 1980.

12. Mechanic, D. Medical Sociology 2nd ed. New York: The Free Press, 1978.

13. Rayman, Paul M. and Barry Bluestone. Out of Work: The Consequences of Unemployment in the Hartford Aircraft Industry. Chestnut Hill, M.A.: Boston College, Social Welfare Research Institute, October 1982.

14. Catalano, R. and C. D. Dooley. "Economic Predicators of Depressed Mood and Stressful Life Events". Journal of Health and Social Behavior 18:292-307, 1977.

15. Liem, R. "Economic Change and Unemployment: Contexts of Illness". In Social Contexts of Health, Illness, and Patient Care. E. G. Mishler, et al., pp. 54 - 78. Cambridge: Cambridge University Press, 1981.

16. Kasl, S. V., S. Gore, and S. Cobb. "The Experience of Losing a Job: Reported Changes in Health, Symptoms and Illness Behavior". Psychosomatic Medicine 37:106-122, 1975.

17. Levi, L., ed. Society, Stress and Disease. Vol. 4. Working Life. Oxford: Oxford University Press, 1981.

18. Elliott, G. R. and C. Eisdorfer, eds. Stress and Human Health. New York: Springer Publishing Co., 1982.

19. Alfredsson, L., R. Karasek, and T. Theorel. "Myocardial Infarction Risk and Psychosocial Work Environment: An Analysis of the Male Swedish Working Force". Soc. Sci. Med. 16, 463, 1982.

20. McLean, A., ed. Mental Health and Work Organizations. Chicago: Rand McNally, 1970.

21. McLean, A., ed. Occupational Stress. Springfield, III.: Charles C. Thomas, 1974.

22. U.S. National Institute for Occupational Safety and Health. Reducing Occupational Stress. Proceedings of a Conference. April, 1978.

23. Kahn, R. L. Work and Health. New York: Wiley, 1981.

24. Gardell, B. and G. Johansson. Working Life: A Social Science Contribution to Work Reform. New York: Wiley, 1981.

25. Berkman, L. F. "Physical Health and the Social Environment: A Social Epidemiological Perspective". In The Relevance of Social Science for Medicine (ed. by L. Eisenberg and A. Kleinman), p. 51. Dordrecht, Holland: D. Riedel Publishing Co., 1981.

26. Gore, S. "Stress-Buffering Functions of Social Supports: An Appraisal and Clarification of Research Models". In Stressful Life Events and Their Contexts (ed. by B. S. Dohrenwend and B. P. Dohrenwend), p. 202. New York: Prodist, 1981.

27. McKinlay, J. B. "Social Network Influences on Morbid Episodes and the Career of Help Seeking". In The Relevance of Social Science for Medicine (ed., by L. Eisenberg and A. Kleinman), p. 77. Dordrecht, Holland: D. Reidel Publishing Co., 1981.

28. Berkman, L. F. and S. L. Syme. "Social Networks, Host Resistance, and Mortality: A Nine-Year Follow-up of Alameda County Residents". Am. J. Epi. 109-186, 1979.

29. Cobb, S. "Social Support as a Moderator of Life Stress". Psychosomatic Medicine 38:300-314, 1976.

30. Barrett, J. E., ed. Stress and Mental Disorder. New York: Raven Press, 1979.

31. Dohrenwend, B. S. and B. P. Dohrenwend, eds. Stressful Life Events and Their Contexts. New York: Prodist, 1981.

32. Neufield, R. W. F. Psychological Stress and Psychopathology. New York: McGraw-Hill, 1982.

33. Justice, B. and D. F. Duncan. "Life Crisis as a Precursor to Child Abuse". Public Health Reports 91:110-115, 1976.

34. Lefcourt, H. M. "Locus of Control and Stressful Life Events". In Stressful Life Events and Their Contexts (ed. by B. S. Dohrenwend and B. P. Dorhenwend), p. 157. New York: Prodist, 1981.

35. Hamblin, R. L., R. B. Jacobsen, and J. L. L. Miller. A Mathematical Theory of Social Change. New York: Wiley, 1973.

36. U.S. Department of Health and Human Services. Coronary-Prone Behavior and Coronary Heart Disease: A Bibliography. NIH Publication No. 80 - 2018. March 1980.

References for economic change model of pathology

37. U.S. Congress. Joint Economic Committee. Estimating the Social Costs of National Economic Policy: Implications for Mental and Physical Health and Criminal Aggression, by M. Harvey Brenner. Washington: U.S. Government Printing Office, October 26, 1976.

38. Brenner, M. H., "Health Costs and Benefits of Economic Policy", International Journal of Health Services, 7:(4) 581-623. (1977).

39. Brenner, M. H., "Mortality and the National Economy: A Review and the Experience of England and Wales, 1936-1976, "The Lancet", 568-573 (September 15, 1979).

40. Brenner, M. H., "Industrialization and Economic Growth: Estimates of their Effect on the Health of Populations", in M. H. Brenner, A. Mooney, T. J. Nagy, eds. Assessing the Contributions of the Social Sciences to Health, 65-115. AAAS Symposium 26, Boulder, Colorado: Westview Press, 1980.

41. Brenner, M. H. and Mooney, A. "Economic Change and Sex-Specific Cardiovascular Mortality in Britain 1955-1976", Social Science and Medicine 16:431-442 (Spring, 1982).

Fig. 1

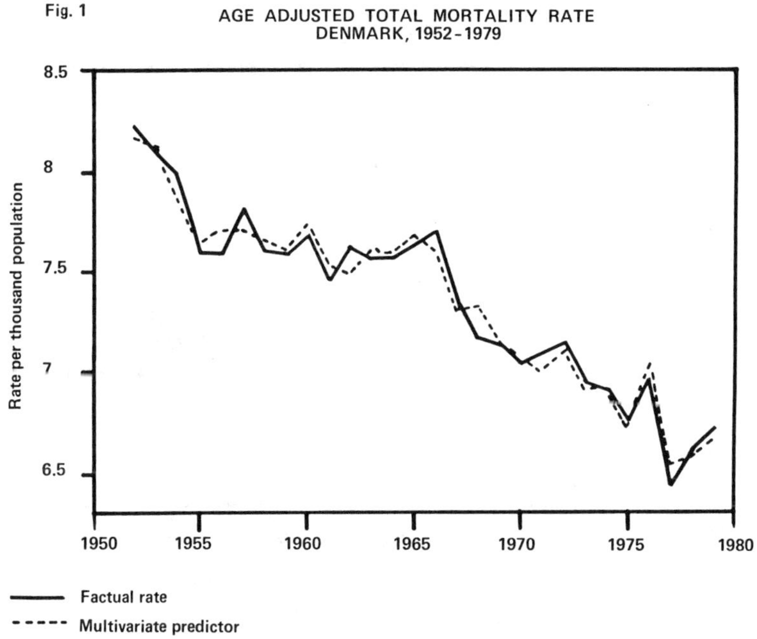
AGE ADJUSTED TOTAL MORTALITY RATE
DENMARK, 1952-1979
Rate per thousand population
8.5
8
7.5
7
6.5
1950
1955
1960
1965
1970
1975
1980
Factual rate
Multivariate predictor

Fig. 2

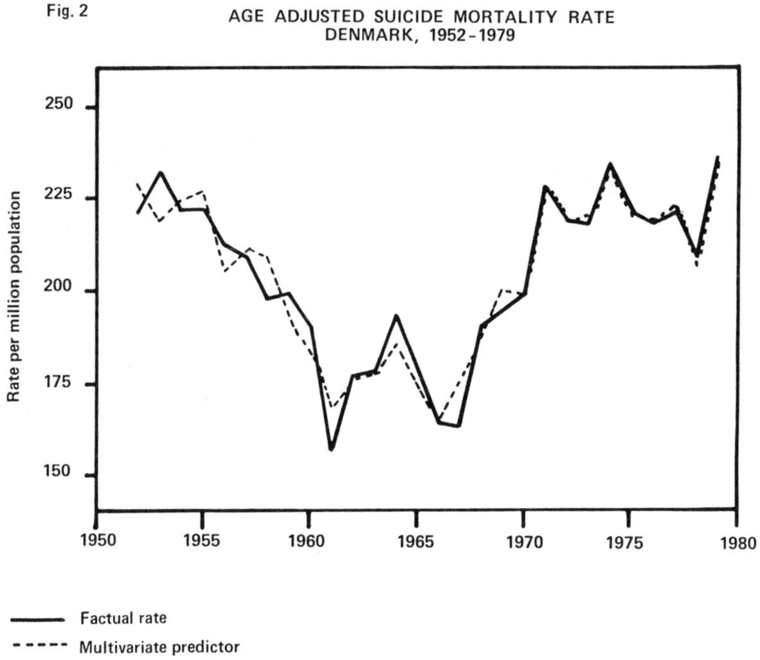
AGE ADJUSTED SUICIDE MORTALITY RATE
DENMARK, 1952-1979
Rate per million population
250
225
200
175
150
1950
1955
1960
1965
1970
1975
1980
Factual rate
Multivariate predictor

Fig. 3 AGE ADJUSTED CARDIAC DISEASE MORTALITY RATE DENMARK, 1952-1979

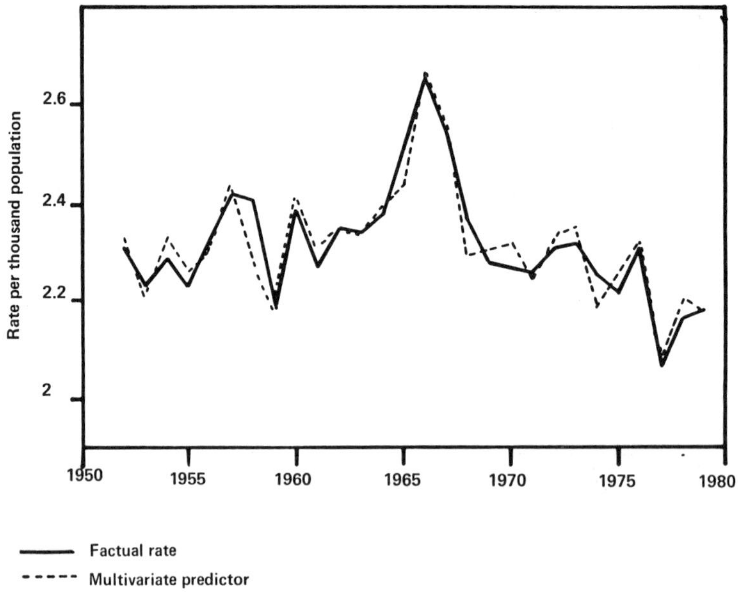

Table 1: Equations for Total Mortality Rate

Country	Australia	Canada	Denmark	England & Wales	Finland	France	Sweden	United States	West Germany
	1955-77	1954-77	1951-79	1954-79	1952-78	1954-78	1952-79	1950-80	1954-78
Economic									
Real income % exp. trend:	-6.017	-0.148	-0.142	-0.214	-20.591	-8.647	-17.592	-0.143E-02	-0.398
t-statistic	(-12.051)	(-15.585)	(-8.826)	(-8.420)	(-18.019)	(-5.433)	(-14.497)	(-34.043)	(-7.769)
Labour force									
Unemployment rate lag:	10 - 15	4	3	1		2 - 3	0	3	2 - 3
	0.121	0.253 E-01	0.441 E-01	36.817		18.552	10.941	5.639	7.068
t-statistic	(7.188)	(3.808)	(3.394)	(4.938)		(6.784)	(4.595)	(4.086)	(4.905)
Unemployment lag:			9	10			5	10	
coefficient			0.391 E-01	13.175			15.256	5.952	
t-statistic			(3.439)	(3.424)			(6.181)	(8.740)	
Unemployment lag:								13	
coefficient								1.665	
t-statistic								(4.632)	
Unemployment rate ann. chg. lag:			2			1			
coefficient			0.654 E-01			46.583			
t-statistic			(4.499)			(3.847)			
Business failures lag:					1				
coefficient					0.104				
t-statistic					(2.536)				
Business failures ann.chg. lag:	2 - 3	2 - 3		0			2	2	3
coefficient	0.119 E-02	0.259 E-02		13.476			0.168	0.125E-01	0.128E-01
t-statistic	(4.933)	(6.538)		(4.791)			(3.741)	(3.175)	(1.988)
Business failures lag:				2					
coefficient				9.886					
t-statistic				(2.714)					
Hours worked lag:				0					
coefficient				-0.504					
t-statistic				(-5.696)					
Hours worked ann. chg. lag:		0							
coefficient		-0.161							
t-statistic		(-4.592)							

Table 1 (continued)

	Australia 1955-77	Canada 1951-77	Denmark 1951-79	England & Wales 1954-79	Finland 1952-78	France 1954-78	Sweden 1952-79	United States 1950-80	West Germany 1954-78
Labour displaced lag:									
coefficient									
t-statistic									
Labour displaced (days) lag:									
coefficient									
t-statistic									
Behavioural									
Cigarettes lag:	4 - 8	14	3	5	14	0	0	5 - 6	0
coefficient	0.119 E-02	0.326 E-03	0.251 E-02	0.108 E-02	0.574 E.01	0.151	0.244	0.433E-03	0.114E-02
t-statistic	(13.151)	(5.624)	(6.955)	(2.698)	(7.478)	(2.348)	(8.299)	(10.390)	(4.542)
Cigarettes lag:			10			16			
coefficient			0.626 E-03			0.145			
t-statistic			(4.028)			(5.814)			
Cigarettes lag:			18						
coefficient			0.402 E-03						
t-statistic			(2.368)						
Total alcohol lag:	1								
coefficient	1.093								
t-statistic	(7.0113)								
Total alchohol ann. ch. lag:									
coefficient									
t-statistic									
Spirits lag:							3		
coefficient							17.366		
t-statistic							(2.576)		
Spirits ann. change lag:							1		
coefficient							31.097		
t-statistic							(3.374)		
Spirits ratio lag:		1					0		0
coefficient		2.987					305.167		11.245
t-statistic		(4.662)					6.259		(3.165)

Table 1 (continued)

	Australia 1955-77	Canada 1951-77	Denmark 1951-79	England & Wales 1954-79	Finland 1952-78	France 1954-78	Sweden 1952-79	United States 1950-80	West Germany 1954-78
Wine lag:									3
coefficient									0.100
t-statistic									(3.584)
Wine ratio:						2			
coefficient						250.034			
t-statistic						(3.770)			
Beer lag:					4				
coefficient					-2.055				
t-statistic					(-7.923)				
Beer ann. change lag:						0			
coefficient						-5.347			
t-statistic						(-2.888)			
Family & Household									
Divorce ann. ch. lag:		0	3					1	
coefficient		0.217 E-02	0.283					0.953	
t-statistic		(2.868)	(2.351)					(5.586)	
Other Controls									
Fat ann. change lag:	0								
coefficient	0.404 E-01								
t-statistic	(4.746)								
Health Services lag:				1					
coefficient				-14.716					
t-statistic				(-4.215)					
Immigratn. ann. ch. lag:									3
coefficient									58.862
t-statistic									(4.080)
Emigration lag:									1
coefficient									-73.233
t-statistic									(-2.119)

Table 1 (continued)

	Australia	Canada	Denmark	England & Wales	Finland	France	Sweden	United States	West Germany
	1955-77	1951-77	1951-79	1954-79	1952-78	1954-78	1952-79	1950-80	1954-78
Rho.	-0.402	-0.673	0.263	-0.762	-0.594	-0.518	-0.665	-0.507	-0.380
	(-2.058)	(-4.369)	(1.440)	(-5.892)	(-3.768)	(-2.967)	(-4.639)	(-3.218)	(-2.012)
Constant	11.586	8.667	6.746	44.165	1171.35	-535.256	560.785	39.	7.074
	(71.597)	(45.850)	(15.853)	(8.110)	(121.498)	(-1.229)	(12.407)	(34.257)	(7.662)
R^2	0.9735	0.9965	0.9518	0.9857	0.9946	0.9847	0.9963	0.9952	
Adjusted R^2	0.9629	0.9949	0.9316	0.9785	0.9936	0.9780	0.9946	0.9937	
F-statistic	73.508	578.533	39.521	137.599	927.116	128.883	535.988	621.937	
d.f.	6,15	7,15	8,19	8,16	4,21	7,16	8,18	7,22	
Durbin Watson statistic	2.2253	2.2589	2.3569	2.2974	2.2900	2.1432	2.0918	2.263	

NOTES: lags given in years
figures following E (e.g. E-02) signify the power of 10 to which the coefficient should be raised

Table 2: Equations for Suicide Mortality Rate

	Australia 1955-77	Canada 1954-77	Denmark 1951-79	England & Wales 1955-76	Finland 1952-78	France 1954-78	Sweden 1952-79	United States 1951-80	West Germany 1954-78
Economic									
Real income % exp. trend:	-0.359 E-01		0.283 E-02	-0.357 E-03	-1.406				
t-statistic	(-8.184)		(-11.201)	(-9.508)	(-9.018)				
Labour Force									
Unemployment rate lag:			0	3	1	2-3	1-2	2	
coefficient			0.146 E-02	0.476	1.476	0.515	0.263	0.104	
t-statistic			(3.653)	(4.556)	(5.344)	(10.726)	(2.397)	(2.754)	
Unemployment rate: lag					3				
coefficient					0.541				
t-statistic					(2.148)				
Unemp. rate ann. ch.: lag		2	2	0					
coefficient		0.198 E-02	0.610 E-02	0.516					
t-statistic		(2.808)	(6.751)	(6.666)					
Unemp. rate ann. ch: lag			3						
coefficient			0.326 E-02						
t-statistic			(3.508)						
Labour displaced: lag =1						0.133 E-01			
t-statistic						(4.473)			
Labour disp., days: lag = 0						0.474 E-02			
t-statistic						(2.357)			
Business failures: lag	3			2				1	3
coefficient	0.501 E-03			0.486				0.150 E-03	0.375 E-03
t-statistic	(13.452)			(12.569)				(3.311)	(4.322)
Business fail. ann. ch: lag	1 - 2								
coefficient	0.952 E-04								
t-statistic	(3.016)								

Table 2 (continued)

	Australia	Canada	Denmark	England & Wales	Finland	France	Sweden	United States	West Germany
	1955-77	1954-77	1951-79	1955-76	1952-78	1954-78	1952-79	1951-80	1954-78
Hours worked: lag				1-2					1
coefficient				-0.457					-0.475
				E-02					E-02
t-statistic				(-5.782)					(-4.927)
<u>Behavioural</u>									
Total alcohol lag						3	0		
coefficient						0.282	1.038		
t-statistic						(6.317)	(10.872)		
Total alc. ann. ch. lag	3		3				1		
coefficient	0.875		0.223				3.214		
	E-01		E-01						
t-statistic	(7.871)		(3.688)				(6.506)		
Spirits: lag				2				0	
coefficient				0.166				0.513	
				E-01				E-02	
t-statistic				(3.726)				(1.811)	
Spirits ann. chang: lag	1				2	0			2
coefficient	0.406				14.495	1.381			0.142
	E-01								E-01
t-statistic	(1.873)				5.579	(3.854)			(3.715)
Spirits ratio: lag	2			0					
coefficient	0.125			0.371					
t-statistic	(2.758)			(10.623)					
Beer coefficient: lag =2				-0.209					
				E-02					
t-statistic				(-16.977)					
Beer ratio coeff. lag =2							-0.735		
t-statistic							(-4.494)		
<u>Family & Household</u>									
Divorce: lag	+1		0		0-1				
coefficient	0.470		0.561		0.677				
	E-05		E-01		E-02				
t-statistic	(2.043)		(17.116)		(12.186)				

Table 2 (continued)

	Australia 1955-77	Canada 1954-77	Denmark 1951-79	England & Wales 1955-76	Finland 1952-78	France 1954-78	Sweden 1952-79	United States 1951-80	West Germany 1954-78
Divorce ann. ch. lag				3	3		0-1	2	
coefficient				0.792 E-02	0.201 E-01		0.194 E-02	0.207 E-01	
t-statistic				(2.446)	(5.452)		(7.830)	(4.791)	
Living alone coeff. (lag = 0)								0.196 E-03	
t-statistic								(2.856)	
Other controls									
Pop. ratio (15 - 24) lag = 0		0.978 E-01							
t-statistic		(22.299)							
Emigration coeff. lag = 0			0.652 E-02						
t-statistic			(5.036)						
Immigration coeff. lag = 0						-0.198			
t-statistic						(-7.149)			
Immig. ann. ch. lag = 1			-0.690 E-02						
t-statistic			(-3.265)						
Rho: coefficient	-0.646	-0.842 E-01	-0.686	-0.758	-0.526	-0.447	-0.[illegible]06	-0.158	0.573
t-statistic	(-3.971)	(-0.405)	(-4.987)	(5.322)	(-3.153)	(-2.451)	(-1.669)	(-0.785)	(3.423)
Constant	0.164	-0.102	0.185	0.832	13.056	8.145	18.073	0.756 E-01	0.323
t-statistic	(16.64)	(-8.082)	(27.255)	(8.989)	(13.430)	(8.075)	(11.554)	(20.151)	(7.554)
R Squared	0.9453	0.9839	0.9722	0.9975	0.9843	0.9285	0.9269	0.9694	0.7528
Adjusted R squared	0.9283	0.9804	0.9605	0.9954	0.9793	0.9032	0.9095	0.9630	0.7157
F statistic	51.8791	245.404	69.8787	392.659	188.020	25.9613	50.[illegible]339	126.755	18.2695
(d.f.)	(5,16)	(4,18)	(8,19)	(9,11)	(6,19)	(6,17)	(5,21)	(5,24)	(3,20)
Durbin Watson stat.	1.8986	2.0457	2.4526	2.5434	2.1906	2.1972	2.1150	2.040	1.706

NOTES: lags given in years
figures following E (e.g. E-02) signify the power of 10 to which the coefficient should be raised

Table 3: Equations for Infant Mortality Rate

Country	Australia	Canada	Denmark	England & Wales	Finland	France	Sweden	United States	West Germany
	1955-77	1954-77	1951-79	1955-76	1952-78	1954-78	1952-77	1950-80	1954-77
Economic									
Real inc. exp. trend	-3.413	-1.470	-0.952	-0.653 E-01	-3.296	-0.484	-1.150	-0.917 E-02	-5.361
	(-25.052)	(-30.536)	(-17.709)	(-10.211)	(-24.677)	(-35.189)	(-14.493)	(18.554)	(-18.228)
Unemp. rate: lag		3	2	1	0			0	0-1
coefficient		0.306	0.162	0.810 E-01	0.718			32.140	18.513
t-statistic		(3.652)	(3.561)	(2.626)	(4.454)			(4.358)	(2.407)
Unemp. rate ann. ch: lag						2	0-1		
coefficient						0.759	0.224		
t-statistic						(3.179)	(2.677)		
Unemp. ratio: fem 20-40 lag				0					
coefficient				1.648					
t-statistic				(2.561)					
Business fail. ann. ch: lag	1	0-2			1				
coefficient	0.209 E-01	0.785 E-02			0.194 E-01				
t-statistic	(2.747)	(2.652)			(3.754)				
Labour force partic. rate: coeff. (20 - 24 male)								-0.270	
t-statistic								(-3.769)	
Hours worked lag				0		0			2
coefficient				-0.521		-1.154			-0.895
t-statistic				(-2.825)		(-18.188)			(-6.020)
Behavioural									
Cigarettes lag				2				0	0
coefficient				0.289 E-02				0.335 E-02	0.430 E-02
t-statistic				(4.240)				(5.935)	(4.046)
Cigarettes ann. ch. lag	2	0-1			0		1		
coefficient	0.266 E-02	0.192 E-02			0.199 E-02		0.280 E-02		
t-statistic	(1.851)	(2.500)			(2.001)		(2.118)		

Table 3 (continued)

	Australia	Canada	Denmark	England & Wales	Finland	France	Sweden	United States	West Germany
	1955-77	1954-77	1951-79	1955-76	1952-78	1954-78	1952-77	1950-80	1954-77
Total alcohol lag				2	0-2				
coefficient				0.676	1.004				
t-statistic				(2.648)	(5.818)				
Total alc. ann. ch. lag = 0	4.434								
t-statistic	(5.466)								
Spirits lag			3					0	
coefficient			5.213					2.242	
t-statistic			(5.873)					(3.995)	
Spirits ann. ch. lag	2					2	1		
coefficient	3.572					1.217	1 110 E-02		
t-statistic	(2.168)					(2.388)	(3.318)		
Spirits ratio lag		0-1				3			
coefficient		26.349				87.847			
t-statistic		(5.270)				(13.152)			
Wine coefficient lag = 0					0.721		1.031		
t-statistic					(2.740)		(5.992)		
Wine ann. ch. coeff lag = 3						0.170			
t-statistic						(6.507)			
Beer coeff. lag = 0								0.512	
t-statistic								(4.457)	
Beer ratio coeff. lag = 1						-2.418			
t-statistic						(4.655)			
<u>Family & Household</u>									
Divorce ann. ch. lag =3									15.271
t-statistic									(4.329)
Living alone ann. ch. lag = 0								0.111	
t-statistic								(4.206)	
AFDC coeff. lag = 0								-0.751 E-01	
t-statistic								(-9.528)	
Birth rate coeff. (lag = 1)									-1.048
t-statistic									(-20.219)

Table 3 (continued)

	Australia	Canada	Denmark	England & Wales	Finland	France	Sweden	United States	West Germany
	1955-77	1954-77	1951-76	1955-76	1952-78	1954-78	1952-77	1950-80	1954-77
Non white birth ratio (lag = 0)								9.233	
t-statistic								(5.349)	
Other									
Health Services (lag = 1)				-71.664					
t-statistic				(-10.552)					
Immigration lag						3	1		
coefficient						-0.255	-0.142		
t-statistic						(-8.772)	(-3.771)		
Jan temp lag = 1							-0.750 E-01		
t-statistic							(-2.927)		
Influenza lag = 0							0.181 E-02		
t-statistic							(3.370)		
Rho	-0.631	0.224 E-03	-0.101	-0.739	-0.712 E-01	-0.483	-0.491	-0.497	-0.606 E-01
t-statistic	(-3.896)	(0.107) E-02	(-0.536)	(-5.024)	(0.371)	(-2.701)	(-2.821)	(-3.137)	(0.291)
Constant	31.760	27.837	43.991	82.587	50.541	101.054	39.635	35.216	157.061
t-statistic	(56.778)	9.482	(34.854)	(7.210)	(53.245)	(33.710)	(30.856)	(6.464)	(15.538)
R-squared	0.9895	0.9971	0.9930	0.9980	0.9918	0.9979	0.9979	0.9990	0.9977
Adjusted R-squared	0.9864	0.9963	0.9921	0.9969	0.9892	0.9995	0.9969	0.9985	0.9968
F-statistic	282.041	1047.41	1126.74	497.138	363.013	3392.31	967.062	1981.93	860.003
d.f.	5,17	5,17	3,24	7,13	6,19	8,15	8,16	9,20	6,16
Durbin Watson statistic	1.9769	1.9628	1.7862	2.3853	2.0651	2.2514	2.1903	2.1759	2.4727

Table 4 Equations for Total Heart Disease Mortality Rate, Age Adjusted

Country	Australia	Canada	Denmark	England & Wales	Finland	France	Sweden	United States	West Germany
Year	1955-77	1954-77	1951-79	1955-76	1952-78	1954-78	1952-79	1951-80	1954-78
Economic									
Real income % exp trend	-1.707	-6.449	-0.709 E-01	-0.840 E-02	-53.889		-0.626 E-01	-0.603 E-03	-0.270 E-01
t-statistic	(-43.817)	(-53.273)	(-8.431)	(-13.143)	(-5.040)		(-9.640)	(-10.520)	(-2.526)
Real income % ann. chg, lag = 0			-0.376 E-01						
t-statistic			(-3.145)						
Unemployment rate, lag:	3	3-4	3	1			3	3	3
Coefficient	0.199 E-01	0.537	0.149 E-01	0.316 E-01			0.456 E-01	4.632	6.128
t-statistic	(4.296)	(3.208)	(3.104)	(8.640)			(3.468)	(5.321)	(11.096)
Unemployment rate lag:	10-15		9	3				10	
Coefficient	0.314 E-01		0.611 E-01	0.159 E-01				1.653	
t-statistic	(26.209)		(11.133)	(4.484)				(3.775)	
Unemployment rate, lag:			17						
Coefficient			0.269 E-01						
t-statistic			(6.779)						
Unemp. rate ann. ch. lag:						1			
Coefficient						5.152			
t-statistic						(4.090)			
Bus. fail ann. chg. lag:	0	3			1-2		2	0	2
Coefficient	0.251 E-03	0.131			0.764		0.806 E-03	0.491 E-02	0.235 E-02
t-statistic	(2.906)	(4.586)			(3.236)		(4.546)	(2.318)	(1.916)
Bus. fail ann. chg lag:	2-3							2	
Coefficient	0.103 E-02							0.114 E-01	
t-statistic	(9.367)							(4.435)	
Hours worked, lag = 0				-0.179					
t-statistic				(-8.278)					
Behavioural									
Cigarettes, lag:	4-8	1-2	3	5	7	5-6	9-14	6	0

Table 4 (cont'd)

	Australia	Canada	Denmark	England & Wales	Finland	France	Sweden	United States	West Germany
	1955-77	1954-77	1951-76	1955-76	1952-78	1954-78	1952-79	1951-80	1954-78
Coefficient	0.380	0.127	0.104	0.326	0.236	0.178	0.119	0.321	0.646
	E-03	E-01	E-02	E-03		E-01	E-03	E-03	E-03
t-statistic	(57.333)	(16.048)	(7.865)	(3.501)	(3.922)	(7.831)	(5.177)	(5.350)	(11.746)
Cigarettes, lag:			10		11-12				
Coefficient			0.985		0.250				
			E-03						
t-statistic			(10.585)		(8.481)				
Cigarettes, lag:			17						
Coefficient			0.702						
			E-03						
t-statistic			(9.325)						
Spirits, lag = 1								0.182	
t-statistic								(2.554)	

Table 4 (cont'd)

	Australia 1955-77	Canada 1954-77	Denmark 1951-79	England & Wales 1955-76	Finland 1952-78	France 1954-78	Sweden 1952-80	United States 1951-80	West Germany 1954-78
Spirits ratio lag = 1				2.171					
t-statistic				(3.635)					
Spirits ann. chg, lag:		3				0	1		
Coefficient		69.985				9.402	0.211		
t-statistic		(3.532)				(2.854)	(5.182)		
Wine lag = 3									0.121 E-01
t-statistic									(2.417)
Wine ratio, lag:						2	1		
Coefficient						59.873	0.285		
t-statistic						(14.176)	(4.619)		
Beer, lag:					3	0		5	
Coefficient					-13.447	-1.486		-0.333 E-01	
t-statistic					(-5.423)	(-11.510)		(-5.434)	
Beer ratio, lag:				2	0				
Coefficient				-0.125	-73.072				
t-statistic				(-4.055)	(-5.219)				
Beer ann. chg, lag = 0									0.134 E-01
t-statistic									(3.938)
Total alcohol lag = 1	0.163								
t-statistic	(12.013)								
<u>Family & Household</u>									
Divorce lag = 2			0.118						
t-statistic			(3.170)						
Divorce ann. chg, lag:							0	1	
Coefficient							0.906 E-04	0.362	
t-statistic							2.535	(3.651)	

Table 4 (cont'd)

	Australia 1955-77	Canada 1954-77	Denmark 1951-79	England & Wales 1955-76	Finland 1952-78	France 1954-78	Sweden 1952-78	United States 1951-80	West Germany 1954-78
Other Controls									
Fat ann. chg, lag = 0	0.133 E-01								
t-statistic	(20.059)								
Health Serv, lag = 0-1				-3.427					
t-statistic				(-5.574)					
Binary var. 1958 ICD	-0.167	-3.779	0.134	0.352 E-01					
t-statistic	(-14.880)	(-2.206)	(3.246)	(1.334)					
Binary var. 1968 ICD	-0.380 E-01		0.584 E-01			9.250		0.522 E-01	0.146
t-statistic	(-3.992)		(1.244)			(4.220)		(1.202)	(3.697)
Binary var. 1961 ICD		-1.044							
t-statistic		(-0.488)							
Binary var. 1979 ICD								0.159	
t-statistic								(2.710)	
February temp. lag = 0				-0.914 E-02					
t-statistic				(-5.758)					
Rho	-0.933	-0.657	-.699	-0.257	-0.357	-0.732	-0.720	-0.865	-0.752
t-statistic	(-12.184)	(-4.176)	(-5.167)	(-1.218)	(-1.948)	(-5.266)	(-5.384)	(-9.263)	(-5.581)
Constant	4.625	311.719	0.332	18.372	3905.89	-201.718	2.950	4.194	0.654
t-statistic	(328.312)	(128.649)	(1.352)	(11.308)	(14.394)	(-6.954)	(41.430)	(15.011)	9.290
R-squared	0.9997	0.9981	0.9669	0.9862	0.9701	0.9880	0.9326	0.9955	0.9890
Adjusted R-squared	0.9994	0.9973	0.9442	0.9723	0.9606	0.9838	0.9077	0.9925	0.9841
F statistic	3120.94	1072.43	29.256	71.236	97.309	164.523	27.655	219.992	179.032
d.f.	(10,11)	(7,15)	(11,16)	(10,10)	6,19	(6,17)	(7,19)	(11,17)	(7,16)
Durbin Watson stat.	2.8791	2.3503	2.5500	2.2302	2.0631	2.1703	2.4817	2.1679	2.1140

Table 5 Equations for Ischaemic Heart Disease Mortality, Rate, Age Adjusted

Country	Canada 1954-77	Sweden 1952-79	W. Germany
Economic			
Real inc % exp trend	-6.452	-5.095	-0.347
t-statistic	(-9.976)	(-0.764)	(-4.168)
Unemployment rate lag:	3-4	4	
Coefficient	0.267	39.617	
t-statistic	(1.942)	(3.878)	
Unemployment rate lag = 7	2.054		
t-statistic	(6.386)		
Bus. fail. ann. chg, lag:	3	2	2
Coefficient	0.141	0.472	0.345 E-02
t-statistic	(6.725)	(2.520)	(2.386)
Behavioural			
Cigarettes, lag:	1-2	13	5
Coefficient	0.172 E-01	0.193	0.651 E-03
t-statistic	(12.452)	(1.861)	(2.951)
Spirits, ann. chg. lag = 1		229.684	
t-statistic		(8.027)	
Wine ratio lag = 1		315.085	
t-statistic		(7.571)	
Beer, lag:	4	6	
Coefficient	-41.746	-6.653	
t-statistic	(-2.590)	(-6.619)	
Beer ratio lag = 3			-0.204
t-statistic			(-5.413)
Family & Household			
Divorce, lag:	0		3
Coefficient	0.117		1.717
t-statistic	(3.994)		(3.456)
Divorce ann. chg. lag:		3	3
Coefficient		0.129	0.722
t-statistic		(5.143)	(2.881)
Other Controls			
Influenza lag = 1		0.201	
t-statistic		(4.409)	
Binary var, 1958 ICD	-4.316	5.064	
t-statistic	(-3.426)	(0.769)	
Binary var 1959 ICD			-0.474 E-01
t-statistic			(-1.301)
Binary var 1968 ICD			-0.416
t-statistic			(-10.190)

Table 5 (cont'd)

Country	Canada 1954-77	Sweden 1952-79	W. Germany
Binary var 1969 ICD	-6.119	-92.023	
t-statistic	(-3.346)	(-3.651)	
Rho	-0.627	-0.769	0.771
t-statistic	(-3.864)	(-6.250)	(5.931)
Constant	249.787	1784.63	5.502
t-statistic	(68.738)	(27.203)	(8.932)
R-squared	0.9988	0.9922	0.8906
Adjusted R-squared	0.9979	0.9865	0.8323
F statistic	805.879	127.744	8.142
d.f.	(9,13)	(11,15)	(8,15)
Durbin Watson Statistic	2.522	2.6328	2.0025

ECONOMIC INSTABILITY AND HEALTH: INFANT MORTALITY AND SUICIDE RECONSIDERED

Jürgen John

INTRODUCTION

This paper reports on a current research project dealing with the influence of economic instability on infant mortality and on suicide mortality. Up to now, the study is in a phase of exploratory data analysis, the findings of which may point to modifications of the explanatory models applied so far and will also clarify the data needs for such research. Because of the present state of the project this report has a rather fragmentary character. This paper presents some preliminary and incomplete results, some tentative interpretations of these results, and some suggestions on possible improvements of the regression models tested so far.

Infant mortality was chosen as the subject of this investigation because it became obvious at an earlier stage of our research in connection with the WHO(EURO) study on the influence of economic development on health that the application of Brenner's model to West German mortality data was not very successful [apart from the case of infant mortality] (John, 1983). Thus, our interest concentrated on a more detailed analysis of the possible relationship between economic instability, or more general: economic change, and infant mortality.

Suicide mortality was incorporated into the study because there is much empirical evidence from aggregate level studies for various Western industrialised countries that economic change and suicide mortality are closely interrelated. There has been no investigation as yet as to whether this aggregate level relationship holds for the Federal Republic of Germany.

The basic approach of the research project is a macro ecological one. It is not the purpose of this contribution to discuss the strengths and limitations of such an approach. But it should be stressed that aggregate level analyses are not only indispensible in their function as exploratory instruments in the generation of hypotheses. If one deals with social phenomena, aggregate level analyses are not only a more or less fruitful starting point of research efforts; it is also legitimate to regard an aggregate level analysis as target of research effort. Maybe the most powerful explanation of societal phenomena is to be looked for within the framework of a theory, perceiving as its object not the individuals but the society.

INFANT MORTALITY

Background

Investigations into the relationship between infant mortality and socio economic conditions have a long history. By and large, most of these studies can be grouped into two categories:

- Studies dealing with the long term relationship between infant mortality and the general socio economic level of nations.

The general empirical evidence collected from these studies is that the secular trend of economic growth has seemed to be inversely related to the long term trend in infant mortality rates.

- Studies dealing with differences in infant mortality rates between different socio economic groups of the population. The general empirical evidence collected from those studies is that there is a declining long term trend in infant mortality rates for all socio economic groups on the one hand, but a persistent inverse relationship between socio economic status and the level of infant mortality on the other hand.

The declining secular trend in infant mortality rates is apparent in all industrialised countries (as far as data are available), but it is also evident that this decline does not take place in a continuous manner. Up to now, only a few research efforts were devoted to the attempt to analyse the causes of these oscillatory movements of infant mortality. Some years ago, Brenner (1973) showed that short and medium term fluctuations of infant mortality in the USA, 1915-1967, can be statistically explained by economic fluctuations, especially by changing conditions on the labour market. A further study of Brenner (1979b), based on time series data for England and Wales, 1936-1976, also indicates a strong influence of unemployment rates on the oscillatory component of the development of infant mortality. A replication of Brenner's approach for the Federal Republic of Germany, 1950-1979 (John, 1983), illustrated too a statistically significant influence of unemployment rates on infant mortality rates.

This result was the starting point for our further statistical analyses. Up to now, major emphasis was given to the following issues:

- A breakdown of total infant mortality into different sub groups, because there are some arguments that the influence of economic instability could be varying in strength for these sub groups.

- An investigation into some critical arguments concerning Brenner's approach, especially the problem of detrending, the problem of lag specification, and the problem of robustness of estimation results with regard to a change of the estimation period.

The standard model

Our attempt to explain infant mortality patterns by changing economic conditions is essentially built upon Brenner's models applied to the USA (Brenner, 1977) and to England and Wales (Brenner, 1979b). In our slightly simplified version this model has three components:

- The long term trend in economic growth, catching all components of socio economic development which might contribute to the declining secular trend in infant mortality rates. This trend is measured in our model by the linear trend of real GNP per caput (LINIGNP);

- the unemployment rate (UR), which according to Brenner (1975b) as a national indicator of recession can be regarded as a global measure of income loss and work stress in employees of firms experiencing economic difficulty. Despite the fact that there are reasonable arguments for including current and lagged unemployment rates, we included in our model, as a first approach, only the current unemployment rate. To some extent this restriction is supported by Brenner's findings for the USA (Brenner, 1973). We will revert to this point later on;

- rapid economic change, measured by the absolute value of the difference between the trend value of real GNP per caput and the actual value (LINIGNPR). This specification implies that rapid economic change in a positive or a negative direction is thought to be similarly harmful.

Assuming a linear and additive structure, our standard model for the statistical explanation of infant mortality (IM) is given by:

$$IM_t = a_o + b_o LINTGNP_t + b_1 UR_t + b_2 LINTGNPR_t + u_t$$

When estimation results are presented, the time indices of variables are omitted for convenience. Current and lagged unemployment rates are indicated by adding the number of the lag periods to the symbol 'UR'; thus, UR_t will be indicated by URO, UR_{t-1} by UR1, etc.

The standard model has been tested for the following sub categories of infant morality:

- Total infant mortality (up to 1 year), male (IMMT),

- total infant mortality, female (IMFT),

- total infant mortality, legitimates, male and female (LIMTT),

- total infant mortality, illegitimates, male and female (ILIMTT),

- early neonatal mortality (1st week), male and female (ENMT),

- later neonatal mortality (7-28 days), male and female (LNMT),

- post neonatal mortality (28 days - 1 year), male and female (PONMT).

In addition, the model was applied to:

- perinatal mortality, male and female (PENMT).

To make comparisons more convenient, for estimation of the model all time series of mortality rates were transformed into index numbers (1952 - 100).

The time series data used for the estimation are annual values of the years 1950 to 1980. The estimates for the variables LIMTT and ILIMTT do not include the years 1960 up to 1962; for these three years the corresponding mortality figures were not reported.

Infant mortality data

It is a well known fact that international comparisons of infant mortality suffer from different definitions for live births, still births and abortions (for a comparison of the relevant definitions in various Western Euopean countries see Beck et al, 1978). Unfortunately, this holds for the time series data of the Federal Republic of Germany as well. The following changes of definitions have to be mentioned:

- Live birth: Since 1957 children have been counted as live births if it is ascertained there are heartbeats, that the navel string pulsates or the natural respiration sets in; before 1957 children were defined as live births if the natural respiration had set in.

- Still birth: Since 1 July 1979 children have been counted as still births if all characteristics for live births are missing but weighing at least 1000g. Before this date children were defined as still births if none of the characteristics applying to live births were found, and if the embryo's length of body amounted to at least 35 cm.

- Abortion: Since 1 July 1979 children are defined as abortions if none of the characteristics for live births can be applied, but with a birth weight below 1000g; before that date the body length was not to exceed 35 cm.

Reliable corrections of the time series are not possible. However, it can be assumed that the fluctuations of the mortality rates around their long term trend are not influenced by these definitional changes.

In view of the mortality rates for legitimate and illegitimate children it has to be kept in mind that a person can change the attributes 'legitimate' and 'illegitimate' in the course of time. The dates decisive for this attribution when computing infant mortality rates are the day of death for the infants died (numerator of mortality rates) and the day of birth for the live births (denominator of mortality rates). The number of subsequent legitimations of children born out of wedlock presumably exceeds the number of successful contestations of children's legitimacy. Therefore the mortality of legitimate children is presumably a bit over rated, whereas the mortality of illegitimate infants is under rated.

The mortality figures used for the estimations are based on two different computation methods. As far as available, weighted mortality figures were used, taking into account the development of births. For a number of the years under observation it was necessary to return to unweighted figures, ie to mortality rates, simply relating the number of infants died during the year under report to the number of live births of the same year. The values stated below show that the differences between weighted and unweighted mortality rates are relatively small:

Year	Total infant mortality, males and females, FRG	
	weighted rates	unweighted rates
1972	22,4	22,7
1973	22,7	22,9
1974	21,1	21,1
1975	19,7	19,8
1976	17,4	17,4

The only slight differences should not obscure the fact that, when using unweighted mortality rates, dependent variables enter into the regression models which are possibly affected by a systematic measurement error.

Estimation results for the standard model

At first the standard model was estimated by using ordinary least squares procedure (OLS). The results are reported in Table 1. As can be seen, the explanatory power of the model, measured by the coefficient of determination (R^2) or the adjusted coefficient of determination (R^{-2}) is rather high for all sub groups of infant mortality rates including perinatal mortality. Looking at the estimators of regression coefficients, it has to be stated that:

- there is a statistically significant influence of the growth trend of GNP in all equations,
- there is no significant influence of the economic change variable in any equation,
- the influence of unemployment rates is significant on a high level ($p < 0.0001$) for all mortality rates except the perinatal and early neonatal mortality rates.

TABLE 1

OLS - Estimation Results for the Standard Model

Infant Mortality, FRG, 1950 - 1980

DEP VAR	INTERC	LINTGNP	LINTGNPR	URO	F	$R^2(R^{-2})$	DW
IMMT	112.53 x (34.18)	-0.0065 x (-22.43)	0.0019 (0.30)	2.0382 x (7.18)	340.5 x	0.974 (0.971)	0.50
IMFT	112.82 x (39.09)	-0.0066 x (-25.95)	-0.0011 (-0.19)	2.1662 x (8.70)	468.4 x	0.981 (0.979)	0.62
LIMITT	114.41 x (27.83)	-0.0064 x (-18.47)	0.0018 (0.25)	1.9947 x (.574)	261.8 x	0.970 (0.967)	0.42
ILIMTT	129.28 x (33.00)	-0.0077 x (-23.32)	0.0056 (0.81)	1.2075 x (3.65)	344.8 x	0.977 (0.975)	0.81
ENMT	131.54 x (39.32)	-0.0073 x (-24.57)	0.0077 (1.17)	-0.0564 (-0.20)	283.4 x	0.969 (0.966)	0.37
LNMT	80.58 x (16.71)	-0.0047 x (-10.98)	-0.0001 (-0.01)	4.7752 x (11.48)	176.3 x	0.951 (0.946)	0.72
PONMT	91.50 x (18.88)	-0.0057 x (-13.29)	-0.0067 (-0.71)	4.6767 x (11.19)	215.1 x	0.960 (0.955)	0.83
PENMT	127.55 x (52.18)	-0.0072 x (-33.22)	0.0044 (0.92)	0.5048 o (2.40)	567.3	0.984 (0.983)	0.40

(.) T values
x $p < 0.0001$
+ $0.0001 \leq p < 0.01$
o $0.01 \leq p < 0.05$
z $0.05 \leq p < 0.1$
standardized coefficients are given

Comparing the magnitude of the regression coefficients for the unemployment rate it is surprising that this coefficient is smaller for illegitimate than the legitimate infant mortality rates. Taking into account that single pregnant women and single young mothers and their infants generally are regarded as especially vulnerable groups, the opposite result could have been expected. Clearly, this difference (as any other difference between the regression coefficients for the unemployment variable or the differences between the significance levels) might be due to a possible misspecification of the reaction time pattern of mortality rates on changes of the labour market conditions. We will return to this point later on.

The Durbin Watson test statistic (DW) indicates a strong first order autoregressive scheme of the residuals. Thus, one cannot exclude that the standard errors of the estimated regression coefficients are biased and that the T statistics are invalid. Therefore, the regression models were reestimated by using the generalised least squares procedure with appropriate weights (GLS). Because of the technical problems, which emerge from the occurrence of missing values in the time series of the variables LIMITT and ILIMTT, a GLS estimation for the equations with these two variables has not been carried out. The results are reported in Table 2. The figures indicate that minimising residual auto regression by using GLS yields no substantial changes of estimation results. As expected the coefficient of determination and the T values are slightly reduced; but with the one exception all independent variables which appeared to be of significant influence on infant mortality when using OLS have statistically significant GLS estimators as well. Only in the case of perinatal mortality the correlation between unemployment and infant mortality seems to be caused by residual auto correlation.

The estimates for IMMT and IMFT further demontrate that, due to the low inter correlation, omitting the statistically insignificant variable LINTGNPR leaves the estimators of the other independent variables fairly stable. It should be mentioned that the F test statistic is of dubious value when applying GLS; therefore this figure has been omitted in all tables reporting GLS estimation results.

The trend problem

One of the major points in the critical discussion of Brenner type analyses for mortality and economic instability has been the issue of detrending. Even if it has to be stressed that in the framework of multivariate regression analysis of time series mortality data the problem is not detrending mortality rates themselves but to determine the trend component in economic growth, one is in need of an explicit conceptual rationale to justify the choice of a certain type of trend (see Kasl, 1979). We must confess that even the most sophisticated techniques of time series analysis can offer such a conceptual rationale only in purely formal sense. On the other hand, there are no substantial theoretical arguments favouring the choice of a certain type of trend in economic growth.

TABLE 2

GLS - Estimation Results for the Standard Model

Infant Mortality, FRG, 1950 - 1980

DEP VAR	INTERC	LINTGNP	LINTGNPR	URO	R^2
IMMT	119.65 x (20.09)	-0.0070 x (-13.82)	0.0003 (0.08)	1.5509 + (3.46)	0.927
IMMT	119.81 x (20.32)	-0.0071 x (-14.08)		1.5415 + (3.52)	0.925
IMFT	116.87 x (22.70)	-0.0069 x (-15.69)	-0.0026 (0.80)	1.8971 x (4.74)	0.947
IMFT	116.95 x (23.18)	-0.0070 x (-16.26)		1.8723 x (4.78)	0.497
ENMT	135.60 x (21.87)	-0.0076 x (-14.27)	0.0027 (1.00)	-0.1979 (-0.46)	0.907
LNMT	87.19 x (11.07)	-0.0052 x (-).67)	-0.0027 (-0.44)	4.3885 x (6.92)	0.893
PONMT	95.18 x (12.65)	-0.0060 x (-9.31)	-0.0043 (-0.62)	4.4577 x (7.21)	0.916
PENMT	131.42 x (28.68)	-0.0075 x (-18.94)	0.0008 (0.42)	0.2501 (0.78)	0.948

(.) T values
x $p < 0.0001$
\+ $0.0001 \leq p < 0.01$
o $0.01 \leq p < 0.05$
z $0.05 \leq p < 0.1$

With this rather unsatisfactory state of the art, we have carried out a small sensitivity analysis by replacing the linear growth trend assumption by an exponential growth trend assumption. Thus, the model included the estimated exponential growth trend value of real GNP per caput (EXPTGNP) instead of LINIGNP, and instead of LINIGNPR, the absolute value of the difference between EXPTGNP and the actual value of real GNP per caput (EXPTGNPR) were included in the model.

In this context it should be remembered that it is the exponential growth trend assumption on which Brenner's models are based. However, it has to be pointed out that (measured by the usual statistical criteria) this assumption is a clear misspecification for the growth of GNP in the FRG, 1950 - 1980.

The OLS estimation results for the exponential growth trend model are reported in Table 3. These figures draw a remarkably changed picture compared with the linear growth trend model:

- All estimators for the coefficients of the growth trend variables are (absolutely) smaller. Assuming an economic development corresponding to the growth trend path from 1950 to 1980 this implies that the marginal contribution of an additional unit of GNP to the decline of infant mortality is smaller compared with the linear trend. Moving on the growth trend path the absolute decline of infant mortality is still much the same; this is due to the considerably greater range of the exponential growth trend variable. Finally, in the case of exponential growth all infant mortality rates corresponding to the growth trend state of the economy are clearly smaller than in case of linear growth.

- If accepting a conventional significance level of 10% in the case of postneonatal infant mortality one would reject the hypothesis that the growth trend residual does not influence mortality rates (Prob > /T/ = 0.065); this is opposite to the linear growth trend model.

- In all equations the estimated coefficients of the unemployment variable are substantially higher (up to three times of the values in the linear growth trend model). Moreover, in the case of early neonatal mortality one would reject the hypothesis that unemployment does not influence infant mortality (Prob > /T/ = 0.0002); this is opposite to the linear growth trend model, as well.

TABLE 3

OLS - Estimation Results for the Exponential Growth Trend Model

Infant Mortality, FRG, 1950 - 1980

DEP VAR	INTERC	LINTGNP	LINTGNPR	URO	F	$R^2(\bar{R}^2)$	DW
IMMT	101.38 x (33.47)	-0.0058 x (-18.18)	0.0031 (0.87)	2.9830 x (9.97)	302.46 x	0.971 (0.968)	0.58
IMFT	101.31 x (36.50)	-0.0060 x (-20.33)	0.0037 (1.14)	3.1196 x (11.38)	380.50 x	0.977 (0.974)	0.71
LIMTT	102.35 x (26.54)	-0.0055 x (-13.38)	-0.0006 (-0.14)	3.0888 x (8.12)	251.43 x	0.969 (0.965)	0.53
ILIMTT	116.77 x (31.59)	-0.0069 x (-17.68)	0.0053 (1.26)	2.2454 x (6.16)	327.23 x	0.976 (0.973)	0.90
ENMT	119.31 (44.45)	-0.0062 x (-21.72)	-0.0022 (-0.71)	1.1280 + (4.25)	333.58 x	0.974 (0.971)	0.47
LNMT	72.13 x (16.67)	-0.0041 x (-8.90)	0.0002 (0.04)	5.5223 x (12.92)	164.62 x	0.948 (0.942)	0.78
PONMT	81.45 x (18.44)	-0.0055 x (-11.78)	0.0100 z (1.93)	5.3333 x (12.22)	194.50 x	0.956 (0.951)	0.85
PENMT	115.26 x (56.53)	-0.0062 x (-28.66)	-0.0009 (-0.39)	1.6528 x (8.21)	615.85 x	0.986	0.55

(.) T values
x $p < 0.0001$
\+ $0.0001 \leq p < 0.01$
o $0.01 \leq p < 0.05$
z $0.05 \leq p < 0.1$

As in the case of the standard model, DW indicates a strong autoregressive scheme of residuals. Table 4 provides the GLS estimation results for the exponential trend model. It is obvious that minimising residual autocorrelation by using GLS does not qualitatively change the results of the comparison between the linear and the exponential growth trend model. Furthermore, the GLS results show that, contrary to the linear trend model, in the case of perinatal mortality the influence of unemployment rates on mortality rates cannot be regarded merely as an effect of residual autocorrelation.

Even this small scale sensitivity analysis demonstrates that estimation and test results react very sensitively to changes of the trend assumption. Thus, the question as to which criteria should determine the choice of a certain type of trend requires an urgent answer.

The Lag Problem

The most complicated problem when applying Brenner's approach to analyze the development of time series mortality data is the choice of the appropriate lag structure. With regard to our problem under investigation Brenner has argued that there are differential lags of fetal and infant mortality behind economic fluctuation which are age specific (Brenner, 1973). According to Brenner's finding for the USA increases in fetal mortality rates generally occur within the same year in which the national economy deteriorates; increases in infant mortality rates under 1 day tend to lag approxiately 1 year behind any given year of an economic downturn; increases in post neonatal mortality rates tend to lag from 3 to 5 years behind any given year of an economic downturn. These results are in contrast with our findings which indicate on the one hand only a weak influence of current unemployment on early neonatal mortality and perinatal mortality and on the other a strong influence of the current unemployment rate on post neonatal mortality rates on the other hand. These results could be supported by the argument that post neonatal deaths are most likely to reflect the infant's post natal social enviornment because at that stage the bulk of congenitally caused deaths will already have occurred and the child is most directly exposed to the circumstances of the parental home. Stillbirths and first week deaths, on the other hand, are more likely to reflect the long term growth and health history of the mother and hence her past social experience (Illsley and Mullen, 1982).

Thus, in the light of these contradictory results and arguments, two further models have been tested. The first of these two models is a simple version of a finite distributed lag model: It includes as additional variable the unemployment rate of the foregoing year (UR1). Due to the high intercollinearity betweeen URO and UR1 this model did not yield statistically satisfactory results. All estimation results can be grouped in to two types: The first and more frequent type, illustrated by an example in Table 5, shows that only one or two coefficients is significantly different from zero. In the second case both coefficients are statistically significant, but one of them has a 'false' sign. Thus, the choice of the appropriate reaction time pattern cannot be based on the estimation results. But judged on the basis of the quantitiative impact of unemployment on infant mortality, this problem is meaningless: Computations of the (mean) elasticities of mortality rates with

TABLE 4

GLS - Estimation Results for the Exponential Growth Trend Model

Infant Mortality, FRG, 1950 - 1980

DEP VAR	INTERC	EXPTGNP	EXPTGNPR	URO	R^2
IMMT	106.40 x (19.40)	-0.0062 x (-12.43)	0.0043 (1.47)	2.4828 x (5.42)	0.918
IMFT	103.99 x (21.42)	-0.0061 x (-13.60)	0.0034 (1.15)	2.8359 x (6.73)	0.937
ENMT	122.96 x (24.38)	-0.0066 x (-14.68)	0.0016 (0.70)	0.7648 z (1.94)	0.919
LNMT	76.85 x (11.03)	-0.0045 x (-6.92)	0.0031 (0.63)	5.1283 x (8.20)	0.889
PONMT	84.89 x (11.90)	-0.0057 x (-8.44)	0.0097 z (1.89)	5.0377 x (7.81)	0.902
PENMT	118.17 x (31.61)	-0.0064 x (-19.18)	0.0016 (0.88)	1.2580 + (4.14)	0.956

(.) T values
x $p < 0.0001$
+ $0.0001 \leq p < 0.01$
o $0.01 \leq p < 0.05$
z $0.05 \leq p < 0.1$

respect to unemployment yield fairly similar (equilibrium) values, whether UR0 or UR1 or URO and UR1 are included into the regression model.

TABLE 5

GLS - Estimation Results for the Finite Distributed Lag Model

Infant Mortality, FRG, 1950/51 - 1980

DEP VAR	INTERC	LINTGNP	LINTGNPR	URO	UR1	R^2
IMFT	115.33x	-0.0068x	-0.0025	1.7068o	0.1532	0.943
	(20.76)	(-14.53)	(-0.72)	(2.44)	(0.22)	
IMFT	116.87x	-0.0069x	-0.0026	1.8971x		0.947
	(22.70)	(-15.69)	(-0.80)	(4.74)		
IMFT	114.89x	-0.0067x	0.0002		1.6653+	0.943
	(21.23)	(-14.79)	(0.04)		(4.07)	

(.) T values
x $p < 0.0001$
\+ $0.0001 \leq p < 0.01$
o $0.01 \leq p < 0.05$
z $0.05 \leq p < 0.1$

The second model is based on the assumption of an infinite geometric lag distribution for unemployment rates and the growth trend variable and the rapid economic change variable. That is, current infant mortality rates are assumed not only to be influenced by the current economic conditions but by all the economic history with lag coefficients declining continuously, following the pattern of a geometric progression.

These assumptions lead to the well known Koyck lag model[a] which includes as independent variables only the unlagged independent variables of the original model plus the dependent variable with lag 1.

(a) We can do here without a formal derivation of the Koyck transformation and without the discussions of the estimation problems related to the Koyck lag model. But it should be mentioned that interpreting the estimation results of the Koyck lag model in the sense of the underlying assumptions presupposes that the estimated regression coefficients of all independent variables are significantly different from zero, and that the value of the regression coefficient of the lagged endogenous variable lies between 0 and 1.

The Koyck lag model proved to be totally unsuccessful; therefore, only one example of estimation results is reported in Table 6. Just as in this example, in all cases the only significant variable was the lagged mortality rate itself. Thus, the only finding from this model is the fact that the time series of the different infant mortality rates can be well described by a simple autoregressive scheme.

TABLE 6

OLS - Estimation Results for the Koyck Lag Model

Infant Mortality, FRG, 1951 - 1980

DEP VAR	INTERC	LINTGNP	LINTGNPR	URO	IMMT1
IMMTO	6.31 (0.48)	-0.0004 (-0.52)	0.0032 (1.08)	0.2364 (-0.22)	0.9117 (8.16)
	F = 608.31x		$R^2(\bar{R}^2)$ = 0.991 (0.989)		DW = 2.02

(.) T values
x $p < 0.0001$
\+ $0.0001 \leq p < 0.01$
o $0.01 \leq p < 0.05$
z $0.05 \leq p < 0.1$

The choice of the estimation period

Brenner's analysis of the relationship between economic instability and mortality in England and Wales (Brenner, 1979b) has been sharply criticised for different reasons by Gravelle, Hutchinson, and Stern (1981). One major point of this criticism was the fact that the period over which Brenner tested his hypothesis was apparently crucial for the reported results. For this reason a further sensitivity analysis was carried out with respect to changes in the sample period. For this, the following simple technique was applied: The sample period was shortened by the stepwise elimination of observations from the beginning and from the end of the original sample period. For each step the linear and the exponential growth trend model were reestimated. Because of the insignificant results for the growth trend residuals this variable was omitted from the model. The growth trend variables used in this procedure are in all cases the growth trend path values of the original sample period 1950 - 1980. The results of this test of robustness are reported in Tables 7 and 8.

TABLE 7

Test of Robustness: Total Infant Mortality, FRG

Model: IMMT, IMFT = f(LINTGNP, URO)
(GLS - Estimators)

Estimation period	DF	IMMT b(URO)	IMMT Prob	IMFT b(URO)	IMFT Prob
1950-80	27	1,54	0,0016	1,87	<0,0001
1951-80	26	1,50	0,0019	1,81	<0,0001
1952-80	25	1,00	0,0360	1,38	0,0029
1953-80	24	0,79	0,1123	1,28	0,0094
1954-80	23	0,53	0,2948	1,04	0,0417
1955-80	22	0,37	0,5324	1,o7	0,0757
1956-80	21	0,21	0,7451	0,85	0,1916
1957-80	20	-0,11	0,8713	0,37	0,5627
1958-80	19	-0,15	0,8266	0,40	0,5458
1959-80	18	-0,27	0,7154	0,38	0,6084
1960-80	17	-0,35	0,6888	o,27	0,7554
1961-80	16	-0,54	0,5710	0,06	0,9482
1962-80	15	-0,83	0,3337	-0,24	0,7658
1963-80	14	-0,91	0,2890	-0,34	0,6766
1964-80	13	-0,99	0,2588	-0,45	9,5869
1965-80	12	-1,06	0,2501	-0,52	0,5498
1950-79	26	1,55	0,0020	1,84	<0,0001
1950-78	25	1,56	0,0021	1,84	<0,0001
1950-77	24	1,61	0,0016	1,86	<0,0001
1950-76	23	1,77	0,0008	1,96	<0,0001
1950-75	22	1,94	0,0004	2,07	<0,0001
1950-74	21	2,28	0,0006	2,36	0,0002
1950-73	20	2,39	0,0014	2,45	0,0006
1950-72	19	2,12	0,0048	2,28	0,0013
1950-71	18	2,16	0,0060	2,24	0,0011
1950-70	17	2,20	0,0040	1,72	0,0044
1950-69	16	1,73	0,0062	1,69	0,0048
1950-68	15	1,44	0,0144	1,40	0,0116
1950-67	14	1,17	0,0458	1,16	0,0400
1950-66	13	1,11	0,1432	1,13	0,1238
1950-65	12	0,56	0,4670	0,77	0,3331

TABLE 8

Test of Robustness: Total Infant Mortality, FRG

Model: IMMT, IMFT = f(EXPTGNP, URO)
(GLS - Estimators)

Estimation period	DF	IMMT b(URO)	IMMT Prob	IMFT b(URO)	IMFT Prob
1950-80	27	2,6859	<0,0001	2,9747	<0,0001
1951-80	26	2,4966	<0,0001	2,7860	<0,0001
1952-80	25	1,9964	0,0003	2,3642	<0,0001
1953-80	24	1,7257	0,0027	2,2232	0,0002
1954-80	23	1,3666	0,0187	1,9022	0,0016
1955-80	22	1,1828	0,0828	1,9220	0,0075
1956-80	21	0,9139	0,2181	1,5941	0,0392
1957-80	20	0,4150	0,5728	0,9002	0,2216
1958-80	19	0,2617	0,7242	0,8595	0,2606
1959-80	18	0,0031	0,9970	0,6994	0,4138
1960-80	17	-0,2109	0,8258	0,4182	0,6727
1961-80	16	-0,4434	0,6583	0,1421	0,8870
1962-80	15	-0,7329	0,3845	-0,1633	0,8453
1963-80	14	-0,7990	0,3263	-0,2535	0,7503
1964-80	13	-0,8638	0,2829	-0,3653	0,6353
1965-80	12	-0,9217	0,2682	-0,4277	0,5880
1950-79	26	2,6378	<0,0001	2,8969	<0,0001
1950-78	25	2,5765	<0,0001	2,8321	<0,0001
1950-77	24	2,5531	<0,0001	2,7830	<0,0001
1950-76	23	2,6572	<0,0001	2,8348	<0,0001
1950-75	22	2,7937	<0,0001	2,9131	<0,0001
1950-74	21	3,1184	<0,0001	3,1923	<0,0001
1950-73	20	3,2583	<0,0001	3,3085	<0,0001
1950-72	19	3,0149	0,0002	3,1529	<0,0001
1950-71	18	3,0512	0,0003	3,1191	<0,0001
1950-70	17	3,0555	0,0002	2,6622	<0,0001
1950-69	16	2,6334	0,0001	2,5950	<0,0001
1950-68	15	2,3302	0,0003	2,2880	0,0002
1950-67	14	2,0335	0,0017	2,0197	0,0012
1950-66	13	2,0964	0,0092	2,0997	0,0066
1950-65	12	1,5560	0,0583	1,7494	0,0352

The figures in these tables indicate that the inclusion of the early fifties is crucial for both models, whereas a shortening of the sample period starting from the end of the original estimation period leads to insignificant results only for the linear growth trend model and when estimations are based on a rather small number of degrees of freedom (DF). The economic data show that the crucial period 1950-56 has by far the highest unemployment rates and the highest growth rates of real GNP per caput in the original sample period.

Of course, there is nothing in Brenner's and our arguments underlying the models tested so far that these models are valid only for specific time periods. But one could argue, on the other hand, that economic instability and insecurity must have a certain level or degree of intensity to exert a substantial impact on the health of the population. The singularity of those economic conditions in the time span 1950-56 makes it impossible to decide this question on the basis of the currently available data for the Federal Republic of Germany. It can be appreciated that the recent and the foreseeable economic development will give the opportunity to make a crucial statistical experiment.

Perspectives

Although the results of the analysis up to now are very unsatisfactory and though we do not see how to overcome some central methodological problems related to an aggregate level approach of Brenner's type, as eg the problem of detrending GNP development or the problem of an appropriate specification of the lag structures, research efforts to investigate the possible impact of economic instability on health should continue on an individual and on an aggregate level, as well.

One of the major problems of our model specifications may be the omission of relevant independent variables, as eg some classical risk factors such as alcohol and nicotine abuse, the liberalisation of the German abortion law in 1976, or the improvement of health care for pregnant women and infants since the mid seventies. In the future we will attempt to control for some influences on infant mortality rates stemming from changes in demographic factors. For example, it is well known that the risk of infant mortality is essentially dependent on the age of the mother, the time span between the births, and the number of foregoing births. In the Federal Republic of Germany the distributions of all these variables have changed drastically in the last two decades. A further problem resulting from demographic factors is the continuous increase of the foreign population in West Germany. For this population group fertility and infant mortality rates are considerably higher than for the German population.

Incorporating those factors in an aggregate level approach either by a further splitting of infant mortality rates or by including appropriate independent variables might change the results of those analyses (perhaps in favour of Brenner's hypothesis).

SUICIDE MORTALITY

Background

The impact of changing economic conditions on the reported suicide rates has, since Durkheim (1897), been the subject of many empirical studies. Some of these studies, like our own investigation, are based on a macroecological approach as eg the studies cited in Platt (Chapter 3).

Up to now a similar aggregate study of suicide mortality has not been carried out for the Federal Republic of Germany. The major emphasis in our investigation is currently placed on discovering whether the empirical relationship found in other countries can also be found in the Federal Republic of Germany.

The models

The basic ideas underlying the specification of the regression models have been developed by Brenner (1977, 1979b) and Marshall and Hodge (1981). Essentially, these authors argue that an attempt to gauge the total impact of the economic environment on suicide should take into account:

- the state (of development) of the economy
- improvement or deterioration of the economy, and
- short term economic fluctuations, per se

Hence, the first model for the statistical explanation of the suicide rates (SUI_t) includes an indicator of the state of the economy (SE_t), a measure of change of this state over the previous year ($Se_t - SE_{t-1}$), and a measure of the direction of that change ($SE_t - SE_{t-1}$). Assuming a linear and additive specification, model 1 is given by

$$SUI_t = a_o + b_o SE_t + b_1 (SE_t - SE_{t-1}) + b_2 (SE_t - SE_{t-1}) + u_t$$

The second model tested so far assumes a lagged adjustment of suicide rates to a change of economic conditions. As in the case of infant mortality, we apply Koyck's geometric lag scheme. Thus, model 2 is given by

$$SUI_t = a_o + b_o SE_t + b_1 (SE_t - SE_{t-1}) + b_2 (SE_t - SE_{t-1}) + b_3 SUI_{t-1} + u_t$$

It should be noted that model 2 can be interpreted in a very different way:

- as with infant mortality the reaction time must be taken into account, therefore, not all elements of the aggregate under investigation might adjust themselves to the changed economic situation in the period in which that change is taking place. Thus, the distributed lag can be regarded as the reaction time pattern of the aggregate under investigation.

- One can assume that people's actions and decisions are influenced not only or perhaps even not primarily by the actual economic conditions, but rather by the expectations with regard to these conditions. Indeed, model 2 can be interpreted this way, as well. However, this interpretation implies that the formulation of expectations takes place in a very rigid adaptive manner, that is, current expectations are formed by gradually modifying previous expectations in the light of current experience.

As indicators of state and change of the economy two different sets of variables have been chosen. The first set of variables emphasizes the growth conditions of the economy: the state of the economy is characterized by the growth rate of the real GNP per caput (GRGNP); improvement or deterioration of the economy is indicated by the first differences of these growth rates (DGRGNP), and the economic change per se is measured by the absolute value of this difference (ADGRGNP). The second set of variables places emphasis on the labour market conditions: The unemployment rate (UR) is regarded as indicator of the state of the economy, improvement or deterioration of the economy and economic change per se are measured by the first difference of the unemployment rate (DUR) and the absolute value of this difference (ADUR) respectively.

The models were applied to four subgroups of suicide mortality:

- suicide rates for the male population in the age group from 15 to 64 years (SUIMLF),
- suicide rates for the male population at the age of 65 and more (SUIMAG),
- suicide rates for the female population in the age group from 15 to 64 years (SUIFLF),
- suicide rates for the female population at the age of 65 and more (SUIFAG).

All mortality rates are age standardised on the basis of the resident population, FRG, 1970. To make comparisons more convenient, for estimation purposes all time series of suicide rates were transformed into index numbers (1952 = 100).

Estimation results

The estimation results for model 1 are reported in Tables 9 (OLS estimators) and 10 (GLS estimators); they can be summarised quite briefly: The explanatory power of the model measured on the basis of the variance explained by the independent variables is very poor: this may indicate that the model is heavily misspecified (of course, we cannot exclude that stochastic factors really are the important explanatory factors). If one looks at the GLS estimators, only five regression coefficients are significantly different from zero, but only three of the significant estimators have the expected sign.

TABLE 9

OLS - Estimation Results for Model 1 (Instantaneous Adjustment Model)

Suicide, FRG, 1959 - 1980

DEP VAR	INTERC	GRGNP	DGRGNP	ADGRGNP	UR	DUR	ADUR	F	$R^2(R^{-2})$	DW
SUIMLF	120.98 x 36.72	-1.76 x (-3.29)	0.71 (0.94)	0.94 z (1.86)				4.1 o	0.33 (0.25)	0.91
SUIMLF	117.45 x (57.61)				-0.14 (-0.23)	4.45 + (2.99)	-1.63 (-0.73)	3.9 o	0.32 (0.24)	0.78
SUIMAG	90.38 x (29.79)	-0.26 (0.53)	-0.38 (-0.81)	-0.30 (-0.44)				0.4	0.05 (-0.07)	0.67
SUIMAG	88.88 x (54.05)				1.39 + (2.84)	1.86 (1.51)	-2.81 (-1.56)	2.8 z	0.25 (0.16)	0.82
SUIFLF	119.15 x (33.06)	-1.09 z (-1.85)	0.35 (0.63)	0.86 (1.05)				1.5	0.16 (0.06)	0.86
SUIFLF	120.24 x (59.26)				-0.69 (-1.14)	3.04 z (2.00)	-1.40 (-0.63)	3.4 o	0.29 (0.20)	0.77
SUIFAG	134.87 x (21.36)	-3.56 + (-3.48)	2.22 o (2.28)	0.54 (0.37)				4.4 +	0.34 (0.26)	0.76
SUIFAG	127.87 x (33.66)				-0.79 (-0.70)	7.64 z (2.67)	-5.31 (-1.28)	4.8 +	0.37 (0.29)	1.06

(.) T values
x $p < 0.0001$
+ $0.0001 \leq p < 0.01$
o $0.01 \leq p < 0.05$
z $0.05 \leq p < 0.1$

TABLE 10

GLS - Estimation Results for Model 1 (Instantaneous Adjustment Model)

Suicide, FRG, 1950 - 1980

DEP VAR	INTERC	GRGNP	DGRGNP	ADGRGNP	UR	DUR	ADUR	R^2
SUIMLF	118.09 x (34.76)	-1.05 z (-1.87)	0.44 (1.09)	0.34 (0.67)				0.14
SUIMLF	116.96 x (36.13)				-0.55 (-0.74)	2.51 z (1.89)	-0.58 (-0.35)	0.16
SUIMAG	88.59 x (29.06)	0.52 (1.09)	-0.63 z (-1.92)	0.27 (0.66)				0.14
SUIMAG	89.23 x (33.84)				1.28 z (2.06)	0.91 (0.80)	-2.48 z (-1.74)	0.19
SUIFLF	114.75 x (31.90)	-0.05 (-0.09)	-0.21 (-0.51)	0.45 (0.85)				0.04
SUIFLF	120.70 x (37.52)				-1.26 (-1.70)	1.[illegible]8 (0.90)	-0.98 (-5.59)	0.18
SUIFAG	122.46 x (20.27)	-0.98 (-1.04)	0.78 (1.21)	0.83 (0.31)				0.12
SUIFAG	127.83 x (25.53)				-2.14 (-1.71)	1.05 (0.42)	-0.95 (-0.29)	0.15

(.) T values
x $p < 0.0001$
+ $0.0001 \leq p < 0.01$
o $0.01 \leq p < 0.05$
z $0.05 \leq p < 0.1$

The estimation results for model 2 were also totally unsatisfactory, (the two 'best' regression equations are reported in Table 11). Only one regression equation (SUIMLFO with DUR and SUIMLF1) could be interpreted in the sense of the hypotheses mentioned above underlying the Koyck lag model. But taking into account the estimation results as a whole it seems to be more reasonable to interpret this equation in the sense of an unexplained autoregressive scheme.

TABLE 11

OLS - Estimation Results for the Koyck Lag Model

Suicide, FRG, 1951 - 1980

DEP VAR	INTERC	UR	DUR	ADUR	SUIMLF1
SUIMLFO	40.86+	0.45	2.61o	-0.99	0.65x
	(2.97)	(1.01)	(2.46)	(-0.67)	(5.53)
	F = 12.18x		$R^2(\bar{R}^2)$ = 0.68 (0.62)		DW = 1.64
SUIMLFO	42.49+		2.37o		0.64x
	(3.24)		(2.33)		(5.63)
	F = 24.70x		$R^2(\bar{R}^2)$ = 0.66 (0.64)		DW = 1.65

(.) T values
x $p < 0.0001$
\+ $0.0001 \leq p < 0.01$
o $0.01 \leq p < 0.05$
z $0.05 \leq p < 0.1$

Perspectives

Up to now, the attempt to explain the development of suicide mortality rates by general economic conditions seems to be a totally misleading approach for the Federal Republic of Germany. In the light of the foreign empirical evidence the results as a whole and especially the fact that the level of unemployment apparently does not influence the suicide rates are rather surprising.

May be that in comparison with the USA, above all, there are radical differences concerning the role and the weight of economic success and economic failure in the process of the individual's evaluation of his social environment and the individual's self assessment. Perhaps the relationship between economic instability and suicide rates holds only for certain special risk groups eg the isolated elderly or the young unemployed; such a relationship could remain concealed within an aggregate level analysis for the whole population.

Restricted to the available data all we can do in the near future is to carry on the analysis for smaller age groups and to characterise economic conditions by age specific variables such as age specific income levels and unemployment rates and/or by additional variables such as public welfare expenditures or the number of cases of persons getting financial aid or other forms of transfers by social support agencies.

REFERENCES

Beck, L., Maier, E., Schmidt, E., Rohde, J. (1978), Mütter- und Säuglingssterblichkeit, W. Kohlhammer, Stuttgart, Berlin, Köln, Mainz (=Schriftenreihe des Bundesministers für Jugend, Familie und Gesundheit, Band 67)

Brenner, M.H. (1973), Fetal, Infant, and Maternal Mortality during Periods of Economic Instability, in International Journal of Health Services 3, 2 (1973), pp.145-159

Brenner, M.H. (1977), Health Costs and Benefits of Economic Policy, in International Journal of Health Services 7, 4 (1977), pp. 581-623

Brenner, M.H. (1979a), Influence of the Social Environment on Psychopathology: The Historical Perspective, in Barrett, J.E. et al (eds) Stress and Mental Disorder, Raven Press, New York, 1979, pp. 161-177

Brenner, M.H. (1979b), Mortality and the National Economy: A Review, and the Experience of England and Wales, 1936-76, in The Lancet, September 15 1979, pp. 568-573

Durkheim, E. (1897), Suicide. Translated by J. Spaulding and G. Simpson, 1897. Reprinted Glencoe, Ill,. Free Press, 1951

Gravelle, H.S.E., Hutchinson, G., Stern, J. (1981), Mortality and Unemployment: A Critique of Brenner's Time Series Analysis, in The Lancet, September 26, 1981, pp. 675-679

Hamermesh, D.M., Soss, N.M. (1974), An Economic Theory of Suicide, in Journal of Political Economy 82 (1974), pp. 83-98

Illsley, R., Mullen, K. (1982), Poverty and Health in N.W. Europe, unpublished paper presented at the WHO Consultation on Poverty, Unemployment, and Health, Aberdeen, 22-26 November 1982

John, J. (1983), Economic Instability and Mortality in the Federal Republic of Germany: Problems and Macroanalytical Approach with Special Reference to Migration, in John, J., Schwefel, D, Zollner, H (eds) Influence of Economic Instability on Health, Springer, Berlin, Heidelberg, New York, Tokyo, pp. 113-138

Kasl, S.V. (1979), Mortality and the Business Cycle: Some Questions about Research Strategies when Utilizing Macro-Social and Ecological Data, in American Journal of Public Health 69, 8 (1979), pp. 784-790

Marshall, J.R., Hodge, R.W. (1981), Durkheim and Pierce on Suicide and Economic Change, in Social Science Research 10 (1981), pp. 101-114

Vigderhous, G., Fishman, G. (1978), The Impact of Unemployment and Familial Integration on Changing Suicide Rates in the USA, 1920-1969, in Social Psychiatry 13, 4 (1978), pp. 239-248

WHY THE ECONOMY PREDICTS HELP SEEKING: A TEST OF COMPETING EXPLANATIONS*

David Dooley and Ralph Catalano

Introduction

The hypothesis that economic instability increases the incidence of behavioral disorder is not new in sociology (Durkheim, 1897). Recent research claims to have supported this hypothesis by discovering time-series correlations between economic indicators and the use of mental health facilities (Barling and Handal, 1980; Brenner, 1973, 1976; Catalano and Dooley, 1979; Catalano et al, 1981; Frank, 1981; Marshall and Funch, 1979; Sclar and Hoffman, 1978). The most common inference from these correlations is that economic instability causes behavioral disorder from previously healthy persons (Albee, 1982). Implicit in this inference is the assumption that a proportion of the newly disordered person seeks professional help, thereby creating a time-series correlation between economic changes and subsequent use of services. The different mechanisms hypothetically linking economic change to help seeking via psychological symptoms are collectively referred to as the "provocation" explanation because they assume the economy provokes new disorder (Catalano and Dooley, 1977).

While the provocation explanation is plausible, there are equally plausible rival interpretations of the time-series correlations. These rival explanations, which also have roots in sociology, assume that economic indicators may be correlated with aggregate use of mental health facilities because the economy affects decisions to seek help whether or not a person is newly disordered.

Empirically pitting the provocation explanations against each other and their rivals could not only further sociological theory but also yield useful knowledge for those who provide mental health services or who desire to influence economic policy (Redburn and Buss, 1982). An attempt to determine which explanation best fits data describing the experiences of 4 144 residents of Los Angeles County is described in this paper.

Provocation Mechanisms

The central tenet of the provocation explanation is that economic instability somehow causes disorder in previously healthy people and that this disorder increases their likelihood of seeking help. Four plausible connections between the economy and disorder are suggested by the literature. The first connection is through the experience of undesirable job and financial events. This explanation draws heavily from the stressful life events research that typically reports that undesirable life experiences are risk factors for psychological and physiological disorder (Dohrenwend and Dohrenwend, 1974). This possible connection is supported by findings that the aggregate incidence of stressful life events is correlated with economic indicators (Catalano and Dooley, 1977) and that job and financial events have been associated with psychological disorder in individuals (Pearlin et al, 1981). Such a connection could not, however, account for the typically strong associations reported by the time-series research. One reason is that stressful life events have seldom been found to be strong predictors of subsequent disorder. A second is that job loss, which is one of the most stressful job and financial events, has not been found to be strongly related to the use of mental health facilities (Cobb and Kasl, 1977). These facts make it necessary to consider additional provocation mechanisms.

A second form of provocation is the possibility that economic contraction leads directly to disorder through the anticipation of undesirable job or financial events. The assumption is that the cognitive process of anticipating an undesirable event can be as stressful as the experience of the event.

A third provocation mechanism is that economic expansion may "potentiate", or interact with, undesirable job and financial events through a cognitive process. Experiencing such an event in an expanding economy may lead to disorder by implying that the individual rather than the environment is at fault (Cohn, 1978). The individual makes a negative assessment of his or her competence or adequacy and becomes depressed and symptomatic.

A fourth possible provocation mechanism is rooted in Durkheim's (1897) theory of _anomie_. This possible connection assumes that economic change _per se_ creates disorder by disrupting the perceived constancy of the physical and social environment (Pierce, 1967; Stokols, 1975). Individuals who perceive unpredictable change in their environments are assumed to be at risk of becoming uncertain as to how to respond to stimuli. This uncertainty and attendant risk of atypical behavior is assumed to increase anxiety and symptoms and, in turn, the likelihood of seeking help. Like the anticipation explanation explained above, the _anomie_ mechanism does not require that individuals experience undesirable job or financial events. The _anomie_ explanation has received support from research reporting a time-series correlation between economic change _per se_ and suicide rates (Pierce, 1967), but attempts to replicate the findings have not been successful (Marshall and Hodge, 1981).

Rivals to the Provocation Explanation

There are at least four rivals to the provocation explanation of the time-series association between economic indicators and aggregate use of mental health facilities. Unlike the provocation mechanism, these rival explanations assume that economic instability can lead to help seeking without causing disorder in previously healthy people. The first rival to provocation is based on a synthesis of elements drawn from labeling theory in sociology and from ecological psychology. Reduced audience tolerance for atypical behavior is assumed to lead to use of mental health facilities whether or not that behavior is new or has been previously treated (Scheff, 1966; Sarbin, 1969). Drawing from ecological psychology it is further assumed that overstaffed organizations are less tolerant of atypical behavior than those that are optimally or understaffed (Barker and Shoggen, 1973; Wicker, 1979). The assumptions are combined to yield the proposition that economic contraction decreases the tolerance for existing disorder by creating overstaffed labor markets. Employers are freer to discharge or not hire persons who are chronically or marginally disordered. This discrimination requires labeling individuals as "ill" and increases their chances of seeking help. This explanation is referred to as the "uncovering" position because it assumes that economic instability leads to the labeling or uncovering of existing, rather than the creation of new, atypical behavior.

A second rival to the provocation position is the possibility that economic contraction leads to anticipation of disorder and, in turn, to the prophylactic use of mental health facilities. This explanation differs from the anticipation form of the provocation position because neither disorder nor stressful experiences intercede between the economic change and the use of facilities. Help is sought when the economy contracts because people want to preclude the onset of symptoms or to cope better with anticipated undesirable job or financial events.

A third rival to provocation assumes, like the mechanism described immediately above, that prophylactic use of facilities can account for the time-series association between economic contraction and facility use. Unlike the simple prophylactic explanation, this mechanism assumes that prophylaxis is initiated by the experience of undesirable job or financial events. Help is sought when the economy contracts because people want to preclude the disorder intuitively associated with experienced undesirable life events. This rival to provocation implies that help seeking will be associated with undesirable job and financial events when variance both variables share with disorder is controlled.

A fourth rival to the provocation hypothesis assumes that _anomie_ can lead to help seeking without the intervening variable of disorder. Economic contraction or expansion supposedly reduces the predictability of the social and physical environment and can lead individuals to anticipate difficulties in coping. This anticipation is assumed to motivate individuals to seek help. Unlike the prophylactic explanations described above, this explanation implies that economic change _per se_ rather than economic contraction will, controlling for disorder, predict help seeking.

Previous Attempts to Resolve the Issue

Only two previous attempts have been made to pit the provocation explanation against its rivals. One test used data from a metropolitan area (Kansas City, Missouri, Catalano and Dooley, 1979) while another was based on the experience of a nonmetropolitan community (Washington County, Maryland, Catalano et al, 1981). Both tests used archival, time-series data to measure economic performance and the use of mental health facilities. Longitudinal survey data, originally collected for other purposes, were used to measure disorder (Langner-22 scores) in the population. The time series yielded by the survey data were short (just 16 months in Kansas City) making the results suggestive at best.

Findings from both tests supported the rivals to the provocation position. While the economy was associated with the use of facilities (in both communities) and with disorder (in Kansas City), the latter two variables were not associated with each other. The association between the economy and use of facilities, moreover, was not reduced significantly when the variance both shared with disorder was removed.

The Kansas City and Washington County tests are less than definitive for several reasons. The first is that the data allow only aggregate, time-series analysis making the findings subject to several inferential problems including the ecological fallacy. A second reason is that the short time series raised questions regarding the stability of the discovered associations. A third problem is that the lack of individual level data describing help seeking precluded discrimination among different versions of the provocation and rival explanations. It is not possible to determine if individually experienced events interacted with the aggregate economic conditions (the potentiation variant of provocation) or if those who used mental health facilities during periods of economic instability had chronic high symptom levels (i.e. were uncovered) or had no symptoms (i.e. used the facilities for "prophylaxis"). Finally, the use of archival treatment records excluded help seeking from informal and nonspecialist sources and threatened contamination of the treatment variable by the supply of services.

HYPOTHESES

Discriminating among the various forms of the provocation explanation and its rivals requires testing the ten hypotheses listed below. Each explanation implies that a unique set of these hypotheses will be supported. According to the first provocation explanation, economic contraction leads to the experience of undesirable job and financial events (hypothesis 1) that, in turn, leads to disorder (hypothesis 2) which leads to help seeking (hypothesis 6). The second provocation explanation holds that economic contraction causes disorder by increasing the anticipation of undesirable job and financial events (hypothesis 4) and that disorder, in turn, causes help seeking (hypothesis 6). The third provocation mechanism assumes that the interaction of undesirable events and economic expansion elicits disorder (hypothesis 3) that then leads to help seeking (hypothesis 6). The fourth or *anomie* form of the provocation explanation assumes that economic change *per se* causes increased symptoms (hypothesis 5) that lead to help seeking (hypothesis 6). The four rivals to the provocation explanations all omit the link between disorder and help seeking. The uncovering explanation expects symptomatic persons to seek help during contraction (hypothesis 9). The prophylaxis explanation assumes that, regardless of symptoms, people will be more likely to seek help during economic contraction (hypothesis 8). The third rival to the provocation explanation links the economy to events (hypothesis 2) and then directly to help seeking (hypothesis 7). The *anomie* rival to the provocation explanation expects change *per se* to predict help seeking (hypothesis 10). These ten hypotheses are as follows:

1. Individuals interviewed during periods of economic contraction will be more likely to experience undesirable job and financial events than individuals interviewed during periods of economic stability.

2. Individuals who experience undesirable job and financial events, will be more likely to report high symptom levels than individuals who do not.

3. Individuals who experience undesirable job and financial events during periods of economic expansion will be more likely to exhibit high symptom levels than individuals who experience such events in periods of contraction.

4. Individuals interviewed during periods of economic contraction, controlling for undesirable job and financial events, will be more likely to have high symptom levels than individuals interviewed during periods of stability.

5. Individuals interviewed in periods of economic change *per se*, controlling for undesirable life events, will be more likely to have high symptom levels than individuals interviewed in periods of economic stability.

6. Individuals who have high symptom levels will be more likely to seek help than individuals with low symptom levels.

7. Individuals who have had recent undesirable job and financial event, controlling for symptoms, will be more likely to seek help than those who have not experienced such events.

8. Individuals interviewed during periods of economic contraction, controlling for events and symptoms, will be more likely to seek help than individuals interviewed during periods of stability.

9. Individuals with high symptom levels during times of economic contraction, controlling for undesirable job and financial events, will be more likely to seek help than individuals with high symptom levels in periods of relative economic expansion.

10. Individuals interviewed during periods of economic change per se, controlling for symptom levels, will be more likely to seek help than individuals interviewed in times of economic stability.

These ten hypotheses are summarized as a causal model in Figure 1. It is possible that more than one of the mechanisms is at work. The above sets of hypotheses can, therefore, be combined to form the logical conditions necessary for more than one of the mechanisms to be supported. It is also possible that none of the mechanisms will be supported thereby raising the possibility that the aggregate, time-series findings are spurious or that altogether different causal processes are at work.

Figure 1

Causal Model Summarizing 10 Hypotheses Linking Economic Contraction or Instability to Undesirable Economic Events, Symptoms, and Helpseeking

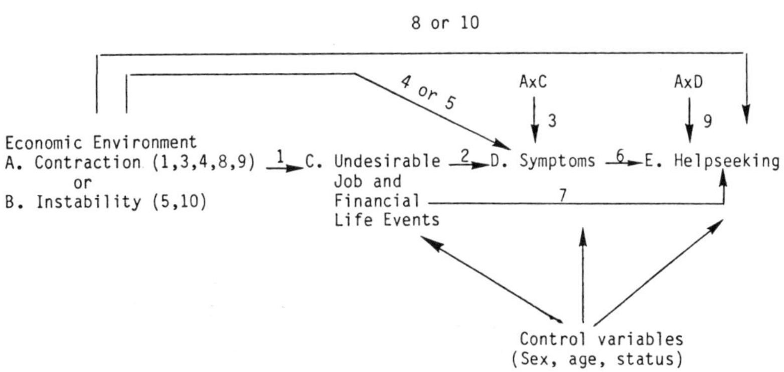

(Note: Numbers on causal paths correspond to hypotheses in text)

METHODS

The data analyzed below were collected through 12 quarterly telephone surveys, conducted from 1978 through 1980, of 500 randomly selected households (new households drawn each survey) in the Los Angeles-Long Beach SMSA (coterminous with Los Angeles County). Interviews were conducted in both English and Spanish. Completion rates (i.e. completions/completions + refusals + terminations) averaged 76 percent for the 12 survey waves. Variation in completion rates from wave to wave was not statistically significant. Compared to the 1980 census, the sample was biased towards females (57% in sample vs. 52% in census) and Anglos (67% in sample vs. 58% in census).

Sample and Control Variables

The following analyses control for four respondent characteristics: sex, age, socio-economic status (SES), and ethnicity. Because the analytic method is based on a multi-way contingency table and because of the number of other factors of interest, it was decided to control ethnicity by limiting these analyses to the largest group (Anglos) rather than creating another multi-level dimension that would have included small samples in several categories. A total of 4,144 Anglos gave responses for the variables of interest. Sex, age and SES were controlled by including them as variables in the analysis. Sex was a naturally dichotomous variable, and age was divided arbitrarily into approximate quartiles: 18-28, 29-39, 40-55, and 56+.

SES was calculated from respondent's education and the occupation of the principal wage earner in the household (using Hollingshead's weights, 1975). Because of incomplete responses or refusals to answer the occupation item, status could not be calculated for 19% of the respondents. In these cases, status was estimated using regression formulae (based on education and several other variables) derived from the respondents with complete information. The continuous SES variable was trichotomized[1]. All three control variables (i.e. age, sex and SES) were included in all analyses before testing the hypothesized relationships.

Intervening and Dependent Variables

The symptom and life event items were adapted for telephone use from existing scales designed for paper-and-pencil or face-to-face administration. The results of the telephone interviews may differ from face-to-face interviews using the same scales. Recent research, however, suggests that telephone survey results would be similar to face-to-face results (Klecka and Tuchfarber, 1978; Rogers, 1976). No differences, for example, were found between scores on a symptom scale, similar to that used in this study when administered by telephone and in person (Aneshensel et al, 1982). Even if telephone interviewing yields more optimistic or socially desirable answers on sensitive questions (Jordan et al, 1980; Groves and Kahn, 1979), this bias should not affect the analysis of interwave variability.

The help-seeking variable was derived from an item asking whether or not the respondent had sought help for an emotional problem in the past three months. Of the total sample, 13.8% reported an emotional problem for which they considered seeking help. Most of these (75.3%) actually sought help. Of those who specified a type of help sought, most sought it from informal sources (friends or family, 61.4%) rather than psychotherapists, doctors, or self-help groups (38.6%). The psychological symptom measure consisted of the sum of 25 items adapted from the PERI Demoralization Scales (Dohrenwend et al, 1981). Each item asked whether the respondent never, sometimes, or often had the symptom in the past three months. Over 12 samples, this 25-item scale achieved an average *alpha* reliability of .90. Given the dichotomous nature of the principal dependent variable and the analytic approach to be used, it was necessary to categorize all variables. The symptoms variable was dichotomized at the median over the entire sample.

The central conceptual difference between the provocation explanation and its rivals is the presence or absence of disorder. The validity of this analysis rests, therefore, on the measurement of disorder. It should be noted that there has not been convergence among psychiatric epidemiologists as to which of the several self-report symptom inventories is the best estimator of true disorder (Dohrenwend and Dohrenwend, 1982). The PERI inventory (a modified version of which was used in this analysis) was considered state-of-the-art when the surveys began in 1978. The problem of measuring disorder through survey methods implies, however, that this, and similar research be carefully interpreted.

The life event inventory included items drawn from the PERI Life Event Scale (Dohrenwend et al, 1978), the Holmes and Rahe Scale (1967) and the Theorell "workload" scale (Theorell and Floderus-Myrhed, 1977) as well as original items devised for this study to provide adequate sampling of job and financial events. The count of life events was used in this analysis rather than the sum of adaptation weights following recent research (e.g. Lei and Skinner, 1980; Ross and Mirowsky, 1979). Of the 30 undesirable events, 15 were considered job or financial events[2]. An event recall period of three months was used following findings that more recent events have more impact (Brown and Harris, 1978; Horowitz et al, 1977; Rahe, 1974) and are recalled more accurately (Uhlenhuth et al, 1977). Because undesirable job and financial events were relatively rare in this sample (55% had none), the life event variable was scored dichotomously as "none" and "one or more" categories.

Economic Independent Variables

Two economic variables were chosen to measure conceptually different types of change. The first type of change, expansion or contraction of employment opportunities, was measured by the unemployment rate. The rate is the proportion, determined by survey, of the population that wants but does not have a job (U.S. Bureau of the Census, 1978).

A second dimension of economic change, change *per se*, was measured by absolute change in the size and structure of the metropolitan workforce. The variable, the formula for which appears in Catalano and Dooley (1977), sums the absolute monthly differences across an 89-sector classification of the metropolitan area's workforce (U.S. Office of Management and Budget, 1972).

The mean of each of these variables was computed for 12 three-month periods corresponding to the 12 survey waves (Unemployment Rate: Minimum = 5.2, Maximum = 7.7, Mean = 6.3; Absolute change: Minimum = 348.7, Maximum = 657, Mean = 490.1). The three-month periods included the month of the survey and the two preceding months. This lag period was chosen based on the research noted above indicating that stressful events have their effect within a few months, and based on aggregate research showing a 2 or 3 month lag between economic change and symptoms (Catalano and Dooley, 1977) and psychiatric admissions (Catalano, Dooley, and Jackson, 1983). Each of the resulting series of 12 values was then divided into a categorical measure with low, medium, and high levels.

Analytic Approach

The hypotheses to be tested imply a multivariate analysis that would measure the main and interaction effects of the economy on events, symptoms or help seeking, while controlling for demographic or socio-economic characteristics. Although the symptom and life event measures were devised to yield continuous scores, their frequency distributions, in fact, were highly skewed. Given the dichotomous nature of the principal dependent variable (Hanushek and Jackson, 1977), the interpretative appropriateness of dichotomizing the other dependent variables (e.g. high/low symptoms), and the large sample size, logit analysis was chosen (Fienberg, 1978). Logit analysis is interpretatively similar to widely used techniques such as multiple regression (Swafford, 1980), and it has been used for analyzing surveys (Goodman, 1978), short time trend models (Clogg, 1979), and cross-level models such as the one tested here (Catalano and Dooley, 1983). While other techniques such as logistic regression were considered, the log linear approach was used here in part because it can better detect curvilinear relationships that could not be ruled-out by *a priori* considerations.

The logit coefficients discussed below were derived from log-linear co-efficients (see Dixon and Brown, 1979) that were converted to their multi-plicative "effect-on-odds" form as described by Swafford (1980). In this antilog form the coefficients describe the nature of the relationships in the original metric rather than the logarithmic form.

Models of association are tested in the following analyses for two purposes. The first is to discover parsimonious models that produce expected cell frequencies that fit (are not significantly different from) the observed frequencies (as indicated by low X^2 values and high probability values that expected vs. observed differences could have occurred by chance). The second is to test the hypotheses listed above by gauging the improvement in fit contributed by adding the hypothesized association to a model including the control variables. The statistical significance of the improvement contributed by a term representing a relationship (e.g. "UL" representing the association of unemployment or "U" and life events or "L") is judged by contrasting two models that differ only by the term in question. The difference between the X^2 of the fit of the two models is distributed as X^2 with degrees of freedom equal to the difference in the degrees of freedom of the two models.

Although the X^2 test may indicate that a term's contribution is reliably greater than zero (as with a small *p* value for the *F*-test in regression), it does not indicate the magnitude of the effect. The extent of the improvement in fit contributed by the term (analogous to change in R^2 in regression) can be gauged by the coefficient of partial determination (or CPD) for degrees of freedom (see Goodman, 1978, pp. 78-80). The overall explanatory power of all the terms added to the baseline model (consisting only of control terms) can similarly be gauged (analogous to R^2) by the coefficient of multiple partial determination (or CMPD).

A potential problem with the log-linear method is that the collapsing of continuous variables into few levels (below 5) can lead to false rejection of the null hypothesis of conditional independence (Reynolds, 1978). This risk can be ruled out if the variables in their continuous forms are independent of at least one of the variables in the studied association. Pearson correlations among the continuous versions of this study's variables revealed such independence.

RESULTS

Tests of the Hypotheses

Hypothesis 1, that economic contraction increases the risk of undesirable job and financial events, is tested in a 5-way cross tabulation of unemployment rate, sex, age, status, and undesirable job and financial events. Support was found for this relationship, but only for middle-status respondents ($p > .10$, CPD = .10). Table 1 summarises the pertinent log-linear models derived from this cross tabulation. There is a large and significant main effect of age (CPD = .65) and significant but smaller interactions of unemployment and sex

(CPD = .08) and of status and sex (CPD = .23). The model containing these terms fits the observations well (CMPD = .76). The coefficients from this model are shown in Table 2. The unemployment-by-sex interaction is curvilinear with males having more events in low and high unemployment quarters but with women having more in middle unemployment quarters. The significance of the interaction term appears to be due primarily to the sex differences in quarters of medium unemployment when women have higher, and men lower, risks of experiencing an undesirable job or financial event. The unemployment-by-status interaction that middle SES respondents' events rise linearly with unemployment while low and high SES respondents' fall linearly[2]. This interaction, however, should be interpreted carefully given that the only log-linear coefficient to exceed twice its standard error was that for middle SES respondents in quarters of high unemployment. In sum, Hypothesis 1 is supported only for middle-SES respondents. While other interactions were found, they are counterintuitive and difficult to interpret.

TABLE 1

Models of Log Odds of Experiencing One or More Undesirable Job or Financial Life Events (L) as a Function of Age (A), Sex (X), Status (S), and the Unemployment Rate (U).

	Model	df	LRx^2	p
1.	L	71	245.71	.00
2.	AL***[1]	68	81.61	.12
3.	AL, XL	67	81.60	.11
4.	AL, SL	66	77.63	.16
5.	AL, UL	66	80.48	.11
6.	AL, SXL, UXL	59	53.53	.68
7.	AL, SXL, USL	57	51.16	.69
8.	AL, UXL, USL	57	60.92	.34
9.	AL, SXL***[8], UXL***[7], USL*[6]	55	45.17	.82

NOTE: The term "AXSU" is included in each model, and .5 is added to each cell. The significance level is determined by contrast between the model with all of the same terms except the one tested (the latter is indicated by the model number in the superscript with asterisks).

*p<.10
**p<.05
***p<.001

TABLE 2

Multiplicative Dummy Logit Coefficients for Undesirable Job or Financial Events: Model 9 in Table 1 (XASU, AL, SXL, UXL, USL)

Term		Coefficients		
Age: 18 to 28		1.00		
29 to 39		.90		
49 to 55		.53		
56+		.26		
Unemployment Rate by Status			Status	
		Low	Medium	High
Unemployment Rate:	Low	1.39	1.00	1.28
	Medium	1.21	1.10	1.26
	High	1.06	1.52	1.04
Unemployment Rate by Sex (includes unemployment main effect)		Sex		
		Male	Female	
Unemployment Rate:	Low	1.00	1.00	
	Medium	.79	1.12	
	High	.93	.86	
Status by Sex (includes status main effect)				
Status:	Low	1.00	1.00	
	Medium	.94	.74	
	High	.62	1.02	
Constant by Sex (includes sex main effect)		.46	.34	

NOTE: To estimate the odds of having one or more events, multiply together five coefficients, one from the appropriate level of each term: age, unemployment by status, and (within the the correct sex) unemployment, status, and the constant.

Hypotheses 2 through 4, in which symptoms are the dependent variables, are tested in a cross tabulation of the unemployment rate, sex, age, SES, events, and symptoms. Symptoms were related to events (hypothesis 2) but not to the unemployment rate (hypothesis 4) or to the interaction of events and the unemployment rate (hypothesis 3). Table 3 summarizes the loglinear models derived from the cross tabulation. All three control variables are significantly associated with symptoms: (age, CPD = .12; status, CPD = .23; sex, CPD - .59). Hypothesis 2, that undesirable job and financial events affect symptoms, is supported by the substantial association of events and symptoms (CPD - .51). The model including these four main effects fits the observations well (CMPD = .69). Table 4 shows the coefficients for this model. The experience of one or more events increases the odds of higher than median symptoms by 148%. Hypothesis 3, that undesirable job and financial events interact with economic expansion to increase symptoms, was not supported. The contribution of the interaction of unemployment and events (the ULP term in model 8) to the model with unemployment (model 7) is insignificant (X^2 M7-M8 = 1.20, df = 2). Hypothesis 4, that economic decline affects symptoms controlling for events, is likewise not supported. The contribution of the unemployment rate (the UP term in model 7 of Table 3) to the most parsimonious model (model 6 in Table 3) is insignificant (X^2 M6-M7 = 3.21, df = 2).

TABLE 3

Models of Log Odds of Symptoms (P) as a Function of Age (A), Sex (X), Status (S), Unemployment Rate (U) and Undesirable Job or Financial Events (L)

	Model	df	LRx^2	p
1.	P	143	393.57	.00
2.	LP, XP, SP	139	137.05	.53
3.	LP, XP, AP	138	155.13	.15
4.	LP, SP, AP	137	199.66	.00
5.	XP, SP, AP	137	240.90	.00
6.	XP^{*4}, SP^{*3}, AP^{*2}, LP^{*5}	136	117.66	.87
7.	XP, SP, AP, LP, UP	134	114.45	.89
8.	XP, SP, AP, ULP	132	113.25	.88

NOTE: The term "AXSUL" is included in each model, and .5 is added to each cell. The significance level is determined by contrast between the model with the term and the model indicated by the superscript beside the asterisk.

* $p<.001$

TABLE 4

Multiplicative Dummy Logit Coefficients for Symptoms: Model 6 in Table 3
(AXSUL, XP, SP, AP, LP)

Term		Coefficients
Age:	18 to 28	1.00
	29 to 39	1.00
	40 to 50	.74
	56+	.76
Sex:	Male	1.00
	Female	1.79
Status:	Low	1.00
	Medium	.80
	High	.61
Events:	0	1.00
	1+	2.48
Constant		.81

NOTE: To estimate the odds of higher than median symptoms, multiply together five coefficients: one selected from each category (age, sex, status, and event, plus the constant).

Hypotheses 6 through 9, in which help seeking is the dependent variable, are tested with the previous 6-way table to which the help seeking has been added. Help seeking was associated with both symptoms (hypothesis 6) and events (hypothesis 7), but not to unemployment (hypothesis 8) nor the interaction of unemployment with symptoms (hypothesis 9). Table 5 summarizes the pertinent log-linear models derived from the cross tabulation. Each control variable is associated significantly with help seeking (age, CPD = .33; sex, CPD = .04; status, CPD = .04). Hypothesis 6, that symptoms affect help seeking, is supported by the significant association of symptoms with help seeking (CPD = .34). Hypothesis 7, that events affect help seeking regardless of symptoms, is supported by the significant association of events with help seeking (CPD = .26). Together these 5 significant main effects constitute a model that fits the observed data and is parsimonious (model 7 in Table 5, CMPD = .65). Events and symptoms are each positively associated with help seeking controlling for the other. The experience of one or more events raised the odds of help seeking by 133%, and having greater than median symptoms raises the odds of help seeking by 159% (see the first column of Table 6 for the coefficient).

Hypothesis 8, that economic contraction affects help seeking regardless of either symptoms or events, is not supported. The unemployment rate-help seeking term (UH in model 8 in Table 5) does not add significantly to the best fitting model (X^2 M7-M8 = 3.28, df = 2). Hypothesis 9, that symptoms interact with economic contraction to affect help seeking, is not supported. The interaction term involving unemployment, symptoms, and help seeking does not add significantly to the fit of the model with unemployment and help seeking (X^2 M8-M9 = 1.95, df = 2).

TABLE 5

Models of Log Odds of Help Seeking (H) as a Function of Age (A), Sex (X), Status (S), Unemployment Rate (U), Undesirable Job & Financial Events (L) and Symptoms (P)

	Model	df	LRX^2	p
1.	H	287	568.42	.00
2.	PH, LH, SH, XH	282	290.88	.34
3.	PH, LH, AH, SH	280	202.24	1.00
4.	PH, LH, AH, XH	281	202.16	1.00
5.	PH, AH, XH, SH	280	262.51	.77
6.	AH, XH, SH, LH	280	291.16	.31
7.	AH**2, XH**3, SH*4, LH**5, PH**6	279	192.50	1.00
8.	AH, XH, SH, LH, PH, UH	277	189.22	1.00
9.	AH, XH, SH, LH, UPH	275	187.27	1.00

NOTE: The term "AXSULP" is included in each model, and .5 is added to each cell. The significance level is determined by contrast with the model indicated by the superscript beside the asterisks. Probability levels of 1.00 are due to rounding.

*p <.01
**p <.001

TABLE 6

Multiplicative Dummy Logit Coefficients for Help Seeking Based on Models with Either the Unemployment Rate of Absolute Economic Change

Term		Model with Unemployment (AXSULP, AH, XH, SH, LH, PH: 7 in Table 6)	Model with Absolute Change (AXSBLP, AH, XH, SH, LH, PH, BH: 8 in Table 7
Constant		.07	.10
Age:	18 to 28	1.00	1.00
	29 to 39	.95	.94
	40 to 55	.54	.54
	56+	.30	.29
Sex:	Male	1.00	1.00
	Female	1.34	1.34
Status:	Low	1.00	1.00
	Medium	1.27	1.28
	High	1.46	1.46
Events:	0	1.00	1.00
	1+	2.33	2.33
Syptoms:	Low	1.00	1.00
	High	2.59	2.61
Absolute Change:	Low	-	1.00
	Medium	-	.64
	High	-	.86

NOTE: To estimate the odds of seeking help, multiply together the coefficients one for the appropriate level of each significant category.

Hypotheses 5 and 10, which are implied by the anomie explanation, are tested with contingency tables that substitute a measure of economic change *per se* or absolute change for the unemployment rate. Absolute change was associated with help seeking (hypothesis 10) but not with symptoms (hypothesis 5). Although no link between absolute change and undesirable job and financial life events was hypothesized, this association is tested in a contingency table that also included the control variables of sex, age, and SES. As with unemployment (see Table 1), life events are associated with age and a combination of sex and SES. In contrast to the unemployment rate, absolute change is unrelated to events in combination with SES or sex. Hypothesis 5, that economic change *per se* affects symptoms regardless of events, is tested in a contingency table including absolute change, sex, age, SES, events, and symptoms. The main effects of age, sex, SES, and life events are all highly significant. Hypothesis 5, however, is not supported. The interaction of absolute change and symptoms does not significantly add to the model with the four significant main effects ($X2 = .81$, df = 2).

Hypothesis 10, that economic change per se leads to help seeking regardless of symptoms, is tested in a 7-way contingency table that includes the same factors as Table 5 except that absolute change is substituted for the unemployment rate. The pertinent log-linear models from this cross tabulation are summarized in Table 7. The results are similar to those in Table 5 in that there are main effects of the control variables of age, sex, and SES and the previously noted effects of life events (hypothesis 7) and symptoms (hypothesis 6). Support for hypothesis 10 is found in that absolute change is linked directly to help seeking controlling for all the previously mentioned main effects. The contribution of absolute change is highly significant as seen in Table 7 (X^2 M2-M8 = 16.62, df = 2, $p<.001$), but it is modest in magnitude (CPD = .07). The model that includes all six significant main effects (model 8 in Table 7) fits the data well (CMPD = .65). The coefficients derived from this model are summarized in the second column of Table 6. Contrary to hypothesis 10, however, help seeking does not vary linearly with absolute change. Rather it peaks in the lowest change quarters, falls to a minimum in the medium change quarters, and rises to a secondary peak in the highest change quarters.

TABLE 7

Models of Log Odds of Help Seeking (H) as Function of Age (A), Sex (X), Absolute Economic Change (B), Undesirable Job & Financial Events (L) and Symptoms (P)

	Model	df	LRx^2	p
1.	H	287	596.95	.00
2.	PH, LH, AH, SH, XH	279	221.03	1.00
3.	PH, LH, AH, SH, BH	278	213.95	1.00
4.	PH, LH, AH, XH, BH	279	214.24	1.00
5.	PH, LH, SH, XH, BH	280	304.13	.15
6.	PH, AH, SH, XH, BH	278	273.85	.56
7.	LH, AH, SH, XH, BH	278	304.26	.13
8.	PH**7, LH**6, AH**5, SH*4, XH**3, BH**2	277	204.41	1.00
9.	LH, AH, SH, XH, BPH	275	201.29	1.00

NOTE: The term "AXSBLP" is included in each model, and .5 is included with each cell. The significance level is determined by contrast with the model indicated by the superscript beside the asterisks. Probability levels of 1.00 are due to rounding.

*p <.001
**p <.001

Tests for Spuriousness

Before discussing results, several threats to the inferences drawn above need to be addressed. The first is that trends or seasonal cycles may lead to systematic sampling error, such as undersampling of one of the socio-economic status groups during the summer surveys due to the vacations. Such time-dependent sampling error of sex, age, or SES is, however, automatically controlled by the inclusion of these variables in the initial interaction term in each logit model. A second risk is that trend or cycle remains or appears in a dependent variable such as help seeking after controlling for the demographic variables. This possibility was tested within contingency tables that include factors for year (surrogate for secular trend), quarter (surrogate for seasonal cycle), age, sex, SES, and the dependent variable of interest. No association was found between any dependent variable and either the trend or cycle variable.

Another potential source of confound is undesirable events other than job or financial experiences. While the life event literature usually portrays events as stochastic processes, there are reasons to expect a relationship of job and financial events with other events. There may be personality characteristics such a "event proneness", willingness to admit events, or ability to recall events, that could produce positive inter-event correlations. The relationships involving job and financial events (e.g. with symptoms) may be the result of the influence of noneconomic events and, therefore, spurious. If so, controlling for noneconomic events would eliminate the associations involving the economic events.

To test this possibility, a 7-way contingency table was composed of the following factors: undesirable noneconomic events[3] (excluding health events to avoid confounding with health-related psychological symptoms), undesirable job and financial events, symptoms, help seeking, and the control variables of age, sex, and SES. As expected, both types of undesirable events were positively related to each other and each was independently, significantly, and positively related to symptoms and to help seeking (even after controlling for the other). In fact, undesirable job and financial events were more strongly related than undesirable noneconomic events to symptoms ($CPD_{Ec} = .56$ vs. $CPD_{Nonec} = .22$) and to help seeking ($CPD_{Ec} = .26$ vs. $CPD_{Nonec} = .11$). The interaction effect of the two kinds of events is nonsignificant with both symptoms and help seeking.

Another possibility is that the effects of the unemployment rate-by-SES and unemployment rate-by-sex interactions on undesirable job and financial events would disappear if noneconomic events were controlled. The test of this possibility yielded negative results. The unemployment rate is not related to noneconomic events, and controlling for noneconomic events does not appreciably reduce the previously reported interactions.

Finally, it is possible that non-Anglo respondents react differently to economic change than do Anglos. Replications of these analyses on the entire sample show little difference in the relationships reported for Anglos. The unemployment rate-by-sex interaction with financial or job events falls below significance in the total sample, but the status-by-unemployment rate interaction, which has a p value of less than .1 in the Anglo sample yields a p value less than .05 in the total sample. The overall unemployment-to-help seeking association that is insignificant in the Anglo sample reaches significance in the total sample. As with the absolute change-with-help seeking relationship, in Anglos, the unemployment rate-with-help seeking relationship in the total sample is U-shaped with more help seeking in the lowest and highest quarters. In sum, there may be ethnicity effects in several of the relationships, but the overall results for Anglos appear to generalize to the total sample. (For analyses that treat ethnicity as a separate factor with levels for Anglos, Hispanics, and Blacks, see Dooley and Catalano, 1982.)

DISCUSSION

Summary and Interpretation

Support for hypotheses 1, 2, 6, 7, and 10 was found in the present analyses (see Figure 1 for a review of the hypotheses). This pattern of findings is consistent with the first provocation explanation and the third and fourth rivals. The first provocation explanation links the unemployment rate to undesirable job and financial events that are linked to symptoms that are, in turn, linked to help seeking. The third rival explanation links the unemployment rate to life events that are connected to help seeking independently of symptoms. The fourth rival or *anomie* explanation is that absolute economic change is associated directly with help seeking controlling for events and symptoms.

One contribution of this study is its conceptualization of numerous causal paths from the economy to treated disorder. As noted above, the eight explanations tested here are not mutually exclusive. In fact, three pathways were supported by the data. An integration of these suggests that economic contraction can lead to increased help seeking by increasing the incidence of symptoms and by increasing the prophylactic (asymptomatic) use of facilities. Economic change *per se* also appears to increase prophylactic help seeking but the relationship is not linear and therefore defies easy interpretation.

These findings support the general proposition that the social environment affects both disorder and help seeking in a systematic and, at least in the case of economic contraction, intuitive way. This support should encourage further theoretical and empirical work that attempts to clarify the mechanisms by which community dynamism affects individual well being. Such work would not only further our understanding of the etiology of disorder but also contribute to the debate over whether and how community change should be managed.

The applied implications of the findings are complex. The findings add support to the argument that cost-benefit analyses of alternative policy options should include the costs of providing mental health services (Dooley and Catalano, 1977). These arguments, however, often assert that the use of facilities is a surrogate measure for pain and suffering that should be included among the accounted costs over and above the cost of providing services (Liem and Rayman, 1982; Sclar, 1982). While this position is logically, and in the authors' opinions, morally sound, the above findings suggest that facility use is not always driven by new symptoms. The cost category of pain and suffering, therefore, should probably be accounted at a fraction of the facility-use category. The size of the fraction cannot yet be estimated. More importantly, the weight given the pain and suffering and facility use, *vis a vis* other cost categories is a political, not scientific issue (Catalano, 1982).

The fact that the relationships among the economy, symptoms, and help seeking can be systematically modeled suggests that both proactive and reactive prevention can be planned. This possibility has been discussed at length elsewhere (Catalano and Dooley, 1980) and need not be developed further here.

This research was intended to identify the intervening relationships that account for the widely assumed overarching positive relationship between undesirable economic conditions and admissions for treatment of psychological disorder. If this overarching relationship exists as inferred by those who cite aggregate time-series analyses (e.g. Brenner, 1973), relatively strong, linear, main effects would be expected in the data analyzed in this study (e.g. between unemployment and undesirable job and financial events). The nature of the associations found here do not, however, support these expectations.

The unemployment rate does not have a main effect on undesirable job and financial events. The relationship varies with sex and status and the variations in events explained by these interactions is relatively small (CPDs less than .10). In some groups, the association is intuitive, i.e. linear and positive as in the middle status group. In contrast, there are also unexpected linear but negative relationships of events and unemployment in the low and high SES groups (although the fact that the coefficient for the middle status, high unemployment group was responsible for the interaction suggests that the two negative relationships in the low and high status groups may be more apparent than real). Possibly the low status group is so economically distressed in the best of times that rising unemployment cannot increase the experience of undesirable economic events. Similarly, the affluence of the high status group may provide an immunity to rising unemployment. It should also be noted that these data were collected in a period of "normal" economic swings rather than during a time of recession. A recession might raise the likelihood that low and high SES persons will experience an undesirable job or financial event.

The other significant relationships that link undesirable job and financial events to help seeking both directly (hypothesis 7) and <u>via</u> symptoms (hypotheses 2 and 6) appear more sensible. They are positive and fairly strong. It must be noted, however, that these variables are measured by the same method at the same point in time. These associations may, therefore, include uncontrolled reverse or reciprocal causation (e.g. pre-existing symptoms may cause increased events) as well as spuriousness due to response or method bias (e.g. tendency to report or remember such things as events and symptoms). The fact, howeverm that controlling for noneconomic events did not reduce the effect of undesirable job and financial events on either symptoms or help seeking reduces the chances of spuriousness due to a response or method bias.

Finally, the association of absolute economic change to help seeking (hypothesis 10) is modest in size (CPD >.10) and curvilinear in shape. From the <u>anomie</u> hypothesis, we would expect a linear increase in help seeking as absolute change increases. Instead, help seeking reaches its maximum in the low change quarters, decreases in middle quarters and then rises to a secondary peak in the high change quarters. A <u>post hoc</u> explanation that involves two processes can be suggested. One is the intuitive effect in which there is slowly increasing level of help seeking from the low through the middle change quarters with a greater increase in the high change quarters. The offsetting process might involve a "catch up" phenomenon in which individuals with a pre-existing interest in psychological help take advantage of the tranquility of low economic change periods to seek help. As the economic activity increases to medium and high, individuals may postpone their help seeking and concentrate on the demands of the economic environment (including those due to desirable events not studied here such as promotions, new employment, etc.). The sum of these two processes could yield the U-shaped results obtained.

In summary, the individual level data analyzed in this study of over 4 000 subjects interviewed over three years suggest that economic contraction provokes increased events and, via events, symptoms and the use of mental health facilities in middle-SES Anglos. Undesirable job and financial events also cause help seeking without the intervening experience of disorder. Economic change *per se* may lead to prophylactic help seeking without the experience of undesirable events or symptoms. The nature of this last relationship is not, however, consistent with *a priori* models.

Relationship to Aggregate Time-Series Research

While these results point to several possible pathways that link the economy to help seeking, they do not match the models often inferred from the most widely disseminated time-series research. Two possibilities must be considered: (a) that the present work does not capture the phenomenon studied in aggregate time-series analysis, and (b) that the aggregate time-series analyses do not imply the strong, linear, positive main effects of unemployment on psychiatric help seeking that are usually inferred from such studies (e.g. Brenner, 1976).

With respect to the first issue, the present study measures processes not reflected in the aggregate time-series studies. Archival measures of psychiatric admissions used in aggregate research apparently do not covary with aggregate surveyed psychiatric symptoms (see Catalano and Dooley, 1980; Catalano et al, 1981) and rarely include comprehensive counts of psychiatric contacts (since they usually exclude private fee-for-service contacts). Archival admissions data cannot measure use of informal or nonspecialist sources of help as do the data in this test. Admissions series are, moreover, suspected of being influenced by supply as well as demand (Marshall and Funch, 1979). The dependent variables employed here (symptoms and help seeking), therefore, could well diverge from whatever is measured in archival admission records.

A second major difference of this research from most time-series studies is time lag. Instead of the usual unit of analysis of one year, the present study employs the quarter. We can offer no theoretical causal process to account for a lag of one or two years from unemployment rise to admission rise (as found by Brenner, 1973). Our work is based on psychological theories of stressful life events and crisis onset that suppose lags of weeks or months from environmental change to symptom rise and help seeking.

A third difference pertains to the independent variable of economic change. By using long, annual time series, analysts enjoy predictors of great reliability (due to the cancelling of random error in the aggregation) and of great variability (due to the inclusion of wide swings in the business cycle). Short trend survey studies such as the present one are less likely to capture extreme fluctuations. Further, quarterly averages of monthly unemployment estimates are subject to substantial sampling error inherent in the limited sample sizes of the Current Population Survey taken in any single SMSA (U.S. Bureau of the Census, 1978). With relatively greater error and smaller true variation, short monthly economic series could lead to attenuated associations compared to longer and more aggregated economic series.

In sum, the present study addresses a set of relationships different from those implicit in aggregate time-series work with respect both to the lag structure and the dependent variables under investigation. Moreover, differences in the independent variables might account for differences in the magnitudes of the measured relationships even if the dependent variables and lag structures were similar.

The other possible explanation for the differences between this study and the usual interpretation of aggregate time-series work is that the latter is mistaken. Reviews of the time-series literature report mixed results (Dooley and Catalano, 1980). Contradictory findings for the relationship of inpatient admissions to unemployment have been reported, both within studies (e.g. Brenner, 1973) and between studies (e.g. Brenner, 1973 vs. Sclar and Hoffman, 1978). Different subgroups reveal positive and negative associations of unemployment to admissions to mental hospitals. Moreover, inpatients and outpatients have been found to exhibit opposite patterns (Sclar and Hoffman, 1978). Other studies reveal few significant associations between the economy and admissions amidst numerous nonsignificant associations (Barling and Handal, 1980; Catalano et al, 1981). The perception that the aggregate time-series literature repeatedly finds a simple positive connection between unemployment and admissions of all kinds for all groups is incorrect. Assuming that the consistent statistical significance of those associations that do reach publication is not an artifact of failure to publish negative findings (i.e. the "file drawer" problem cited by Rosenthal, 1979), the associations present a rather confusing picture. It seems likely that the black box of aggregate time-series research contains the kind of complex relationships revealed in the present individual level study, including subgroup differences, inexplicable signs, and, possibly, curvilinear relationships.

FOOTNOTES

[1]Descriptively, the three SES levels were well differentiated. About half of the low SES group reported family income under $15,000 (48.7%) and less than high school education (44.6%), and none reported having administrative or professional occupations. In contrast, in the highest SES group, less than one-fifth reported making less than $15,000 (19.7%); just 1.4% reported less than high school education; 94% reported having administrative or professional occupations.

[2]The 15 undesirable job or financial life events used for this index are: mortgage foreclosed; car, furniture or other item repossessed; decrease in wages; financial loss; moved to a worse residence; go on welfare; difficulty paying bills; change to worse job; demoted at work; fired from job; laid off from work; unemployed more than 30 days; trouble with boss; trouble with fellow workers; and business loss or failure.

[3]The 15 items used to calculate the index of undesirable noneconomic nonhealth life events are: lost house through disaster; robbed; involved in law suit; arrested; went to jail; convicted of crime; marriage/engagement broken; separated; divorced; relations with spouse worsened; trouble with in-laws; spouse died; child died; other family member died; and close friend died.

* Reprinted from the Journal of Health and Social Behaviour 1984, vol. 25 (June), pp. 160-176

REFERENCES

Albee, G.W. 1982 — "Preventing Psychopathology and Promoting Human Potential", American Psychologist, 37:1043-50.

Aneshensel, C., Frerichs, R.R., Clark, V.A., and Yokopenic, P.A. 1982 — "Measuring Depression in the Community: A Comparison of Telephone and Personal Interviews", Public Opinion Quarterly, 46:110-21.

Barling, P., and Handal, P. 1980 — "Incidence of Utilization of Public Mental Health Facilities as a Function of Short Term Economic Decline", American Journal of Community Psychology, 8:31-9.

Barker, R.G., and Shoggen, P. 1973 — Qualities of Community Life, San Francisco: Jossey-Bass.

Brenner, M.H. 1973 — Mental Illness and the Economy, Cambridge: Harvard University Press.

1976 — "Estimating the Social Costs of Economic Policy: Implications for Mental and Physical Health, and Criminal Aggression", Paper No. 5, Report to the Congressional Research Service of the Library of Congress and Joint Economic Committee of Congress, Washington D.C.: U.S. Government Printing Office.

Brown, G.W., and Harris, T. 1978 — Social Origins of Depression: A Study of Psychiatric Disorder in Women, New York: The Free Press.

Catalano, R. 1982 — "Psychology Amid Economic Madness", Behaviorists for Social Action Journal, 3:4-7.

Catalano, R., and Dooley, D. 1977 — "Economic Predictors of Depressed Mood and Stressful Life Events", Journal of Health and Social Behavior, 18:292-307.

1979 — "Does Economic Change Provoke or Uncover Behavioral Disorder: A Preliminary Test", pp. 321-46 in Ferman, L., and Gordus, J. (eds.), Mental Health and the Economy, Kalamazoo, MI: Upjohn Foundation.

1980 — "Economic Change in Primary Prevention", pp. 21-40 in Price, R.H., Ketterer, R.F., Bader, B.C., and Monahan, J. (eds.), Prevention in Community Mental Health: Research, Policy and Practice, Beverly Hills: Sage.

1983 — "The Health Effects of Economy Instability: A Test of Economic Stress Hypothesis", Journal of Health and Social Behavior, 24:46-60.

Catalano, R., Dooley, D., and Jackson, R. 1981 — "Economic Predictors of Admissions to Mental Health Facilities in a Non-Metropolitan Community", Journal of Health and Social Behavior, 22:284-297.

1983 — "Selecting a Time-Series Strategy", Psychological Bulletin, 94:506-523.

Clogg, C.C. 1979 — Measuring Underemployment: Demographic Indicators for the United States, New York: Academic Press.

Cobb, S., and Kasl, S.V. 1977 — Termination: The Consequences of Job Loss, (Report No. 76-1261), Cincinnati, Ohio: National Institute for Occupational Safety and Health, Behavioral and Motivational Factors Research, June.

Cohn, R.M. 1978 — "The Effect of Employment Status Change on Self Attitudes", Social Psychology, 41:81-93.

Dixon, W.J., and Brown, M.B. (eds.) 1979 — BMDP Biomedical Computer Programs: P-Series, 1979, Berkeley: University of California Press.

Dohrenwend, B.P., and Dohrenwend, B.S. 1974 — Stressful Life Events: Their Nature and Effects, New York: Wiley.

1982 — "Perspectives on the Past and Future of Psychiatric Epidemiology: The 1981 Rema Lapouse Lecture", American Journal of Public Health, 72:1271-9.

Dohrenwend, B.P., Oskenberg, L., Shrout, P.E., Dohrenwend, B.S., and Cook, D. 1981 — "What Brief Psychiatric Screening Scales Measure", pp. 188-198 in Sudman, S. (ed.), Health Survey Research Methods: Third Biennial Conference, Washington D.C.: National Center for Health Services Research.

Dohrenwend, B.S., Krasnoff, L., Askenasy, A.R., and Dohrenwend, B.P. 1978 — "Exemplification of a Method for Scaling Life Events: The PERI Life Events Scale", Journal of Health and Social Behavior, 19:205-59.

Dooley, D., and Catalano, R. 1977 — "Money and Mental Disorder: Toward Behavioral Cost Accounting for Primary Prevention", American Journal of Community Psychology, 5:217-227.

1980 — "Economic Change as a Cause of Behavioral Disorder", Psychological Bulletin, 87:450-68.

1982 — "Economic Change and Primary Prevention: Ethnicity Effects", unpublished manuscript.

Durkheim, E. (1897) 1966 — Suicide (tr. Spaulding, J., and Simpson, G.), New York: Free Press.

Feinberg, S.E. 1978	The Analysis of Cross-Classified Categorical Data, Massachusetts: MIT Press.
Frank, J.A. 1981	"Economic Change and Mental Health in an Uncontaminated Setting", American Journal of Community Psychology, 9:395-410.
Goodman, L.A. 1978	"A General Model for the Analysis of Surveys", pp. 57-109 in Goodman, L.A., and Magidson, J. (eds.), Analyzing Qualitative/Categorical Data: Log-Linear Models and Latent-Structure Analysis, Cambridge, MA: Abt.
Groves, R.M., and Kahn, R.L. 1979	Surveys by Telephone: A National Comparison with Personal Interviews, New York: Academic Press.
Hanushek, E.A., and Jackson, J.E. 1977	Statistical Methods for Social Scientists, New York: Academic Press.
Hollingshead, A.B. 1975	"Four Factor Index of Social Status", unpublished mansucript (available from 1965 Yale Station, New Haven, CT 06520).
Holmes, T.H., and Rahe, R.E. 1967	"The Social Readjustment Rating Scale", Journal of Psychosomatic Research, 11:213-18.
Horowitz, M., Schaefer, C., Hiroto, D., Wilner, N., and Levin, B. 1977	"Life Event Questionnaire for Measuring Presumptive Stress", Psychosomatic Medicine, 39:413-31.
Jordan, L.A., Marcus, A.C., and Reeder, L.G. 1980	"Response Styles in Telephone and Household Interviewing: A Field Experiment", Public Opinion Quarterly, 44:210-22.
Klecka, W.R., and Tuchfarber, A.J. 1978	"Random Digit Dialling: A Comparison to Personal Surveys", Public Opinion, 42:105-14.
Lei, H., and Skinner, H.A. 1980	"A Psychometric Study of Life Events and Social Readjustment", Journal of Psychosomatic Research, 24:57-65.
Liem, R., and Rayman, P. 1982	"Health and Social Costs of Unemployment: Research and Policy Considerations", American Psychologist, 37:1116-1123.
Marshall, J.P., and Funch, D.P. 1979	"Mental Illness and the Economy: A Critique and Partial Replication", Journal of Health and Social Behavior, 20:282-89.

Marshall, J.R., and Hodge, R.W. 1981 — "Durkheim and Pierce on Suicide and Economic Change", Social Science Research, 10:101-14.

Pearlin, L.I., Lieberman, M.A., Menaghan, E.G., and Mullan, J.T. 1981 — "The Stress Process", Journal of Health and Social Behavior, 22:337-56.

Pierce, A. 1967 — "The Economic Cycle and the Social Suicide Rate", American Sociological Review, 32:457-62.

Rahe, R.H. 1974 — "The Pathway between Subjects Recent Life Changes and Their Near-Future Illness Reports: Representative Results and Methodological Issues", pp. 73-87 in Dohrenwend, B.S., and Dohrenwend, B.P. (eds.), Stressful Life Events: Their Nature and Effects, New York: Wiley.

Redburn, F.S., and Buss, T.F. (eds.) 1982 — Public Policies for Distressed Communities, Lexington, MA: D.C. Heath.

Reynolds, H.T. 1978 — "Some Comments on the Causal Analysis of Surveys with Log-Linear Models", American Journal of Sociology, 83:127-43.

Rogers, T.F. 1976 — "Interview by Telephone and In Person: Quality of Responses and Field Performance", Public Opinion Quarterly, 40:51-65.

Rosenthal, R. 1979 — "'The File Drawer Problem' and Tolerance for Null Results", Psychological Bulletin, 86:638-41.

Ross, C.E., and Mirowsky, J. 1979 — "A Comparison of Life Event-Weighting-Schemes: Changes, Undesirability, and Effect-Proportional Indices", Journal of Health and Social Behavior, 20:166-77.

Sarbin, T.R. 1969 — "Schizophrenic Thinking: A Role Theoretical Analysis", Journal of Personality, 37:190-206.

Scheff, T.J. 1966 — Being Mentally Ill: A Sociological Theory, Chicago: Aldine.

Sclar, E.D. 1982 — "Social-Cost Minimization: A National-Policy Approach to the Problems of Distressed Areas", pp. 15-25 in Redburn, F.S., and Buss, T.F. (eds.), Public Policies for Distressed Communities, Lexington, MA: Lexington Books.

Sclar, E.D., and Hoffman, V.J. 1978 — "Planning Mental Health Service for a Declining Economy", (Final Report to the National Health Services Research), Waltham, MA: Brandeis University, January.

Stokols, D. 1975 — "Toward a Psychological Theory of Alienation", Psychological Review, 82:26-44.

Swafford, M.
1980
"Three Parametric Techniques for Contingency Table Analysis: A Nontechnical Commentary", American Sociological Review, 45:664-90.

Theorell, T., and Floderus-Myrhed, B.
1977
"'Workload' and Risk of Myocardial Infarction: A Prospective Psychosocial Analysis", International Journal of Epidemiology, 6:17-21.

Troldahl, V.C., and Carter, R.E.
1964
"Random Selection of Respondents Within Households in Phone Surveys", Journal of Marketing Research, 1:71-6.

Uhlenhuth, E.H., Haberman, S.J., Balter, M.B., and Lipman, R.S.
1977
"Remembering Life Events", pp. 117-34 in Strauss, J.S., Babigian, H.M., and Roff, M. (eds.), The Origins and Course of Psychopathology, New York: Plenum Press.

U.S. Bureau of the Census
1978
The Current Population: Design and Methodology, Technical Paper No. 40, Stock No. 003-024-01490-4, Washington D.C.: U.S. Government Printing Office.

U.S. Office of Management and Budget
1972
Standard Industrial Classification Manual, Washington D.C.: U.S. Government Printing Office.

Veroff, J., Kulka, R.A., and Douvan, E.
1981
Mental Health in America: Patterns of Help-Seeking from 1957 to 1976, New York: Basic Books.

Wicker, A.W.
1979
An Introduction to Ecological Psychology, Belmont, CA: Wadsworth.

Part II

The health effects of unemployment: new studies

B: Cross-sectional studies of individuals and communities

EMPLOYMENT, UNEMPLOYMENT AND HEALTH IN FAMILIES IN LEIDEN (THE NETHERLANDS)

Ingeborg P Spruit

INTRODUCTION

In the Spring of 1982, a number of employed and unemployed persons living in the Leiden region were interviewed in detail with respect to their feelings about their life situation and their health. The main objective was to obtain units of analysis and variables required for a comparative study to detect differences in subjective health between the employed, the unemployed, and their families. Accordingly, the study had an exploratory character and the interviews were open. The themes to be explored were chosen on the basis of a review of the literature, but with two main conditions: that each interview could deal extensively with the importance for the respondents of factors related to being employed or unemployed (ie for their reaction to being unemployed or employed and the subjective evaluation of their situation), and that the respondents themselves be able to introduce factors of importance to them with respect to being employed or unemployed and to their own health. This was expected to yield a description of aspects considered important by the respondents and to lead to an evaluation of these items.

To this end, a small scale study was set up, with special attention to the individual respondent. The intention was to give precedence to the reflection of flesh and blood people rather than to relationships between abstract factors and characteristics of people who were categorised according to unclear standards. It was hoped that the results would depict something of the actual conditions under which unemployed people live, serving as an empirical point of departure for a quantitative follow-up study in 1983.

Families

A total of 35 families and four unemployed married women participated in the study. 56 interviews were held with them. The respondents included 11 unemployed men and the partners of nine of them, and 11 employed men and the partners of nine of them. They were or had been married and all of them had children (some no longer living with them). There were seven unemployed and six employed women who had been married (divorced or widowed) with children at home or living elsewhere. All of them were employed or seeking office work and were between 30 and 50 years of age. They had given active consent to the interview in response to a letter sent to them by the investigator via the Regional Labour Exchange Job Centre.

Since the study was concerned with families, no unmarried people were included in the sample of either the employed or the jobless. The 22 unemployed respondents accounted for 27% of the number of registered married or formerly married unemployed in this age and occupational category in the Leiden region.

The employed and unemployed individuals were matched for occupation and educational level.[a]

Themes

The interviews covered eight clusters of variables assumed to be relevant on the basis of the literature.[b] The main concern was to arrive at a description of the meaning of the cluster of unemployment factors (duration of the unemployment, how the last job was lost, the financial situation, reaction to unemployment, experience with social assistance, and expectations of the future).

In a comparative way, attention will be given to the employed with respect to the experience of the job (level of the work, nature of the work and the company, management quality and atmosphere among collagues, stability of the function and job security).

(a) Matching with employed individuals was based on the last occupation of the unemployed. The employed subjects were selected from the respondent population of the Dienst Sociaal Wetenschappelijk Onderzoek van de Universiteit (Social Science Research Service of the University of Leiden), after a short telephone survey in which the questions concerned age, marital status, and occupation.

The interviewed unemployed men were reasonably comparable with the indicated category as to marital status but were relatively younger and had been unemployed for a relatively slightly longer period. The interviewed unemployed women were reasonably comparable to the category in question as to age and duration of unemployment, but more of them had once been married. The group with a secondary school education is slightly underrepresented. Because so few unemployed married women were willing to participate in the study, no married employed women were included in the match group. For the women the age composition was the same for employed and unemployed, but for the men the employed category had a slightly higher average age than the unemployed.

The partners of the men who were married or living together were interviewed separately but usually simultaneously. All of the women were interviewed by the author; the men were interviewed by a specially trained interviewer in close collaboration with the author. All of the interviews were recorded on tape.

(b) See Spruit, I P _Unemployment, the unemployed and health, an analysis of the Dutch situation_ in John, J, Schwefel, D, Zollner, H (eds), 'The influence of economic fluctuations on health', Heidelberg, New York, Springer Verlag 1982, pp 387-426.

Demographic factors (age, marital status, children living at home or elsewhere, educational level, employment of the partner) are of importance, because they can exert an influence on the chance of becoming unemployed as well as on the health status and the reaction to being jobless or to work itself.

If unemployment may be seen as a life event, assessment of its significance relative to other life events (nature and number, time of occurrence, coping, present worries) would be important. On the one hand, joblessness could be a specific type of event, and on the other hand, the coincidence of a number of events (including the loss of work) could influence the effect of unemployment.

Social support (belonging to a network of social contacts, practical support, emotional support, and reciprocal emotional relationships) is currently considered important because it can form a buffer against negative influences associated with the reaction to unemployment on health.

Health was dealt with as two subject clusters, one comprising a number of health factors (physical complaints, mental and social wellbeing, medical consumption, number of days of feeling ill, and accidents) and the other covering risk factors which can influence health in the long run, ie the life style (diet, addictions, physical exercise, relaxation). The theme disease history (chronic diseases, hospitalisation, sick leave) was included because of the potential influence on unemployment as well as on the meaning of unemployment and health complaints.

THE REACTIONS TO UNEMPLOYMENT AND EMPLOYMENT

Attention will be given first to factors related to employment and unemployment, focussing on the reaction to both and what both mean to the respondents. The employed and unemployed men and women will be described separately on the basis of their reaction to their situation.

The jobless men and their partners

The unemployed respondents form a pluriform population[c], and the reaction to unemployment was also divergent. All but one of the men had been on a payroll. Ten of them were married or living with a partner.[d] (There were few divorced men among the Leiden unemployed.) Three of the wives or partners of these men were themselves unemployed; the others had a job.

(c) Spruit I P, Definities van werkloosheid en analyseproblemen (Definitions of Unemployment and Problems of Analysis). Sociol. Gids, 21, 1984, 80-95.

(d) One man was not living with his partner. This partner was present at the interview but did not wish to be interviewed herself.

The reaction to being unemployed ranged from pleasurable to highly problematic, the group in between being able to put up with the situation.

A. Half of the men (5 individuals) found being jobless extremely difficult. Their training and occupational levels ranged from intermediate to high, and they were among the oldest respondents. All of the men older than 40 years fall into this category. They had been jobless for between six months and a year. For three of them unemployment was the dominant problem; for two of them other problems played an important role too. These two men were the only ones who had been in the same job for a relatively long time.

B. Three men found unemployment unpleasant but could manage, and were capable of visualizing alternative ways of living. All three had been on an intermediate occupational level, had had temporary jobs, and had been unemployed before. On average, they were slightly younger than the preceding group. One of the men had only finished primary school, was partially disabled, and had a disability allowance but urgently wanted to work, and had started evening classes for retraining to acquire another trade on his own initiative.

C. Two of the men were voluntarily unemployed and had initially found being jobless a relief because they had had many problems at work. One of them had built up a new existence and enjoyed it very much, the other had been less successful, according to his own feeling. His positive reaction to unemployment disappeared and became negative after a year. The occupational level of these two men had been intermediate.

Questions about the feelings evoked by unemployment, about the advantages and disadvantages and subjective consequences, about being sacked, the financial situation, and the like, almost always receive a reasonably straightforward answer. In many cases people were glad to be able to talk frankly for once. The socially desirable answers were known, and they were referred to when their own reaction was different. Two questions were often difficult for them to deal with. The question about the respondents occupational identity and the one about expectations of the future, were experienced as a confrontation, the latter even as threatening and almost impossible to answer.

In general, the wives confirmed to a great extent their husband's feelings about having been declared redundant and the experience of being unemployed. All but one of them were well aware of their husband's feelings and were even able to put them in the same way into words, whether at length or briefly and to the point. One woman reacted to her husband's unemployment almost more strongly than he himself; the others had reached a variable degree of acceptance. Their shared experience concerned mainly the wife's empathy with her partner and the rearrangement of her life according to the demands of the situation. For them, the most important thing was to support their husband in his adjustment to unemployment. They were, however, better able than the men to see advantages of the situation, such as caring for the children together or being able to take a job themselves. Four of the women had first met their partner after he became unemployed or shortly before that.

Differences in reaction among unemployed men

A. Unemployment as a nightmare

For three of the men who experienced being jobless as horrible, the lack of work dominated their thinking completely. They could not conceive of a positive aspect, and saw looking for work as the only thing worth doing with their time. They could also verbalise the most negative feelings: 'your image of yourself takes a real beating, the emotional blow is the worst', 'it is a terribly emotional experience, hits you from all sides and eats up your nerves', 'one feels figuratively almost castrated, and I have noticed it literally too'.

Life seemed to have lost its meaning; they felt discarded and had a sense of growing inertia. Feelings of frustration and impotence, of being humiliated and besmirched recurred repeatedly in the interview in cases where the statutory dismissal process had been far from elegant (2 cases). All three had the feeling that they would go crazy if the situation continued. Other activities gave them little satisfaction: 'hobbies leave a bad taste in your mouth', 'its not satisfying, no one cares whether you do it well', 'you do it to keep busy, but you can't keep it up forever'. One of them spent all his time job hunting, worried, and brooded; the other lay on the livingroom couch all day daydreaming in despair; the third said: 'I have managed a way of survival for myself by maintaining a strict daily schedule'.

It was difficult to talk with these men about the consequences of unemployment and even more difficult to bring up the subject of the future. They invariably returned to the work they used to do, the day they were fired, their extremely negative feelings about the authorities and official bodies they have to deal with, and their attempts to obtain work. Topics outside 'work' were avoided and warded off under a flood of emotions. The interviews offered a chance to unload preoccupations.

The men revealed that they had become vulnerable, their tolerance very low. The situation affected their contacts with friends and acquaintances, with authorities, and with their family. 'Is there anything you think is worse than being jobless?', 'Yes, I'm jumpy and tired, terribly tired, I could sleep the whole time'. 'The most frustrating thing is to have to go to the district office of the Gewestelijk Arbeids Kantoor (GAK = DHSS) every week .... fill in a form to say that I still have not found work. That's humilating, as if I'm an evader, and the lady looks down her nose at me as if I were dirt .....'. They felt socially isolated and stigmatized: 'people don't see any difference between unemployed men .....', and they do not receive adequate assistance: 'you're thrown in a bin and left to save yourself', 'you're driven into a corner where you can't move in any direction and then you're number eight thousand seven hundred and thirty five'. Contacts are avoided. Questions such as 'How are you?' are experienced as painful, embarassing. They can never relax. 'Everything seems to be in a mist; carefree enjoyment never seems to be possible', said one of them, the only one who was able to cope to some degree. The other two felt defeated. The one who had been longest without work was the most exhausted. One of these men survived a suicide attempt a few weeks after the invterview.

For two of the men the role played by unemployment among their other problems is not clear. They had considerable difficulty in describing the effect it had had on them. At first it had in a way seemed pleasurable, but that did not last long: 'Your body rhythm is upset, you no longer have a goal, inertia takes over'. 'By nature I'm very lively and active' said a benumbed man who had been jobless for a month. He had been overwrought due to problems with his children for two months shortly before he was sacked, and the day on which he was dismissed coincided with a crisis in his family problems and financial difficulties. The other man was ill and did not know whether he could stand an interview. The tranquilizers he had been given had reduced his ability to concentrate. For more than a year he had worked hard helping with the winding up of the company he had been employed by: 'Helping .... well, of course, helping, but I was working in a morgue .... in the end I walked out gasping with misery, I was completely exhausted'. He had been unemployed for two months at the time of interview: 'I was the last to go except for the manager, I saw them all leave', but he could not conceive that he was jobless. Both men were pursued by their problems even in their sleep, and they felt that they were looked down on by their neighbours and an amorphous social environment.

They had no idea about the future: 'I have to finish with those medicines first, be rid of the tensions, then I'll see ....', or 'I'm going to apply for rent support, my applications for work are not going well'. Life had entered a timeless temporary phase of problems, one in which they did not even know what they wanted. 'Normal work' did form their frame of references, but seemed an ephemeral possibility in a chaos of ideas. They spoke of alternatives as though they did not believe in them: 'I've talked about going back to school .... or perhaps of doing something in the welfare sector'; or 'walk a lot and avoid fantasies about achievements'.

The other three men too had an extremely short projection of the future, which had shrunk to a very short span. 'If I get this job' and 'If I don't get this job' prefaced their answer to any question about the future. 'I have now reached a critical point .... if I get this job I'll have ground under my feet again ....'. Applying for work was itself a precarious undertaking, especially if there was even a spark of hope: 'and every time you don't get the job you're overwhelmed by despair again'.

At the time of the interview all three were waiting to hear about an application about which they felt both intense hope and intense doubt. They could not see a future without work of some kind. 'I'll have to take a job that pays less .... I think I'll be promoted again, that's what I want of course'. But even if he were to get the job, life will have had a 'lost period': 'I'm back at the beginning again and I'll never be able to catch up. I won't have enough years to'. A life without work would be: 'a very painful situation, if I even imagine it it breaks me up, it would be a catastrophe, I would have a nervous breakdown, become unfit for work: I'd go to pieces'.

One man even refused to talk about the possibility, ignored the questions, and returned systematically to the topic of his current application for work. During a three hour conversation, he only uttered two sentences about how he saw life without a job and the threat of the future: 'I can't sit in a chair until I am 65' and 'Nothing is done for people of our age. If the economy improves in five years it will be too late for me, my life will have been lost by then'. There was even something threatening about finding work: 'I'd never stop being scared of getting into the same situation again ....'. Only one of these men could even vaguely imagine a life without work, but that idea was very distant, very vague, and, in particular, would happen somewhere else: 'move away and become a farmer or something'. Only the role played by his wife kept him from becoming overwhelmed by despair: 'It is only because of her that I can keep going'. They have not known each other long and are very much in love.

The women empathise deeply with their husbands and consider their supportive role so important that they arrange their life accordingly. Two of the wives have the same negative ideas about unemployment as their husband: 'It was terrible what they did to him'. Both had been to see their doctor because they had reacted to the tensions in the family with physical complaints. They felt they should spare their husband, 'but the wife has to bear a lot and must not talk about it, because you can't burden him with your own feelings'. They complained of lack of privacy, always being overheard and seen by the other. One of them (37 years old, young children) was glad that she had a chance to work because her husband was at home, and explicitly considered that to be a positive point, but the other one (47 years old, adolsescent children) was tired of the double load of working outside and being a housewife. If her husband were to find another job with lower pay: 'The worst problem would be solved for him but not for me, because I would have to go back to my old life and now that I'm older I couldn't manage it any more'. Both of these women were afraid of the future. One of them was attempting to obtain a certificate so that she and her husband could set up a business. She was afraid to work full time because she feared that he would become aggressive toward the children, as she had seen happen in friends' families. 'The only thing that can pull you through unemployment is a good marriage', they say, 'and to talk a lot, a whole lot, with each other'. But at the same time they felt that they were left holding the bag.

Another woman said she didn't know whether she could give her husband adequate support. He was so extremely reserved that he did not even show irritability. She said that she had suspected several times that he had problems. She was the only one of the wives who did not know how her husband felt about being unemployed. For herself and her work she found it convenient that he was at home. Their shared worries were more concerned with serious problems with children from a previous marriage and financial difficulties, the latter exacerbating the problems with the children. Still another woman consciously underlined positive aspects of unemployment. As a couple they had more time for each other and he could find himself: 'He was always in a hurry and so impressed by status, now he's learning to see life in a different way and becoming more aware of real values'. She was not bothered by the idea that he might never work again: 'After all, the roles can be reversed'. But in that case she, as well as he, would want to move: 'People don't know what kind of attitude to take toward you, they act as though you had a contagious disease'.

The wives did not have the same sharply reduced view of the future, but the two who had many problems were quite dejected. 'If my husband doesn't find work again the world will fall apart, and I don't know how to cope with that'. 'I'm broken, I've always worked terribly hard, and for what? What I built up is gone and I have to work even harder. Even if he finds work again, everything is destroyed for me'. Those who found the situation less difficult were also less depressed about the future: 'If he finds a job, good: if not, we'll move and start another life', or 'When the time comes, we'll see what happens'.

B. Unemployment as something that can be accepted.

Three of the men found being jobless unpleasant, but not to the degree that their world had collapsed. 'I do my best, but the feeling of being able to do whatever I want doesn't last'; 'Sometimes I find it really difficult, your upbringing means that you tend to aim at achievement, but if it's not possible then its not'; 'Its not agreeable, I keep busy but in a way it's forced'.

In this group the reaction to unemployment was much less emotional and the feelings were sometimes contradictory. These men were able to talk with animation about topics other than work and unemployment, unlike those who saw joblessness as a catastrophe. All three of them spent much time and thought on their hobby (sport, art) and saw this as distinctly positive, but: 'Because of a social evil I can suddenly do something positive, there must be something wrong in that'. The extra time they had for their wife and growing children was also experienced as positive, but being dependent on the dole was a problem: 'I know that I have paid for it out of my wages and that it is a kind of right, but somewhere inside me there's a feeling of independence, I want to do something for my money'; 'Sometimes I feel hopeless and uncertain, am I always going to be dependent on the dole?', 'I don't want the unemployment allowance, it must be possible to get along; so far, I've been able to manage'.

Their view of the future had not shrunk, they were only somewhat uncertain. They could also imagine ways to fill their life. Two had made considerable progress in this direction. None of them expected to find a job doing the same kind of work they had done before, and this did not receive priority either. 'I'll take anything I can get, of course, but my chances are small, I'm too old'. (Actually, they all felt too old and thought that younger men would always be preferred.) Two of them had chosen alternatives and were working toward them: 'I've been told that I'm good [in art] .... I expect it to work. I'm going to make contacts and have exhibitions, perhaps that will lead to sales'; 'My greatest wish is to succeed with my music, we play well, I want to go on with it till I'm 65 and I hope my wife will be able to earn some additional money'. The third was uncertain: 'I have ideas but don't know what to do with them'. He has no home: 'Most of all I want a house and not have to stay with other people all the time. Then I could write a book, for instance, make work for myself'.

The wives of these men had no problems at all with their husband's unemployment. The only drawback was the limited income but they took that as part of the whole situation. However, they refused to see the situation as permanent: 'I can't believe things will never improve'. They saw the time they had for each other within their relationship and the sharing of the bringing up of the children and the housekeeping as positive, but they also found it important to have some things they did alone, as well as their husbands did. So they created outside-the-home activites for themselves. They thought their husband would ultimately devise a future in his own way: 'He'll make it in the end, he's good'. They themselves were unemployed and made a considerable effort to find work.

C. Unemployment as a positive experience

For two men unemployment had been desired and their reaction to it remained positive for a long time. 'I had made a serious attempt to judge whether the work I was doing was right for me and had come to the conclusion that it wasn't'; 'I couldn't take it any more'.

One of these men had a vocation as an artist and was glad he could now work at that. His artist's career offered perspectives, he received recognition, and saw it as his new occupational identity. The other man had had no success, was 'his own psychotherapist' for two years, and now felt himself in a vacuum and was looking for a job again. Thus, although both men had been pleased with becoming unemployed, because they were 'unable to fit themselves into work that did not suit me' and had made use of the 'free' period to discover themselves and their abilities, their experience of the consequences of unemployment was not the same. One had succeeded in constructing a new social identity, the other had fallen back on his old occupation, but this had been as a last resort, because he did not really enjoy it. His comment was: 'There is no purpose in what I am doing. One goes through the world without an aim, without work .... I feel as though I am in a vacuum'. His social contacts had become superficial, he found that they had no meaning and wanted to 'do things that would also have some point for others'.

Both of these men have a chance to work. One expected to develop an income with his new work (art) and anticipated the future with great confidence. The other had a chance of getting a temporary job, and was wrestling with his feelings about it: 'It's a kind of an experimental field, a test area .... I have no real problems, there must be possibilities ....'. At first he seemed able to consider a future without paid employment: 'Then I'll go on as I do now, with the certainty that I will no longer have to go on doing things I have to do now ....', but he nevertheless refused to talk about the chance that he would fail again in the work he found and wrestled with the difficulties he anticipated.

The wives shared their partner's world intensely. One of them was unable to see her husband as unemployed or to talk about it in that way: 'It's a whole new idea to me. I've never seen it that way'. She did not find being unemployed herself so terrible either. If she did not find work: 'there are plenty of other things I enjoy doing'. The other wife had given up her job because she could not manage the load any longer, and had many personal problems. But she had started shortly before to look for work again. Like her husband, her thoughts about the future were confused: 'Its unpredictable, things can happen that I know nothing about'. The couple had never been in a situation in which they were both working, and she was more concerned about the effect on their relationship than about the effect of unemployment on herself: '.... it would be better if we didn't both have a full time job, then you only see each other at night in bed and just have time to say 'Hello, are you still around?'

The employed men and their partners

All but one of the employed were wage earners.[e] As for the unemployed, husband and wife were usually interviewed at the same time but separately. Ten of the men were married or living together; one partner refused the interview. The majority of the partners (n = 6) were working part time or full time, the others (n = 3) were housewives and were not looking for work.

Just as unemployment can give rise to problems, so some can have problems in or with their work. Like the unemployed, the employed were first asked about their general reaction (what do you think about your work, or what do you think about being jobless?). In addition, various items were used to explore feelings. For the unemployed these items included, for example, the reason for the loss of work and how the discharge had occurred, the duration of the unemployment, the degree of the financial loss, the possibilities for giving life purpose without paid employment, and ideas about the future. The employed were asked about the atmosphere at work with respect to the management and fellow workers, the degree of pressure associated with the job, the work load, whether they did heavy work, the wish for other work, and whether there were worries about keeping the job and how the future was visualized.

Among the unemployed, differences in reaction were mainly observable via the reaction to the very general question ('what do you think of it?'). In addition, the possibilities for giving life meaning without paid employment and the ideas about the future were also important. Among the employed, all of the respondents were entirely satisfied with their occupation (what do you think of it?). They liked their work, and the interviewer ran the risk of being supplied with extensive explanations and details about the occupation in question. Differences began to appear with the questions about the atmosphere at work, but particularly those about the wish for other work and worries about holding the job. In three respondents a moderately to strongly negative opinion about the atmosphere (particularly the quality of the management) was accompanied by the wish for other work and worries about holding the job.

The experienced pressure of the occupation and the experience of having a heavy or light workload varied and had no relationship with any of the other

---

(e) One of them was self employed and also had disability allowance. Among the unemployed there also was one man with a disability allowance.

items. Many of those who stated that their workload was heavy (even very heavy) said that this did not create problems for them and was just as enjoyable as it was heavy. All but two of the men said that it would be terrible to be unemployed. They used various superlatives to qualify this: 'dreadful', 'horrible', 'I'd go crazy'. A few found the idea so awful that they could not even think about it, could not imagine themselves being jobless. 'I would peel bulbs, sell apples, I'll never be without work because it would be impossible for me'. The main reason for this reaction was always the thought of enforced idleness: 'I have no hobbies'.

Two of the men could imagine finding something to do with their time. One of them disliked his job so much that he wouldn't mind being unemployed; the other had mixed feelings: 'In the first instance I would find it quite awful, but on the other hand I would be able to train for something I would like to do'.

Three men had been briefly unemployed a long time ago, and at that time it had not been a problem. For one man it had happened quite recently (5 to 6 years ago): 'It was the most humiliating experience I have ever had. But while I was stll unemployed I wouldn't have been able to tell that to you or anyone else. Perhaps I didn't even know myself'. At the time of the interview he was in the process of being dismissed again.

On the whole, fewer problems were found among the employed than among the unemployed people interviewed during the study. As in the case of the unemployed, all of the women but one confirmed their husband's reaction to his work. One woman (who considered her marriage to have problems) gave rather divergent information. The women were less involved in their husband's experiences than the wives of the unemployed were, their involvement being roughly comparable to that of the wives of unemployed men with few problems.

Differences in reactions among employed men

A. Problems at work

Three of the men were highly satisfied with their occupation but only moderately so with the atmosphere among their colleagues. Two of them were not satisfied with the management, although it cost them some effort to talk about it. They were constantly more reserved on this point than those who found the management satisfactory. The third man was dissatisfied to such a degree that it dominated the entire interview. He had even requested legal assistance to enable him to protest against unjustifiable work demands. Of all of the men he was the only one who said he would not mind at all losing his job. He would prefer to become self employed and no longer have to bear the atmosphere at work. All three of the men would prefer to have different work, but two of them felt themselves too old to change (they were over 40). One of them was in the process of being dismissed, but did not wish to talk about it. The other two no longer felt certain that they would be able to keep their job and worried about it frequently. There were no concrete indications that they might be fired, and in the companies for which they worked there had not been more cutting down of the work force, failure to fill openings, or similar signs of retrenching than in the companies the others worked for. The majority of the men were working for reasonably stable companies or for the government. A few reported increasing work loads due to economic pressure on the firm, which affected the atmosphere among the employees and had given others, but not themselves, a feeling of being overloaded.

One of the women did not share her husband's concern. She thought he tended to see the dark side and was a worrier. Another wife found it impossible to judge the situation. An earlier period during which her husband had been unemployed (which he himself had not mentioned in the interview) had been a nightmare for her. She felt very insecure about the future and had the feeling that everything was changing again just when she had thought she could see how it would be.

B. Enjoyment of work

The majority of the men (8) said they were very satisfied about all aspects of their work. They did not want another kind of work, and felt reasonably secure about their job. One man still felt 'homesick' for an earlier occupation and the atmosphere associated with it, but could no longer perform that kind of work because of his heart. After being disabled by a heart attack he was given an office job in the same company. It was difficult at first, but schooling at a more advanced age had led to supplementary certificates.

The women shared their husband's opinion. Few of them wished to think about the long term future, because: 'You can't do anything about it and things are getting worse, no one can do anything about that. We just hope that everything stays as it is now for us'.

<u>The unemployed women</u>

Among the unemployed women in Leiden there are almost as many married as formerly married women. The interviewed women included six who were living alone or with their children (divorced, widowed) and four who were married or living with a partner. The women who were formerly married had had a full time job, and two of the married women had a full time and two a part time job. All of the interviewed divorced women had started to work as wage earners because they saw no other solution. They did not want to be dependent on welfare or alimony. They had wanted to 'prove that I could manage alone'. They enjoyed working as long as they could work in the occupation they were trained for. Gradually they acquired more than one reason for wanting to go on working. The interviewed married women (including partners of employed and unemployed men) were more often employed part time, had not started to work until they felt their children to be old enough, and had gradually begun to work more hours as their children became older. One wife of an unemployed man had started to work full time, but that was only possible because the husband was at home. All of these women said that they would have to return to part time work if their husband found a job. The divorced women had not themselves chosen the time at which they started to work; this had been determined by the situation at home and they had begun with full time work from the start.

Most of the women had only finished primary school or a lower level occupation school and were rather poorly informed about their rights and legal position. Four women had given up their job voluntarily or had accepted dismissal (under intimidation), which meant that they had lost their right to unemployment insurance (80% of their basic wages for 6 months) at a time when their financial situation was already difficult. Other women who did know their rights had often been unable to defend them because of the many problems at home. The women who had left work voluntarily had had personal problems which made the work too much of a load. Three of them were self supporting women with children at home.

Being a one parent family was an important factor in the reaction to unemployment but did not dominate it completely. None of the married women with children found it possible to work full time, and reported having broken down finally because they had tried to. Formerly married women with children not living at home became more isolated than others and considered this the most important element in the reaction to unemployment.

In the Netherlands there are relatively few women in the labour force (compared to other countries). Working women are not a unanimously accepted feature, whereas housewives still are. In public opinion women's unemployment is often considered far less important than men's unemployment. The women had divergent and sometimes complex reasons for working, and they also showed a more complex picture in their reaction to unemployment. Seven of the women (almost two thirds) had a negative reaction to the unemployment itself or its consequences (deterioration of the legal position and the financial situation). For five of them, other problems besides unemployment played an important role. It is also noteworthy that many of them mentioned a number of personal problems which had a strong effect on their life in addition to being jobless.

The women were unanimous in feeling that the loss of contacts was the most negative aspect of being unemployed, an item which was seldom mentioned so explicity by men.

A. Problems with being unemployed are encountered equally among married women and formerly-married women. For two of the married women, being unemployed was a terrible situation not only because they were without a job but also because working had made it possible to escape family problems. For three of the formerly-married women caring for one or more children, financial difficulties and problems with respect to their legal position played a major role in addition to family problems. For two formerly-married women with children no longer at home, being without employment itself and/or being alone were in particular experienced as extremely negative.

B. Two women, one married and the other formerly-married, had mixed feelings about being unemployed. Both preferred to work but could manage without it.

C. Two women found or had found unemployment desirable. One of them had originally had mixed feelings and had been deeply pained by the dismissal procedure in particular, but now had very positive feelings about being unemployed. The other started with positive feelings, but had then solved her personal problems and found a partner, and now had mixed feelings.

Because no employed married women were intereviewed, the formerly-married women (divorced, widowed) and the married women will be described separately.

Differences in reaction among formerly-married unemployed women

A. Unemployment as problem

Three formerly-married women still had one or more of their children to care for: 'I was working to the point of exhaustion, I had no strength left at all'. They felt that as a result, they had failed their children. Two of them were therefore ambivalent about not being employed, but were affected most by the financial limitations inherent in the situation and by the dependence on government assistance. 'I don't know what I think about it, I work to have money, I want to work, but part-time, but most of all I'd like to have a husband who respected me and I could lean on', said a woman who had not got over either her marital problems or the divorce, was drinking a lot, and whose youngest son had the same name as an earlier child who had drowned while playing outside. She felt extremely lonely and very worried about her income.

One woman who had given up her job because of guilt feelings toward her children wanted to start working again because her children had grown up and left home, and she was becoming increasingly isolated. 'You're sidetracked, completely out of everything'. But the main reason was that she wanted to be independent: '.... of every agency. You have to keep demanding, keep on fighting for things you have a right to'. She could not have her handicapped child, placed in an institution, with her as often as she would like, because she could not afford the taxi fares. Otherwise, she found being unemployed 'bearable if you keep yourself occupied'. In that she had been successful, having taken course after course to increase her chance of getting a job. Her plans to do volunteer work had been postponed repeatedly during the last five years because: 'I won't start that until I'm certain that I can't get a job'.

Personal problems loom large for these women. A job had been given up (two cases) after a painful experience, such as the institutionalization of the handicapped child, about which the mother still felt doubts: 'I did it with my head, not my heart', or the death of the husband, after which the wife had left her job to return to her own country: 'so as not to have to cope with everything alone'. She was not certain that she had made the right decision and had very poor housing. She was unable to say what being unemployed meant to her. One the one hand: 'The financial situation is not bad, and I see the children a lot and can help them with their homework', but on the other hand: 'I've never been a housewife and need work and contacts'. Her view of the future was very short: 'I hope I can stand it', was her answer to the question about coping with unemployment, but she meant her cramped living quarters, which bothered her more. She preferred not to talk about the future: 'I find that very hard to do'. Many emotions and problems that were not immediately urgent were masked, and she felt great insecurity about the future. She was surprised at the ease with which other women could accept being confined to the home: '....but I want to work, that seems perfectly normal to me but I cannot talk with them about that'.

The other two also confined themselves to the very near future and had not formed a clear picture of it. This situation can make a job just as threatening as unemployment: 'I can get a job, but it's full time. I might be able to get someone to take care of my little one, but I can't really afford the money. But I can't leave my child alone, he clings to me so .... I'd feel guilty. The adolescent children have been upset by the situation too ....'. She had to decide about something that she couldn't decide about, sometimes lay all night brooding about it and then took a sleeping pill, and would prefer to have a husband and work part time. For these three women the future was '.... dark and gloomy, I can't see a glimmer of light anywhere'.

The two formerly married women with children no longer at home experienced the negative aspect of unemployment itself particularly strongly, and barely mentioned financial or legal aspects. They did not show the complex combination with severe personal problems. Unemployment itself was experienced as negative: 'Its terrible, really awful. At first it seems wonderful, because you can catch up with your housekeeping, but then you want to be able to get out, because you're so alone'. She was ashamed of being unemployed, and particularly when she had to go to the official agency. 'I'm always afraid they think I don't do my best to find work'. Thinking about the future was difficult. One woman said repeatedly: 'I just hope I get work again'. It cost her intense effort to consider the possibility that that would be impossible: 'I'd find it interesting to learn to do some other kind of work, dietician or something, but I'd rather keep on with the old one, I really enjoyed it'. The other woman (the only one with a high educational level) described herself as aimless and apathetic, and she too refused to consider the possibility of never working again: 'I'd move to some small town or village and invent work for myself, but I'm really a city person' or '.... for my salvation I could turn into a 'useful' housewife, that's a way of justifying not working, makes you more certain of yourself .... in the world .... people start to find you pathetic so soon but I do not want to be a housewife'.

B. Unemployment as something that can be accepted

'I've been through so much in my life .... it has made me able to take care of myself .... this isn't so bad after all'. This woman who could accept the situation drew positively on what she had learned from her negative experiences and the capacities she had developed in the process. Her children had left home, but she thought she could cope with unemployment because of the course her life had taken, because she liked to be alone but also can get along well with people, and also because she herself felt a bit guilty about being unemployed. She had taken a 'really enjoyable' but unfortunately temporary job. Her life was coloured by the fact that as an unwanted child she had been allowed to visit her parents and the other children but never to live at home. After that she had held out for years with a husband who beat her several times a week. One of the questions discretely typed on a card, to be answered 'yes' or 'no' and placed in an evelope without discussion, was: 'Would you like to beat someone up, just like that?'. She looked up and read it aloud, laughing. 'Yes!' she said wholeheartedly, 'and I mean my ex husband'. He still threatened her. She hoped intensely to obtain work, especially to have a chance of having her old job back, where the atmosphere among the employees had meant a great deal to her, but she also saw how many young people are trying to find work and thought she could 'manage' if she did not succeed.

C. Unemployment as a positive experience

One woman was forced by intimidation to quit her job, another did so voluntarily. In both cases the loss of work had occurred after personal problems. One of them had sole responsibility for the care of her children. She found it impossible to combine a full time job with adequate attention to her family. 'Shall I tell you the truth? I love it, I'm terribly happy to be at home', she said. A son had died very young and a daughter had first been in a home, then with a grandmother, and after her death with a neighbour. The 'voluntary' giving up of the job had followed a quarrel with the neighbour. This was only the tip of the iceberg of her problems, 'I've had my share'. She regarded the future with mixed feelings. 'I'll be going on the dole soon, even less money, but I'm going to go on breathing, and for the rest I'm not going to think about things'. As the lesser of two evils she preferred to live on the borderline of poverty than have to take a full time job.

The other woman had given up her job because of 'a personal crisis' in which her divorce played an important role. She had been unable to go on, had had the feeling that her work was 'draining the life out of her'. Now that she had found both herself and a (jobless) partner, she wanted to work again but had ambivalent feelings: 'If you work you have no time to do interesting things for yourself. If you don't work you have no money to do them'. But staying home all day meant that '....you have more time for worrying, you can't stop thinking about things'.

Differences in reaction of married unemployed women

The women who hated being unemployed (2) mentioned the opportunity for worrying as one of the most bothersome consequences. They disliked staying at home and missed the activity around them, the appreciation of their performance at work, and the distraction from domestic problems that the job brought with it. They now had unlimited time to worry about the children and also being unemployed.

One of them had had to accept shorter working hours and a form of supplementary assistance. She wept while telling about the problems of her (adult) children. She thinks with abhorrence of a previous but recent period of unemployment: 'My family loved it .... "Oh, Ma, I'm going to come and have coffee and a chat with you", said my children. But I got worse and worse, I wanted to hit my head against the wall'. She finally had to go to the doctor, who prescribed valium.

The second of these women was so seriously ill (heart damage) and confused that a reasonably adequate interview was almost impossible. Despite the documents she showed, it was not clear whether she was receiving disability benefits or unemployment benefits, and it was small wonder that she did not know either. It was also not clear why she was registered as unemployed: 'At the time, the health authorities said I had to register because at the end of the (sick leave) year I would be transferred from health insurance to unemployment insurance'. She was extremely depressive and afraid that she did not give the impression of being sufficiently willing to work. It was evident that she was considered to be a malingerer: '.... under all that pressure from the doctors I started to work again'. She also had problems with her children and gave the impression of being very nervous and confused. She had gone to work: 'to be out of it all for a while, not to have to think about all those things'. Now she had plenty of time to worry.

One woman reacted with indifference to being unemployed. She said she missed the contacts most: 'You don't see people as much'. Unlike an earlier period of unemployment, when the family needed her earnings badly, she reacted equably: 'In these times we're just glad my husband is still working ....'. Although she was still looking for work, she had a busy life and saw many opportunities for volunteer work in her neighbourhood.

The working women

Because so few married women agreed to participate in the study, only divorced or widowed working women were interviewed. But even more problems were encountered in assembling an appropriate matched group. One problem concerned the validity of a comparison of working and unemployed women if some jobless women prefer not to work but are compelled by the statutory provision for assistance to register as seeking work. This was the case of two of the women. Therefore, the sample of working women includes two who preferred to be a housewife and were dependent on social insurance, but not unemployment insurance.

The four women who worked outside the home had very different motives for doing so. One had always worked and was also the breadwinner when she was married, was now self supporting and worked overtime. One had started to work because '.... otherwise it would have been necessary to live so economically that it would have been absolutely impossible'; she considered the assistance payments too small to support her family. One had started to work on her doctor's advice because she had become too isolated. One gave the same reason as the unemployed women: 'After my divorce I had to earn my own living'. The same questions about the reaction to work were posed to the housewives and the other women. The women with a job were considered as women with two jobs and they were questioned about how they felt about the effect of the double load. Two employed women and one housewife enjoyed their work and would not want to change it. The other working women and housewife felt ambivalent. One of them had started retraining for another kind of work closer to her own level. The other two did not feel able to support the effort of retraining, but were not really satisfied with the situation. However, they felt tied by circumstances and inclined to make the best of things.

The heaviness of the work was estimated in different ways. Five women reported being very tired at the end of the day. A full time job and children was considered too heavy a load by both of the women with full time jobs. One of them was planning to work fewer hours, which had been made possible by a new relationship.

All of the women were highly satisfied with the atmosphere among their fellow workers. Those with a job 'didn't even want to think about' becoming unemployed. The self employed woman thought she would always be able to create something for herself to do. The other three considered the worst circumstances of unemployment to be the loss of contacts and (to a lesser extent) the financial disadvantages. One woman was in the process of being made redundant because her employer was cutting down. 'I'm afraid I'll push myself too hard', she said. If she could not find part time work she would take a full time job, 'even though I know I couldn't keep it up'. Being without a job seemed even worse to her than being overworked. Three of the women had positive ideas about the future, one was ambivalent, and two very pessimistic. Four of the women admitted to worrying frequently.

COMPARISON OF ASPECTS OF THE REACTION

The reaction to unemployment and the degree to which being unemployed is felt to be a problem (thus, a stressful life event that might have an effect on health) differed widely, not only between men and women but also among men and among women. One of these differences concerns the reasons they gave for not liking to be jobless. The women almost invariably mentioned missing the contact with other people as one of the main reasons. This is not necessarily to be understood as missing friends or acquaintances. The women said as often as the men did that they did not see fellow workers outside of work. It was more a question of feeling 'no longer part of the world' or being 'outside society', as they put it. The men, however, missed the identity their work provided, the occupation as means of self realization and source of prestige, income, social positon, and so on. They were thrown back on an existence without a social identity. The women were thrown back on a housewife status they did not want and that also did not do justice to them or their abilities. This confrontation, furthermore, did not offer any possibilities that might make it easier to cope with unemployment.

Men and women had different reasons for working. Men worked because it is self evident, women tended to have a specific motivation more often. The wives or partners of unemployed men more often considered it self evident that they find a job than did the wives/partners of employed men. The reaction to working itself differed more among women than men.

For both men and women, a strongly negative reaction to unemployment was accompanied by entering into a temporary timeless existence in which there is no future to look forward to. Men who can revise their idea of the future were found to have fewer problems with being unemployed. This revision means the achievement of what is for them a recognisable and acceptable social status, in other words having a goal in sight to be reached in a positive way. Many men who could do this, already had the capacity to realize it, in the form of a creative talent that had already had an important place in their life as a hobby. Because of the enforced idleness, they developed it further: 'not because I really want to, but to stave off the problems'. The problems do not subside until this activity yields real perspectives.

The ability to revise the future was for the women less effective as a way of ameliorating the negative reactions to being unemployed. The women, especially those who had no partner, were an extremely vulnerable group. When their children left home they became lonely rapidly and severely. Very few of them had found a new partner, whereas rather many of the men had done so. Women with children still at home had little choice if they were divorced: either living on the minimum income provided by assistance, with the feeling of being dependent on official agencies and exposed to constant checks to see whether they were living with a man, the fear of financial penalities, and feelings of guilt because they were not working, or the expectation of many years of the very heavy work load of a full time job combined with caring for the family, until they became exhausted and so guilt ridden about the children that they accepted all the problems of living on a small income or felt trapped in a blind alley. Part time jobs are not only inadequate but also offer little financial perspective for a one parent family if that parent does not have a very high educational level.

In addition, the women were found to have more complex problems than the men did, and among them there was a higher proportion of individuals with other problems besides those associated with unemployment.

THE ROLE OF PROBLEMS RELATED TO EMPLOYMENT AND UNEMPLOYMENT AMONG OTHER PROBLEMS

Reference has been made several times to coincidence of reactions to being unemployed and to other life events and the role of others (the partner, the neighbourhood). These financial constraints themes were dealt with in some depth in the interviews. The observed differences did not permit subdivision of the categories as had been the case for the reactions to employment and unemployment. Therefore, a general discussion will have to suffice.

The role of the financial situation among the disadvantages of unemployment

All of the families had had to cut down and make sacrifices; it was often difficult to make ends meet. Frequent mention was made of being 'dead tired' because even the smallest indulgence had to be resisted. In some cases there were incidental supplementary earnings, but these did not contribute substantially to the family's income. In many cases it was possible to differentiate between problems due to unemployment and financial problems, but not always. For the latter cases this was due less to the actual income than to problems caused by the heavy demands on that income to pay for the house. In two families where it was questionable how long they could continue to make payments on the mortgage, even if they were to 'go hungry to do it', the financial problems weighed as heavily as other conequences of being unemployed. A separation cannot be made within the general reaction, and the finances took up a large part of the interview time.

In the families of formerly married women the reaction to financial problems, as an important component of the unemployment problems, was closely related to the actual amount of the assistance payments. These women were found to have a lower income, to have a relatively unskilled occupation more often, and to be unemployed longer. When they have a combination of financial and immaterial problems, the main concerns are on the level of the daily needs and/or their life style.

Life events

Among both the employed and unemployed there were few individuals who said they had not had undesirable life events. The formerly married women reported the largest numbers of such events. The number and nature of the events differed little between employed and unemployed. Both men and women who were unemployed mentioned problems with children and being temporarily without housing. The employed made no mention of such problems. They were also more often able to mention pleasant life events and were more often of the opinion that they had had relatively more good than bad experiences in their lives.

Divorce and unemployment

Among the men, almost the entire difference in the experience of life events lay in the greater number of divorces (n = 6) among the unemployed. A divorce was felt to be a radical encounter and worse than the loss of work. A number of the men said that it had led to weight change, somatic or mental complaints, or changes in drinking and smoking behaviour. They themselves did not ascribe these changes to unemployment.

Three of the six divorced men did see a relationship between their divorce and their loss of work, 'I started to have trouble with depressions, sleeplessness, and a feeling of paralysis in my limbs. Severe difficulty in concentrating made it impossible for me to work. I've never really gotten over these problems'. 'There were so many problems at home I couldn't give my work the attention it needed, especially because things weren't going so well between me and my boss. I can see myself that I shared in the blame. The divorce cost me years of my life'. 'I met my husband shortly after his divorce. Not long after that I went abroad on vacation. All of a sudden he was standing there in front of me and saying he wanted to marry me. He simply hadn't turned up at work that day, and was, of course, sacked immediately!

Two of the women had given up their job in connection with their divorce, one because she had too many personal problems and the other because her work involved too much contact with her ex-husband. Almost all of the other women had started to work or to look for work after the divorce if they had not been working before that.

Coping with life events

Among the men (and most of all among the jobless), resistance to discussion of this theme sometimes arose. Some of them simply refused at first: 'I've gone through so much, you'd need a whole tape just for that'. Their wives were less reserved, but did not really like to talk about it. The majority of divorced unemployed women, to the contrary, brought up a wide variety of experiences themselves and went into them in detail as a way of explaining what being unemployed meant to them. Where they had not been able to cope they saw an accumulation of effects. Only one unemployed woman reported having been strengthened by having had to cope with difficulties. The employed women without a partner also showed the urge to draw connections between life events they had experienced and their present situation, but said more often that these events were 'over now' and had been coped with, that is, they were less bitter about their marriage and divorce and they had made more attempts to start a new relationship.

With the exception of divorce, many of the unemployed considered relational problems less serious than unemployment: 'You can do something about them yourself, but this you can't fight against, only try to pull yourself through'. Problems with children were considered to be of another order and impossible to generalise. Divorce, serious illness, and death were usually considered more serious, but it is also socially desirable to think so. A few individuals, mainly men, seemed confused on this point: 'I think being unemployed is the worst possible thing .... disease is of course worse, that gives you the feeling that the world has collapsed. But we got over that; this unemployment has hit us really hard. Its as though you aren't part of the world any more'.

Social networks, social support, and help seeking behaviour

'You can't do anything in return and you can't explain that either; you just need them ....', said the wife of an unemployed man in explaining how the network of women she was friends with had been lost. Both employed and unemployed reported loss of friends or disappointment in the quality of friendships. It was among both categories most mentioned by divorced people. The most mentioned cause of loss of friends was divorce and migration. Two of the wives of unemployed men were the only ones who blamed the loss of friendships on unemployment.

Support from the partner

More than half of the jobless men looked in the first instance to their partner for emotional support. In most of the families the more difficult it was for the husband, the more unemployment was talked about. For those who were employed, this situation was less topical, less acute. The majority of them thought that they would turn first to their wife if problems arose. A more striking difference between the two groups is that the employed referred more explicitly and spontaneously to the reciprocality in the relationship. Few of the unemployed men mentioned that their wives also turned to them with their problems, and most of them gave rather uncertain answers when asked how their wife reacted to unemployment, (although they usually did give the same answer as the wife herself had).

For most of the unemployed men the subject was difficult to talk about, because they could not order their thoughts about it. They did not want to speak critically about their wife and appreciated her doing her best to help them cope with the situation. How can you then admit that besides her support you need support and recognition from the world outside the family? How can you admit that you wife's support is not adequate while she is doing her best but the world humiliates and excludes you? 'There's no sense in keeping on talking', many of them said, 'talking doesn't solve anything'. 'My wife never leaves me in the lurch, her solidarity is complete, but I don't care for going on about things, you see'; 'You manage to survive by changing your point of view, your ideas, and your values; that's the only way you can really save yourself'. Much more often than the employed men, they said proudly that they were 'very reserved by nature', kept their problems to themselves, solved their problems themselves, and that it was their wife who started to talk about things: 'she sees from my face that something is wrong and then she gets me to talk about it'.

Support from others

Unemployed men and their partners said more often than their employed counterparts that they had few friends and acquaintances. In particular, the network of individuals they could go to with personal problems or pour out their heart to was smaller. The unemployed mentioned fewer family relationships, and of course no longer had fellow workers. Although both unemployed and employed and both men and women usually said that they did not see the latter outside work, these fellow employees nevertheless offered possibilities for talking matters over that no longer existed after the job had ended. Many of the unemployed deliberately avoided contact with former fellow employees; a few attempted to maintain such relationships, but seldom succeeded: '.... they've got their work to do and can't spend the day thinking about you'. Almost half of the unemployed men avoided contact with others more or less consciously, especially talking with others about being unemployed: 'Must be shame after all, huh; acting the ostrich a bit'; 'Friends? Luckily not; I'm rather realistic'; or: 'They're not sitting around waiting to hear about my problems'. Some of the unemployed even refused to comprehend questions about the need for emotional support. Practical support, on the contrary, is missed, and that is for some a source of disappointment. Such differences make it clear that the only help they can see as really helpful would be finding a job '.... and no one can help you that way'. A minority of the unemployed knew others who were unemployed, and almost all of them said they especially avoided contact with such people, because it was depressing: '.... they put me into a tailspin', '.... always the same drivel'.

Three families felt very bad about the attitude of the neighbourhood or public opinion. They felt themselves to be victims of discrimination, prejudice, and disrespect.

The size of the network of contacts differed little between the employed and unemployed women. Almost all of the unemployed women (both married and formerly married) considered these contacts too shallow, however: 'I can't have a personal conversation even with someone I'm close friends with'; '.... they think I can't stop complaining'; '.... they simply don't understand'. This can even include the husband: 'He's as kind as he can be, but he doesn't understand me'. The women did not avoid contact either consciously or unconsciously, but assigned great importance to solving their problems independently, although they felt the need to ask others' advice. It was especially the women without a partner (all of the unemployed and half of the employed women) who complained about loneliness.

Need for professional help

Not only the employed men and their partners but also the unemployed women were reasonably certain about where they would go for professional help with problems if they felt the need to talk about them. For most of them this was the family physician, for others a minister or priest, a social service, or a union advisor. In only two families professional help was a priori rejected by both husband and wife.

Almost the reverse holds for the unemployed men. The majority of these men rejected professional help, and the same was the case of a minority of the women. The partners of the unemployed men were the most in favour of professional help. Most of them would be willing to go to the family doctor, a minority to a psychotherapist or social worker. In reality, two partners of unemployed men and one unemployed woman had consulted the family doctor. One couple were already being helped by a social worker when unemployment began, and could continue to receive this help. The reasons for this rejection of assistance were stated explicitly: 'It doesn't help me to find work'; or even more sharply: 'They don't know anything about the realities of life'; 'a bunch of bunglers ....'; 'stupid asses'. Others were less sharp: 'They really do their best, and they're necessary, but ....'; 'a valium pill doesn't give you a job'; 'that doesn't solve anything, its just a pacifier'. Solutions they had thought up themselves were hampered by regulations, and lack of interest had undermined their confidence about finding a solution together with some professional helper. The wish for help was oriented towards the finding of solutions. The idea of learning to 'live with the situation' was rejected. When this was thought to be the approach of the person who was to provide help, many of the respondents (men more so than women) preferred to avoid the request altogether.

Only two persons (wives of unemployed men) would have liked to participate in a self help group.

EMPLOYMENT AND BEING UNEMPLOYED, WELL BEING AND SICKNESS

Life styles

The life style was dependent on the income of the unemployed and the fixed expenses that had to be reduced. Some were only forced to economise on the large amounts, others had to cut down on the daily outlays as well. With respect to eating habits, smoking, drinking, physical exercise, and body weight, the families of the men and the women showed roughly the same picture. More than half of them reported no change, either because they had already had to economise to the utmost or because they could manage if they cut down on the large expenses. A minority said that positive changes had occurred such as walking more often, smoking and drinking less, fewer frills, and cooking at home more often. An almost equally large minority mentioned unfavourable changes such as less physical exercise, more smoking and drinking, and poorer quality of the food. A minority were able to fill up the day satisfactorily; another minority were completely unable to do so, and about half could do so with some effort. For a minority of the men and women the atmosphere in the family had become more disturbed, whereas a little less than half of the women reported improvement in this respect, the most important factor being that they had more time for the children and had begun to be better at cooking.

Physical, mental and social well being

Standard scales were used for the estimation of well being. Physical well being or the subjective assessment of health was measured on the basis of the 13 item VOEG (Vragenlijst Onderzoek Ervaren Gezondheid), a questinnaire designed for this purpose in The Netherlands.[f] Although it is considered by some as an indicator of stress, it is generally taken as a good indicator of the health status, able to predict consultation of a doctor and sickness.

(f) Dirken, J M, Het meten van 'stress' in industriele situaties, een multi disciplinaire ontwikkeling van een algemeen diagnosticum (The measurement of stress in industrial situations, a multi disciplinary development of a general diagnostical instrument). Thesis, Amsterdam 1967.

Jansen, M E, Sikkel, D, Verkorte versies van de VOEG-schaal (Short versions of the VOEG scale). Gezondheid and Samenleving, 2, 1981, pp 78-82.

Visser, A Ph, De VOEG: een indicator van ervaren gozendhein (The VOEG: an indicator of experienced health), Gezondheid and Samenleving, 4, 1983.

Verkley, H, Spruit, I P, Selecting a health indicator for comparative health surveys among different social categories, using unemployment as an example. Effective Health Care, 1, 1984, 251-257.

The VOEG includes questions about minor complaints such as headache, insomnia, palpitation, and so on.[g] For psychological well being, use was made of Bradburn's Affect Balance Scale,[h] which has been applied in The Netherlands before and for which a good translation is available.[i] The estimation of social well being was based on Nooy's social discomfort test,[j] a Dutch scale.

Physical wellbeing

Shorter and longer versions of the VOEG are available, the 13 item version being more suitable for small populations than a longer version. The average number of complaints for each category was as follows:

Unemployed women (divorced/widowed)[k]	5.42
Unemployed men	4.27
Partners of unemployed men	3.89
Employed men	3.64
Partners of employed men	3.44
Employed women (divorced/widowed)	3.17

(g) A few examples of VOEG questions:

Do you have pains in the chest or heart region rather often?	yes/no
Do you often feel tired?	yes/no
Do you have dizzy spells?	yes/no

(h) Bradburn, N M, The structure of psychological well being. Chicago, Aldine Publishing Co, 1969.

McDowell, I, Praught, E, On the measurement of happiness: an examination of the Bradburn scale in the Canada health survey. Am J Epid, 116, 1982, pp 949 - 958.

(i) Ormel, H, Moeitie met leven of een moeilijk leven (Difficulty in living or a difficult life). Thesis, Groningen University 1980.

(j) Nooy, A T J, De Boerenpartij, desorientatie en radicalisatie onder de boeren (The Farmers' Party, disorientation and radicalisation among farmers). Boom, Meppel 1969.

(k) The married women are not included in the comparison, because there is no match group.

The unemployed felt less healthy than the employed did, the differences being greatest for the women and smallest for the partners of the employed and unemployed men.

For the men there is a distinct correlation between the number of complaints according to the VOEG and the reaction to unemployment. The men for whom being without work was terrible, scored higher than the men who could manage or had a positive attitude to unemployement. The first of these three groups said that they worried frequently and did not find life worth living. The highest scores were obtained by the men who besides being unemployed had serious problems of other kinds. A correlation between the VOEG score and worrying was also found for the employed men. The men who wanted to change to another kind of work or worried about the possibility of losing their job had much higher scores than the other men. The differences were more extreme for the employed than the unemployed men. Those who could manage without work or reacted positively to unemployment scored on average two complaints; with increasingly negative reactions the score went up to 5.5 complaints; and those who had multiple problems had on average 7 complaints. Among the employed, those with worries about work had on average 7.3 complaints and the others on average 1.9.

Neither the wives or partners nor the employed and unemployed women showed correlation between the VOEG score and the report of frequent worrying. Only a few of the wives had more than three complaints. This low average was in line with a generally low score. No relationship was found between the VOEG score and the severity of the reaction to their husband's unemployment.

The women who were not looking for work (working women and housewives) had on average the lowest VOEG scores, and the scores were equally distributed. No correlation was found with any of the items concerning the reaction to work or the situation in which they lived.

The unemployed women had the highest VOEG scores. (This also holds for the unemployed married women, on average 4.75 complaints, who were not included in the comparison.) In this category, too, there was a distinct relationship between problems and health complaints, ie both personal problems and problems associated with unemployment. The women with only the latter (formerly married, children living elsewhere) had the most health complaints, closely followed by the women with many worries and problems and life events they had not gotten over. Almost all of these women had 7 or more complaints. The women who could get along without a job or did not find unemployment a negative experience scored very low: on average 1.5 complaints. Thus, marked differences were also found within the group of women.

Mental wellbeing

Bradburn's scale consists of positive and negative statements[(l)] about mental wellbeing (positive and negative affect). Denial of a positive feeling and recognition of a negative feeling can yield a maximum of 8 affect scores, indicating the degree of well being or happiness. The average numbers of complaints for the various categories were:

Unemployed women (divorced/widowed)	4.43
Employed women (divorced/widowed)	3.83
Unemployed men	3.73
Partners of unemployed men	2.67
Employed men	2.56
Partners of employed men	2.36

On this scale the formerly married women had the most negative scores. Whereas unemployment was found to have the strongest influence on physical well being, for the women being divorced (or widowed) had more influence on mental well being. (The unemployed married woman had an average score of 3.00). This point could not be determined for the men, because there was only one divored man in each category. Within the categories of married and formerly married people, however, the unemployed scored higher than the employed. The results show clearly that the levels of both physical and mental wellbeing were lower for the unemployed than for the employed, and that the women, especially those not married anymore formed an extremely vulnerable group.

Social wellbeing

The correlations found for physical and mental well being were not detected with respect to social well being. With Nooy's social discomfort scale[(m)], a maximum of 5 feelings of discomfort can be expressed. The values

---

(l) A few examples of questions from Bradburn's scale:

During the past few weeks, have you ever felt very lonely or remote from people?	yes/no
During the past few weeks, have you ever felt pleased about having accomplished something?	yes/no

Two of the ten questions included in this scale are usually omitted in The Netherlands because they do not seem entirely appropriate for the Dutch context.

(m) A few examples from Nooy's cale:

When you get down to cases there are very few people who really care what happen to you?	yes/no
There are so many different ideas about what's right and wrong that you don't know what to think.	yes/no

Nooy's and Bradburn's scales were filled in by the respondents, and the VOEG was done by the interviewer.

obtained for various categories were:

Employed women (divorced/widowed)	2.66
Unemployed men	2.45
Unemployed women (divorced/widowed)	2.28
Partners of employed men	2.22
Partners of unemployed men	1.88
Employed men	1.63

The results do not yield a clear picture. Unemployed men scored appreciably higher than employed men, but neither their partners nor the other women showed a relationship with unemployement or living alone (the unemployed married women even scored the highest of all: 3.0).

Medical consumption, illness, and illness behaviour

The unemployed not only scored more negatively with respect to feeling well or subjective health but also assessed their own health more negatively than the employed did. The answers to this question of opinion gave the same picture as the VOEG.

The employed, both men and women, reported slightly more frequently about a handicap, a chronic disease (eg anginal heart condition, rheumatism, gout), or a chronic disorder (eg migraine, varicose veins, extremely high or low blood pressure), but the differences are not great. On the other side among the unemployed, there had been an accident in more families during the year preceding the study, but the difference is small there too. A greater difference was found for the consumption of medicines that can be purchased without prescription, or prescribed drugs, and being under treatment for a chronic or acute disease or disorder. This behaviour too was reported more frequently by the employed (men, women, and wives) when asked about the month preceding the interview. The unemployed, however, had spent more days in bed because of sickness (in the month before the intereview). Usually they had flu, a heavy cold, or a severe headache.

Among the interviewed men and women there were almost no differences in absenteeism due to sickness. For one divorced woman a distinct relationship was found between this kind of absence and the loss of her job, although she preferred not to admit this to herself. For the other men and women it seemed unlikely that such a relationship had existed.

It would not be difficult to conclude that the unemployed experience illness differently than the employed do, that their complaints are mainly attributable to reduced well being, and that for these complaints they go to bed slightly sooner and tend to be slower to take drugs or consult a doctor. This conclusion might well be correct, but it is premature on the basis of the present findings, and not only because of the size and composition of the sample.

Complaints due to chronic disease or disorder (eg pain in limbs caused by gout, heart palpitation or pain in the chest caused by anginal complaints) reached expression in the VOEG and in some cases this also holds for side effects of drugs (eg tiredness due to psycho active drugs). Nevertheless, the unemployed had higher VOEG scores than the employed, who had chronic diseases or disorders slightly more frequently and used medicines more.

Furthermore, the unemployed probably have a tendency to under report complaints and to show patient delay. For example, two of the unemployed men were handicapped by the severity of their psychological complaints, and one of them had even been placed in a protected workshop before his discharge. Neither of them considered himself to be ill, and both thought themselves moderately healthy. Others had had chronic complaints for many years but considered them as repetitive incidents (in contrast to the attitude of the employed) and tended to take them less seriously. A few mentioned in passing that they could not get themselves to go to the doctor. 'If I was working I would have gone long ago, because I wouldn't have been able to keep up the pace', said a man who had had back complaints for many years, 'but now I keep postponing it'. A woman with a spinal curvature said, 'This back does bother me, but the doctor would send me to a physiotherapist to straighten it out and that would cost eighty guilders which I don't have'.

It is clear that the subjective health of the unemployed was poorer than that of the employed, and that anxiety about job security can also be a threat to the health of the employed. This might also explain the more frequent use of drugs for 'minor complaints'. The findings do not justify further conclusions about health and illness. Even if we were to define health in terms of the absence of medically defined diseases (which, incidentaly, does not give better prediction as to help seeking behaviour or mortality than the subjective health does), it would not be possible to conclude either that the unemployed are healthier than the employed or that they are less healthy. Both would be premature because the findings suggest that a change occurrs in illness behaviour and ideas about illness after unemployment.

SUMMARY AND CONCLUSIONS

There are marked differences in the reaction to being unemployed, not only between men and women but also within both categories. Although there were men and women who thought it agreeable to be unemployed (a minority) and to whom it was a stressful life event, the picture is slightly clearer for the men. The men who considered unemployment abominable lacked the aspects known from the literature concerning the meaning of work, work as a means to acquire a social identity, as a means to acquire an income and prestige, work which regulates activity and contacts, and so on. A strongly negative reaction to unemployment coincides with the lack of perspective on the future and time itself. Existence takes on an ephemeral quality whose duration is unknown.

Past life events have no distinct relationship with the reaction to unemployment. Some men, however, saw a relationship between divorce and unemployment. Although many of the men felt their wife (partner) to be supportive, this support was not sufficient to alleviate the negative effects of being unemployed. These men had a tendency to close part of themselves off from the outside world, partially because they felt humiliated and partially because of irritability and uncertainly, or because these contacts were felt to be the opposite of support.

In the unemployed women the picture of the reaction to unemployment is more amorphous. Women living alone showed a strong tendency to become lonely. Many of them had not coped with earlier life events, and had many other worries as well. Some of them reported unusually many or unusually serious undesirable life events in their family. In particular there was somewhat more clustering of negative life events among the unemployed women living along. Unemployment and its consequences form part of a series of negative experiences. For this reason work is not always a solution, especially for those who still have children living at home. For some, a 'choice' between working and being unemployed is a 'choice' between two evils which it is beyond their ability to make. The women had very few supportive contacts.

A rather distinct relation was found between the degree to which being unemployed and/or the consequences of unemployment are experienced negatively and the number of health complaints. Other problems can strengthen this relationship. Women had more complaints than men, and many of them carried a double load for many years. However, it was also found for the employed men that the response to the atmosphere at work and the reaction to job insecurity were negative to strongly negative in those who scored high with respect to health complaints, and that this negative effect was greater than that of, say, the actual load imposed by the work.

Potential differences between employed and unemployed in the reaction to or ideas about illness and in behaviour during illness and when help is needed, impose heavy demands on the instruments used to measure illness and/or on the composition of the sample to be investigated.

The differences in the reaction to being unemployed and in the degree to which the employed feel uncertain about keeping their job and uncomfortable in their job or workplace, mean that neither group may be seen or analysed as a homogeneous population. Both the employed and the unemployed can include risk groups and groups without problems, which can influence the relations in the categories themselves as well as disturb or mask such relationships. Therefore, the importance of the detection of differences and points of agreement cannot be overestimated.

THE EFFECT OF UNEMPLOYMENT ON THE HEALTH OF WORKERS IN A UK STEEL TOWN: PRELIMINARY RESULTS

Gill Westcott

1. Introduction

The interviews for this survey were conducted in Scunthorpe, a town where the steel works have dominated the labour market and have halved their labour force in the last five years. Unemployment is therefore of recent origin but relatively severe, with the bulk of the increase in 1980 and 1981. Up to Spring 1981, most of those leaving the steel works were "voluntary" redundancies where workers had the option of retaining some job in the steel works, in the short term at least. Then and after, they left on relatively favourable terms paid for by the EEC fund. There are, however, a large number thrown out of work from other enterprises as a result of the steel cutbacks who have no such redundancy payments. The financial status of the unemployed in Scunthorpe thus varies greatly. Altogether, about 30% of the male workforce is unemployed, and in the first half of 1982 a large proportion of them had been out of a job for 12 to 24 months.

As described in another paper[(1)], the objective was twofold:

i) to discover whether any differences in health status existed between the employed and unemployed, controlling for age, class and sex;

ii) to discover the factors that were responsible for any differences observed, and to explain differences in health among the unemployed. Thus it was hoped to identify "maximum risk" factors and protective mechanisms.

The present sample (95) is too small to fulfil the latter task, but some evidence is available on the first question.

2. Methodology

2.1. The sample

Subjects were selected randomly from the electoral register (every 275th). Thus the sample was automatically stratified by residential area. Introductory letters were written to the subjects selected suggesting a time on which the interviewer would call, asking for a reply if this was not convenient.

In most cases the respondents forgot about the letter and were prepared to be interviewed at that time if they were at home. Interviews were done in 102 of the households, of the 177 selected.

---

(1) 'Proposed Research on the Effects of Unemployment on Health' in J. John, D. Schwefel and H. Zöllner (eds) "Influence of Economic Instability on Health", Springer Verlag, 1983.

This represents a response rate of 72% of those who were actually contacted. Table 1 shows what happened about the rest.

TABLE 1 Sample characteristics.

177 individuals selected -	102	interviewed
	23	out
	16	refused
	9	moved
	2	died
	25	not contacted due to lack of time
	177	

TABLE 2 Employment status of adults in households where interviews were carried out.

	M.	F.	Total
Fully employed (excl. MSC)	68	19	87
Part time employed	26	4	30
Part time unemployed (5 of which were employed part-time)	2	8	10
Fully unemployed	27	11	38
of which, registered:	(26)	(4)	
MSC schemes	4	1	5
Full time training - following redundancy	3		3
Not in labour force	18	54	72
	146	94	245

It was possible to interview fully 45 employed, 15 part time and 25 unemployed workers. Additional people were selected randomly from the electoral register and those who were unemployed and responded positively were interviewed, to increase the number of unemployed in the sample to 35.

Most of the interviews were carried out by the author, the others by two volunteers, both of whom were themselves unemployed. The spouses of first respondents were also interviewed whenever possible, though it was not always possible to do this separately.

2.2. Measures of health

A number of subjective measures of health status were used:-

i) Self-reported chronic illness or longstanding symptoms

ii) Self-reported symptoms within the last 3 years

iii) Self-reported changes in health within the last 2 years

iv) General Health Questionnaire (GHQ)

v) A version of the Cornell Medical Index (CMI) (used by Leonard Fagin [2])

vi) Daily Health Record (used by Kasl, Cobb et al [3])

These measures have been described in full and tested in a pilot study for this project [4]. However some comments are in order.

Self-reported illnesses and symptoms are necessarily a crude indicator of health status in the absence of medical qualifications of both the respondents and interviewers. Complaints were reported on a symptomatic basis, in answer to a large number of specific questions

The General Health Questionnaire has been found to detect psychiatric disorders among subjects interviewed from a general practice waiting room [4], and though it has been much used in studies of this kind [5] it has also been found less successful in predicting psychiatric disturbance in a community setting. Gibson et al found that using the 20 item GHQ and a (high) cutoff score of 516, less than half of those interviewed who scored above the cutoff point were found to have a clinically identified psychiatric disorder [6]. Half of those found having a psychiatric disturbance scored high on the GHQ. The correlation would have been greater had not those known to be suffering psychiatric illness or a recent emotional disturbance been deleted from the same by GP's, but nevertheless the GHQ misses a high proportion of those suffering chronic psychiatric illness because of its form of words. It may still, however, be a good indication of the relative frequency with which new psychiatric disturbances will be found in a particular group. The proportions of employed and unemployed having high GHQ scores when unemployment is of recent (ie. within 2 years') origin appears still to indicate propensity to new mental illnesses.

---

(2) "Unemployment and Health in Families", Dr L. Fagin, DHSS, UK, 1981.

(3) 1981 S.V. Kasl and S. Cobb "Termination: The Consequences of Job Loss", US, DHEW, National Institute for Occupational Safety and Health, Cincinnati, Ohio, June 1977.

(4) D. Goldberg "Detection of Psychiatric Illness by Questionnaire", Oxford University Press, London, 1972.

(5) eg. E.M. Stafford, P.R. Jackson & M.H. Banks "Employment, Work Involvement and Mental Health in less qualified young people" J. Occupational Psychology, 1980 53 291-304.

(6) A.J. Gibson et al "Antecedents of Emotional Distress: Community Prevalence" Paper presented at the Annual Conference of British Psychological Socy, University of Surrey, April 9th-13th 1981.

The Cornell Medical Index, on the other hand, does reflect chronic conditions as well as short term psychiatric disturbance, although some of the questions are very similar to those of the GHQ and have not been duplicated in the final questionnaire.

2.3. Health Risk Factors

Information was also collected on:

- housing
- smoking
- alcohol consumption
- social contact and support
- financial status (income and redundancy payments)
- life activities

as well as any changes in these factors over the last 2 years. (Thus changes connected with other life events were also recorded.)

The respondents' attitudes to their unemployment was also explored: whether their redundancy had been technically 'voluntary' or not, and whether they had desired it or not.

3. Results

3.1. Self-perceived Health Status

Too few of the respondents reported a change in their general health to identify systematic differences between employed and unemployed. However such differences did emerge in an analysis of reported symptoms suffered in the last two years.

For the purpose of this analysis, only those having occurred since the last change of employment status were counted, although anxieties related to redundancy had clearly contributed to the symptoms of at least two of those who were not in the unemployed sample. (One had developed very high blood pressure but had regained employment after redundancy, and one suffered worsening diabetes and was still registered sick over a year after his redundancy.)

The symptoms were grouped according to whether or not the respondents attributed them to work. (Most of the attributions were in respect of injuries sustained at work, burns, gassing, etc.)

Table 2 (over) shows that the unemployed reported proportionately more symptoms than the employed, but the difference was only marked in the case of new symptoms which were not work-related. This was despite the shorter average period (of unemployment) over which symptoms were counted; and the difference remained when the sample was split into two by geographical area.

This finding suggests that any excess morbidity in the unemployed is not mainly due to their greater general propensity for reporting symptoms, otherwise this would also have been manifested in chronic and work-related symptoms.

TABLE 2: Self-reported symptoms in employed and unemployed men and women

	Currently suffered symptoms			
	Average no. per person Attributed to work		Average no. per person Not attributed to work	
	Old*	New*	Old*	New*
Employed (N = 45)	.133	.111	.444	.222
Part-time workers (N = 13)	.154	0.0	.538	.308
Unemployed				
i) Random sample (N = 27)	.148	.037	.666	.666
ii) With extras (N = 36)	.194	.250	.611	.694

* New symptoms were defined as those originating within the last two years, or since the last change of employment status, whichever period was the shorter. Old symptoms were defined as those originating prior to that but still being suffered.

Sometimes respondents themselves reported contradictory changes in health over their period of unemployment; for example, Mr. P. He said that he had had migraine but that it had faded away when he stopped having to look at the flames in the furnace and eased off reading. He also said that he got depressed. For the first few months, he used to drink heavily, but had recently given this up.

> "I never got pills. Mind you, I've thought about doing things. There are some folks committed suicide over it .... I've felt a bit chesty lately. I had a bit of pain, but the X-ray showed nothing".

He had also gained in weight and was in the habit of waking up at 4 or 5 in the morning if he didn't retire very late. His dermatatis has subsided since he left work.

Among other unemployed men over 45 these kinds of changes seemed not uncommon, though depression and drinking were rarely referred to.

Table 4: Measures of health for employed and unemployed men

a) Reported recent symptoms

	Employed	Unemployed
None	37	8
Up to 1 episode a year	25	5
More than one episode a year	8	10

X^2 = 11.405 Significance= 0.0033

b) Days' complaint in fortnights' health record

	Employed	Unemployed
None	46	13
1 - 3 days	2	2
4 - 14 days	10	5

X^2 = 2.113 Significance = 0.3477

c) General Health Questionnaire score

	Employed	Unemployed
0 (low)	25	4
1 - 5 (medium)	13	12
6 - 20 (high)	8	6

X^2 = 8.0669 Significance = 0.0177

d) Cornell Medical Index score

	Employed	Unemployed
0 (low)	18	4
1 - 5 (medium)	22	15
6 - 15 (high)	6	3

X^2 = 3.1560 Significance = 0.2064

Tables 4a to 4d have been used to test the significance of the differences in health experience between employed (full and part-time) and unemployed men. The association between employment status and recent symptoms was found to be significant at the .01 level. The relationship with GHQ score was also significant ($p < .02$); but with othervariables the relationships were not significant.

The same tests indicated somewhat less significant differences in health measured by recent symptoms between manual and nonmanual workers, but more significant differences in the number of days' complaint recorded. This suggests that men in manual work were sometimes more reticent to report their symptoms than to put crosses on a fortnightly health record. This would be understandable with a female interviewer. If so it indicates that the former measure, at least, will have underestimated symptoms relatively in those classes.

As one would expect, older workers also reported significantly more symptoms.

An examination of the age and class distribution of the respondents showed that somewhat more of the unemployed tended to be older and in lower class occupations than the employed, though both were heavily in the skilled manual classes. To see whether the apparent association between health and employment status was due to these factors, two groups matched for age, sex and class were chosen from the sample. A comparison of health indicators using these groups is shown in Table 5. The conclusions derived from the larger sample are borne out in that significant health differences appear in the average number of symptoms reported per year, and in the number scoring 4 or more on the GHQ. The employed in the matched groups had slightly more days' complaint than the unemployed, and the other differences were in the expected direction but insignificant.

Table 5: Indicators of health in a matched sample (men)

Indicator	Employed	Unemployed
Average no. of chronic illnesses reported	0.333 (N=18)	0.375 (N=16)
Average no. of recent illnesses reported	0.422 (N=18)	0.750 (N=16)
$X^2 = 1.668 \quad 0.05 < p < 0.10$		
Average days' complaint	1.75 (N=16)	1.533 (n=15)
Average days on which medicine taken	1.00 (N=16)	1.933 (N=15)
Av. days on which a doctor was seen	0.313 (N=16)	0.375 (N=16)
GHQ No. scoring < 4	9	2
≥ 4	6	12
$p < 0.025 \quad X^2 = 4.63$		
CMI No. scoring ≥ 4	2	6
< 4	10	9

3.2. Health Risk Factors

A study of health risk factors showed that in the matched sample (22 pairs) the unemployed appeared more often to be smokers, and on average to smoke more. This was borne out by results from the sample as a whole. (see Tables 6 and 7). However a greater number of the unemployed had both increased and cut down their smoking in the last two years. Those who had cut down had done so mainly because of the expense, and it was the better off unemployed who smoked more.

It is questionable whether alcohol consumption in the amounts admitted here is in fact a health risk factor, particularly when it is so frequently associated with social contact. However the results are given in Tables 8 and 9. They show that on average, alcohol consumption by the unemployed was higher than by the employed in the matched sample, and lower in the whole sample.

Both results again conceal a disparity, between 14 who cut down their drinking, and two who increased it, both in the matched sample, and both brewing or making their own beer, wine or spirits.
The results of this question are also thought to be particularly suspect. Nevertheless the overall results are not incompatible with the observation that beer sales drop during a recession like those of other consumption goods.

It has already been noted how much the financial status of the unemployed varied. BSC redundancy payments of up to £15,000 and over were made, depending on age, salary and period of work at BSC, together with make-up pay of 90% of the former salary for 12 months and 80% for a further 6 months. For men under 55 this was conditional on having another job.

These payments certainly postponed the financial stress which was experienced by other unemployed people. Many had used their money to buy houses, thus achieving a permanent effect on their financial situation. (It should be added that house repairs were often a major worry among council tenants and unemployed home owners).

In men on make-up pay, anxiety was still evident about the time when it would run out - an anxiety often submerged by a determination to enjoy what they felt they had earned with a long working life.

However the redundancy payments were also extremely divisive. Compared to the feelings of melancholy and uselessness of those who had them, there was sometimes anger among those who did not and had exhausted savings and were living from one bill to the next. An acute dilemma was posed to those who wanted to travel to look for work but couldn't afford the financial risk.

A few of those on very low incomes had aquired a distinct pattern of adaptation. Most of the men were middleaged and older, unskilled workers. Their wives were at home, but the extended family or social network of the older council estates provided social support. Local clubs or pubs allowed the traditional separation of mens' and womens' environments to continue. It is not possible even to guess whether this affected illness or not. If advantageous to the men it was not necessarily so for the women. But it certainly eased acceptance of more straightened financial circumstances, and in two cases was known to provide a network for exchange of skills (and maybe some extra remuneration).

The skilled workers more often had working wives, and were more isolated socially. In one very new part of an estate, not one call elicited a response. This was explained by a Yorkshire woman living there who said "They think you're the rent collector. I don't know why they're so stuck up around here - they're all in arrears".

External links were not always of a direct socializing or family nature. One unemployed man had been a jockey in his youth in Ireland, and lived a comparatively isolated life on a council estate, making a daily small investment on the horses. In addition to his wife, who was a radiant personality, his love of nature and specualtive thoughtfulness about the world kept the isolation from being total.

3.3. Attitudes to unemployment

Some had accepted redundancy genuinely glad of a chance to retire early on relatively good terms. These reasons were mainly to do with their own or their spouse's health, or their nearness to retirement making the deal financially irresistable. Others were pressured by the suggestion that there would be future redundancies on poorer terms, or by the closure of their plant and the offer of alternative jobs which they thought unsuitable. A few accepted redundancy for the sake of younger workers. In all of these groups it was not apparent that the formal 'voluntariness' of their redundancy made any difference to the way they felt about being unemployed, if no other pressing reasons were present.

There was a surprising degree of self-blame apparent in the unemployed towards their situation, both in a collective sense - very many thought that overmanning and pressure for higher wages were responsible for the levels of joblessness - but also individually in that they felt they should be doing something, such as being compelled to do work in the community interest from time to time. (Even though some recognized the conflict between this and believing that people ought to be paid proper wages for socially useful work.) Their views about the causes of unemployment, and their suggestions for ways of improving the situation in Scunthorpe indicated a hopelessness and passivity which would also inhibit any initiave on their part, either collective or individual, to relieve or reduce unemployment. This will be described separately.

4. Conclusions

Unemployed male workers in Scunthorpe experienced significantly more symptoms in their period of unemployment than employed workers of the same age and class. The differences between the two groups in the average number of days' complaint and treatment in the fortnight's health record were insignificant. The symptoms which accounted for this difference were mainly of recent origin.

A contributing factor to this finding may have been the higher proportion of unemployed who smoked, and the more intensive smoking. The evidence on alcohol consumption was ambiguous. As with smoking, the averages conceal important differences due to varying financial and social circumstances, with the conflicting influences of stress and boredom, and expense. It is unfortunate that the sample size was too small to identify the impact of these underlying variables.

As reflected by the larger proportion with high GHQ scores, the likelihood of unemployed respondents developing psychiatric disturbances was greater than that of employed workers. Scores from the CMI (reflecting more chronic states of distress) did not differ significantly though the average score of the unemployed was higher.

TABLE 6 Smoking in a matched sample (men)

	Employed (N=18)	Unemployed (N=17)
Av. smoking (cigarettes per day) per person	9.89	16.88
No. who smoked (%)	10 (55%)	12 (71%)
Av. cigarettes per day per smoker	17.8	23.2

TABLE 7 Smoking in whole sample

	Employed (N=45)	Unemployed (N=33)
Av. smoking (cigarettes per day) per person	8.8	24.5
Av. cigarettes per day per smoker	18.8	32.3
No. who smoked (%)	21 (46%)	25 (75%)
Increased in last 2 years	3 (6.6%)	5 (15%)
Cut down in last 2 years	10 (22.2%)	13 (39%)

TABLE 8 Alcohol consumption admitted in a matched sample (men)

	Employed (N=18)	Unemployed (N=17)
Av. No. of pints, glasses of wine, or tots of spirits per day	1.278	2.00

TABLE 9 Alcohol consumption admitted in whole sample

	Employed (N=45)	Unemployed (N=33)
Av. no. of pints, glasses of wine, or tots of spirits per day	1.51	1.39
Av. no. who increased over last 2 years	3	2
Av. no. who decreased over last 2 years	7	14

5. Further Research

The present sample was interviewed again in 1983 and early 1984, together with a much larger sample of 843 employed and unemployed people and their spouses. Preliminary analysis of this data confirms that both unemployed men and women were more likely to have high GHQ and CMI scores ($p < .001$) when age structure and occupational class were controlled, and those with prior illnesses were excluded. Women had higher scores than men, both among the employed and the unemployed. Among the unemployed, those who had cut down on expenditure the most and were most worried about money were significantly more likely to have high GHQ and CMI scores and to report more new physical symptoms, even when those with any illness or symptom prior to unemployment were excluded.

Further analysis of associations between health variables and possible 'risk' and 'protective' factors mediating the effects of unemployment upon health is in progress. The results of second interviews, from a year to 18 months after the first, should also provide information on any changes in health status associated with changes in employment. However evidence from this study would still need to be treated with caution. Health risks arise from a person's entire history, and job loss and re-employment could have a cumulative effect.

The results from this project do nevertheless support the findings of many other studies which suggest that there are systematic, significant and sometimes serious health consequences of unemployment. In communicating these findings to policy-makers and to the general public, it is also perhaps important to remember the number of unemployed people in this audience, and that it cannot be suggested from these results that there is anything inevitable about the health hazards of being jobless from the point of view of the unemployed individual.

HEALTH PROBLEMS IN THE INITIAL PHASE OF UNEMPLOYMENT

Some Research Findings and Policy Implications

Christian Brinkmann

Methods

In mid November 1981 the Institute of Employment Research, which is part of the Federal Institute of Labour, started a new longitudinal survey of newly registered unemployed in order to obtain more detailed information about labour market risk factors, reemployment difficulties and the use of labour market policy instruments. In 25 (out of nearly 150) local Labour Offices all over the Federal Republic of Germany about 8,000 German nationals were selected and reported to our institute, together with some information about the unemployed (including main reason for dismissal and self reported health problems considered relevant for reemployment efforts).

After about 5/6 weeks, in three different sub samples first interviews took place: postal questioning of all unemployed under 25 years of age, and postal or oral interviews with unemployed 25 years or older. The more extensive personal interviews contained a number of questions on health problems. The first results from this sub sample (nearly 2,000 interviews with unemployed 25 years or older) will be presented here. Since a global assessment of health status was also included in the postal interviews, a comparison of results was possible.

One year after drawing the sample, in November 1982, further information was gathered from Labour Offices about the unemployed (employment status, if still or again unemployed, reemployment difficulties, use of labour market policy instruments). A second largely standardized interview had been planned for the spring of 1983. The group selected for personal interviews again were to be asked in detail about health problems, using the same indicators.

The study includes a large number of work related and unemployment related factors, some of them (assumedly relevant to health problems) are listed in Table 4.

To measure health problems, some indicators especially developed and validated for use in population surveys by the Medis Institute in Munich were included (Peter Potthoff 1982):

- Global assessment of health status in the past 2 weeks (GAH)
- Global rating of chronic impairments lasting for several years (used as explanatory factor in the following analysis only)
- Common Complaint Scale (CCS) using 11 items referring to somatic or psychosomatic complaints and dysfunctions (compare Table 2)
- Scale on Psychical Balance (PSB) using 9 items mainly derived from a depressivity scale (compare Table 3).

For those indicators Medis Institute kindly supplied structurally adjusted data from their population survey in the city of Munich (1981/82).

Psycho social strain factors (1-10) are the same used in the IAB follow up study of unemployed (1974/76) reported in Brinkmann (1983). One statement ("I feel absolutely useless sometimes") was excluded from the analysis because it overlapped with the newly introduced Scale on Physical Balance.

Four questions on social support available for unemployed (in case of financial or psycho social problems) are translations from the questionnaire of Gill Westcott (see ch 10) thus making possible some comparisons.

To measure work orientation, the statements and procedure of Dieter Frohlich were adopted (Dieter Frohlich 1983) (ratings of 6 statements according to personal preferences).

Some limitations have to be kept in mind when considering the following results:

- some questions can only be dealt with when reporting the results of the second interview.

- Model building has just begun. The overview presented here relies on tree analyses (reduction of variance by diverse independent variables on subjective health indicators by successively splitting up the population of unemployed into two subgroups).

However, because of the poor measurement of many variables, more refined multivariate methods of analysis have severe limitations in any case.

- In some cases more complex variables have still to be constructed (for instance weighting strain factors of the last workplace with the time actually having worked in this place).

- Group specific analyses still have to be undertaken (for instance for unskilled workers only).

- The time of the first interviews (5/6 weeks after becoming unemployed) is far from being ideal for dealing with the problem of isolating influences of unemployment on health from other influences. For organisational reasons it was not possible to have intereviews prior to that time. Yet, this is the first time in the FRG that a representative survey has covered the initial phase of unemployment; memory problems and perceptual distortions may be less impotant than in former surveys. And, at least one set of health data originates from the very beginning of unemployment: health problems considered relevant for reemployment at the time of registering were reported from local Labour Offices at that time.

- All results of the survey necessarily refer to subjective health only. As far as the Medis indicators mentioned above are concerned, however, selection and validating procedures "seem to assure that they are meaningful and valid operational definitions of health" (Peter Potthoff 1982). (Included were ratings of a group of physicians and patients about the importance of the items for the description of the person's health status, correlations with drug consumption and contact with physicians in the past two weeks, number of chronic conditions in the past year and other comparisons).

First results on physical health

Statistics about the pool of unemployed people and former surveys in Germany all show a large overrepresentation of people with health problems. For severely handicapped persons it could be shown that their unemployment rate was roughly twice the overall unemployment rate (Brinkmann 1981). This may be due to:

- negative selection processes when losing jobs/entering unemployment,
- reduced reemployment chances for those having health problems, and finally to
- damaging effects of unemployment itself to be dealt with here.

The great reduction in reemployment chances has already been clearly demonstrated (Brinkmann 1978).

The entrance "barrier" to unemployment does not seem to have much of a discriminating effect, however: flow statistics available since May 1980 show that the proportion of people already having health problems (relevant to reemployment efforts) when becoming unemployed is only about half the proportion in the stock of unemployed.*

How far unemployment in the long run produces (additional) health problems for the unemployed is one of our major research questions to be answered when the follow up interviews are available (Brinkmann 1984). As far as the first weeks of unemployment are concerned, results of the present survey show that contrary to our prior expectation unemployment itself does not affect physical health status to a great extent.

The global assessment of health status (GAH) and items used in the Common Complaint Scale (CCS) show that in the initial phase of unemployment, people have just as many or even fewer physical health problems than people in employment (Tables 1 and 2). The fact that the comparison was made only with population of one city does not seem to be a major problem. The 'control group' were standardised for age and sex structure, and the influences of some other factors (like qualification level) are marginal.

Differences in GAH results between oral and postal interviews should be noted. (Only this question was used in both subsamples of unemployed 25 years or older). In oral interviews the health status appears more positive, people obviously hestiate to admit such problems in the usual interview situation.

---

* In September 1981, 30,5% of the stock of unemployed had health problems relevant to re-employment efforts, as compared to 16,3% of entrants of May 81 and 13,8% of the entrants of May 82. (Such statistics are available for these times of the year only.)

Thus a direct comparison of interview data on health is possible only if data were collected the same way. Postal interviews of unemployed and employed people yield very similar GAH results.

In our unemployment survey CCS items (as well as items on Psychical Balance, see below) were included in personal interviews only. However, these parts were self administered, unemployed writing down their responses by themselves. Thus a rough comparison with data of a postal population survey should be possible. The somewhat more positive results of the unemployed on CCS items may nevertheless be influenced by the remaining difference in method and therefore should not be overinterpreted.

Additional results of the survey give indications as to why, in the first weeks of unemployment, the physical health of unemployed people at least on the average compares favourably with that of people in employment. Consider the following assessments of the health effects of the last job and of becoming unemployed (referring to unemployed with previous job experience only):

How did you feel in the evening after work? Were you usually in the evening		
	very "worn out"	21%
	somewhat "worn out"	26%
	a bit "worn out"	36%
	not at all "worn out"	17%
		100%
		n = 1 762

Did your last job affect your health negatively?		
	yes, that is true	24%
	no, that is not true	76%
		100%
		n = 1 762

In general: Do you consider your health today (without this job) better, about equal, or worse?		
	better	22%
	equal	61%
	worse	17%
		100%
		n = 1 762

Obviously, in the opinion of the unemployed themselves health hazards connected with the last working place compensate or even overcompensate health hazards connected with the initial phase of unemployment. Which subgroups of unemployed think more about improvements than about deterioration of health in this phase still needs to be analysed.

Additional information results from tree analyses with GAH and CCS as dependent variables and dichotomous splits on the basis of maximal reduction of inter-group variance due to independent factors (demography, work history, work orientation, factors connected with the last working place and factors connected with the unemployment situation itself). Table 4 contains the reduction of variance of all variables considered (first level of analysis; the higher the percentage, the stronger the association), Figures 1 and 2 contain the final 'trees'.

As can be seen, financial strains, psycho social strain due to unemployment, and prospects of finding a new job do have an influence in GAH and CCS, but only a very moderate one, in this initial phase of unemployment (their influence on mental well being is quite high, however). Factors related to the time prior to unemployment dominate the GAH and CCS scores. There might be some perceptual distortion with the highest loading factor ("did last job affect health negatively", variable no 27). But other variables indicating bad health prior to unemployment (reason for last dismissal; a past change in occupation because of health reasons; self reported health problems at the time of registering (nos) 10, 15, 20, 21) should not be contaminated; all of them are more highly associated with GAH and CCS than strain due to unemployment.

Dichotomizing GAH in a different way such that a hard core of unemployed with poor health or acute illness within the last two weeks is separated from all others and then using the remaining scores as independent variable leads to some modification: Work orientation, financial problems and psycho social strains connected with unemployment reveal some additional influence on health, but only in 3rd and 4th level splits. Including Psychical Balance (PSB) in this part of the analysis leads to splits on account of this factor. Such an influence, however, may only partially be interpreted as a consequence of unemployment.

First results on mental well being

Even if on the average the first weeks unemployment do not change physical health very much, almost half of the unemployed (44%) strongly feel strain when becoming unemployed. Of those laid off (not having quitted by themselves) 41% also felt acute strain in the time between dismissal and registering unemployed, 45% said they "waited to see" what happened.

As may be expected, there is a relation between the global assessment of strain (GAS) felt in the initial phase of unemployment and financial problems. But psycho social problems play an evermore significant role, especially the uncertainty about future work prospects and the boring questions about the reason for having become unemployed (Table 4). In tree analysis with GAS as dependent variable, all splits are along the index of psycho social strain, single strain factors and the subjective chance of finding a new job.

As an indicator of mental well being, the Psychical Balance Scale (PSB) of the Medis Institute, roughly measuring depressivity, was included in our survey. Unlike the physicial health indicators, scores on the items of PSB are more negative for unemployed people than for employed (Table 3). For instance, 20% of the unemployed say they are most of the time or always afraid of the future, as compared to 6% of people in employment. 12% of the unemployed say that most of the time or always they cannot sit quietly because of restlessness, as compared to 5% of people in employment.

A rather strong influence of unemployment on PSB in the first weeks of unemployment shows up in multivariate analysis also. Psycho social strain on various dimensions as well as financial strain are associated with PSB most clearly, physical health (whether or not affected by unemployment) also playing a major role (Table 4 and the tree analysis of Figure 3).

The relationship between physical health and mental well being partially concerns health problems prior to unemployment, but only partially since the overall association between GAH and CCS with PSB is high (9% reduction of variance). Since PSB is both associated with strains due to unemployment and with physical health, one would expect (in a dynamic model) a deterioration of physical health as a consequence of long term (or repeated) unemployment, mental health being an intervening variable in this relationship*.

Policy related questions

For a number of reasons not directly linked with health problems, steeply rising unemployment in many countries calls for fundamental changes in economic and labour market policy. Involuntary unemployment always means a loss in private and public welfare, and it may also destabilize political systems. Some such consequences may in the long run influence the health status of a population, too (rising number of homeless, cuts in health service budgets etc).

Due to a rising labour force potential and a long run decline in economic growth rates a sizable reduction of unemployment in the medium term, at least in Germany, cannot be achieved without a massive reduction in hours of work of one kind or another. Selection processes in the labour market unfavourable for unemployed with health problems (as well as for other groups of unemployed, for instance older workers) call in addition, for selective labour market policy measures. Whether or not health problems arise in direct connection wih unemployment, they reduce reemployment chances considerably. In Germany, the Labour Promotion Act of 1969 provides a number of instruments to improve chances for occupational reintegration:

- work creation especially for long term unemployed
- vocational training and retraining
- 4/6 weeks courses to improve information and motivation of unemployed
- wages cost subsidies

There has been a tendency, however, to cut spending on these measures, to a large extent, to neglect the costs unemployment implies for unemployed people as well as for the public, and to neglect the alleviating effect some of these selective measures (work creation schemes) also have on the overall employment situation.

On a more prophylactic level, apparently there is an urgent need for more counselling, information and coordination of help within labour offices and in relation to other institutions. 44% of the unemployed in our sample (not back in employment after 5/6 weeks) would like to have more information and counselling on a large variety of topics including (several responses possible):

- how to fill in application forms (7%)

---

* Results of the follow-up survey (Summer 1983) indeed revealed such a deterioration of physical (and more so of mental) health (Brinkmann 1984).

- how to cope with rising job requirements (8%)
- how to cope with personal problems (9%)
- how to cope with the problem of unemployment in general (17%)
- at help or financial support may be obtained by institutions other than the Labour Office (22%)

In contrast the rising demand for counselling (due to rising numbers of unemployed as well as to the more problematic situation each unemployed person is confronted with) counselling capacities within Labour Offices were even reduced recently in order to ensure punctual payments of unemployment benefits.

At least for sizable groups of unemployed stigmatization and isolation are real problems. 25% of the unemployed (25 years or older, 5/6 weeks afterwards still or again unemployed) did not find it "easy to tell friends and acquaintances about it" (23% undecided, 51% no problem). 20% of them did not visit friends and acquaintances as often as before (23% undecided, 56% no problem). As with other psycho social strains, these factors are clearly linked to mental well being and also to physical health (moderately within the first weeks of unemployment, but probably more so in the long run).

Asked about "social support", the following results were found (again referring to persons 25 years or older (still or again unemployed), 5/6 weeks after registration:

If you are in financial difficulties are there any friends or relatives you could go to to help you out?	yes	36%
among them:		
Would you actually go to ask them?	yes	24%
	no	64%
		100%
		n = 1680

If you are feeling down, or want some company, are there friends or relatives you could go to?	yes	65%
among them:		
Would you actually contact them?	yes	49%
	no	35%
		100%
		n = 1680

In relation to strain felt in the initial phase of unemployment there is a slight but statistically not significant tendency to have less support available for those feeling such strain.

Insufficient "social support", stigmatization and isolation call for more efforts towards the integration of the unemployed into the social network of friends and neighbourhoods as well as in social institutions and society at large. In Germany, until recently even labour unions were very hesitant in this respect.

Recent experience with large scale lay offs in Germany may change public opinion towards the unemployed and the way they cope with their situation. More participation in local "unemployment initiatives" and a first central meeting of unemployed in Frankfurt early December of 1982 are perhaps steps in this direction. Much more seems to be necessary, however, to influence in any substantial way fundamental relationships between unemployment and health dimensions.

In international comparison, financial regulations for unemployed are very different. Effects of this on the association between unemployment and health have to be assumed. Not all the strains connected with unemployment by far, but a considerable proportion of them, are directly or indirectly linked with the question of financial security, as can be seen from the influence of financial indicators (variable no 33 and 34) on health in Table 4.

In Germany these regulations are more favourable for the unemployed than in some other countries (roughly 68% of net earnings as insurance benefits for one year, if previous employment was long enough; afterwards up to 58% unemployment benefits depending on total family income). Nevertheless, for a great number of unemployed these regulations prove inadequate. Even in the first weeks of unemployment, 30% of them have "great financial difficulties", 49% "moderate" ones. A certain relief, partial at least and for a limited time, may come from savings of their own; but only 17% of unemployed say they can rely on this. 5% of unemployed received social welfare benefits at the time of questionning. As a recent study on pauperism in Germany shows, the number of people entitled to social welfare is probably twice the actual figures (Helmut Hartmann 1981) many for various reasons not taking advantage of it.

According to an earlier unemployment study the proportions of welfare recipients is as high as about 25% when unemployment lasts for 2 years or longer. At present, in Germany the average duration of unemployment rose to 6 months in 1982, as compared with 5 months in 1981 and about 2 months around 1970.* In connection with this ongoing development a deterioration of the financial status of unemployed in Germany has to be expected.

Furthermore, recent legislation reduced unemployment insurance benefits by some technical means (not counting special payments etc). Still more restrictions

---

* One period of unemployment may be interrupted up to 13 weeks (due to sickness, a period of work or other reasons) and still be considered as one period, times of interruptions not being counted when computing the duration. The figures cited refer to a completed period of unemployment.

are on the way (changing the requirements concerning previous time of employment etc). In view of these political efforts there should be a public awareness of the existing link between financial security and health.

Bibliography

Brinkmann, Christian, (1978) 'Strukturen und Determinanten der beruflichen Wiedereingliederung von Langfristarbeitslosen', in, MittAB 2.

Brinkmann, Christian, (1983) 'Health Problems and Psycho-Social Strains of Unemployed', in J. John, D. Schwefel, H. Zollner (eds.), Influence of Economic Instability on Health, Proceedings of a Symposium in Munich, September 1981, Springer Verlag, Berlin, Heidelberg, New York, Tokyo, 1983 (no. 21 of Lecture Notes in Medical Informatics).

Brinkmann, Christian, (1984) 'Physical Health and Mental Well-being - Results of a Longitudinal Survey in the Federal Republic of Germany', in W. V. Eimeren, R. Engelbrech, Ch. D. Flagle (eds.), Third International Conference on System Science in Health Care, Springer Verlag, Berlin, Heidelberg, 1984.

Frohlich Dieter, (1983) 'Economic Deprevation, Work Orientation and Health - Conceptual Ideas and Some Empirical Findings', in J. John et al, op. cit.

Hartmann, Helmut, (1981) Sozialhilfebedurftigkeit und 'Dunkelziffer der Armut;, Stuttgart, Berlin, Koln, Mainz, 1981 (Schriftenreihe des Bundesministeriums fur Jugend, Familie und G sundheit).

Potthoff, Peter, (1982) 'Subjective Health Status components in a General Population Survey', in R. R. O'Moore, Medical Informations Europe 82, Berlin, Heidelberg, New York, 1982, (vol. 16 of series 'Lecture Notes in Medical Informations').

Table 1: Global Assessment of Health Status in the Past Two Weeks (GAH)
Results from Unemployment Survey and population Survey, in %

	German unemployed of Nov. 1981, 25 years or older 5-6 weeks after becoming unemployed		Inhabitants of the city of Munich; Bavaria, 25 years or older, in employment, adjusted to age and sex structure of unemployed** post interviews, 1980/81
	a) oral interveiws	b) post interviews*	
Please think about your health within the last 2 weeks: Which of these statements about health would you agree to most?			
A In the last 2 weeks my health status was excellent	32.8	21.7	19.5
B In the last 2 weeks my health status was good	36.2	30.8	35.5
C In the last 2 weeks I had some occasional complaints, but in general my health was satisfactory	20.1	26.7	26.1
D In the last 2 weeks I was in a state of poor health	8.0	12.3	8.7
E In the last 2 weeks I was ill for a shorter or longer period	2.9	8.5	10.2
Sum	100	100	100
Base (n)	1887	1297	930

* provisional results, weighting procedure still pending

** unpublished results, kindly supplied by P Potthoff, Medis-Institute, Munich

Table 2: Common Complaints - Selected Items* Used in Common Complaints Scale (CCS)
Results from Unemployment Survey and Population Survey, in %

How much do you suffer from the following complaints?	German unemployed of Nov. 1981 25 years or older, 5-6 weeks after becoming unemployed (self-administrated part within oral interview					Inhabitants of the city of Munich, Bavaria, 1980/81, 25 years or older, in employment, adjusted to age and sex-structure of unemployed**, (postal inteviews)				
	not at all	scarcely	moderately	strongly	sum	not at all	scarcely	moderately	strongly	sum
1 Feeling of heaviness and tiredness in the legs	66.0	13.8	13.5	6.7	100	56.4	20.2	17.4	6.0	100
2 Sleeplessness	63.3	17.6	11.9	7.2	100	56.5	24.2	14.3	5.0	100
3 Feeling of dizziness, feeling giddy	72.2	13.7	10.1	4.0	100	61.5	24.4	11.5	2.6	100
4 Headache, pressure in the head, pains in the face	58.0	20.0	14.6	7.4	100	47.7	26.9	18.8	6.6	100
5 Complaints in connection with seeing and hearing	75.5	10.3	11.3	3.0	100	67.1	15.3	14.4	3.2	100
6 Heart pain or arhythmia	73.7	12.3	10.0	4.0	100	64.6	20.6	12.1	2.7	100
7 Body pains (including stomach pains, abdominal pains)	75.5	12.5	8.8	3.3	100	64.7	20.2	11.8	3.3	100
8 State of inner tension, restlessness	64.0	15.9	14.5	5.7	100	49.7	28.0	15.9	5.6	100
9 Allergy, skin diseases	85.4	6.0	5.3	3.2	100	(59.5)	(18.8)	(15.3)	(6.3)	100
10 Spinal affection	54.9	14.9	16.4	13.8	100	(28.1)	(27.9)	(31.9)	(12.1)	100
11 Pains in the joints	69.5	10.9	10.4	9.2	100	(59.9)	(18.4)	(16.1)	(5.6)	100

* selected in co-operation with Medis-Institute, Munich
** unpublished results, kindly supplied by P Potthoff, Medis-Institute, Munich

Table 3: Psychical Balance: Items used in the Psychical Balance Scale (PBS)
Results from Unemployment Survey and Population Survey, in %

How often are the following statements true of you?	German unemployed of Nov. 1981 25 years or older, 5-6 weeks after becoming unemployed (self-administrated part within oral interview)						Inhabitants of the city of Munich, Bavaria, 1980/81, 25 years or older, in employment, adjusted to age and sex-structure of unemployed**, (postal inteviews)					
	never	seldom	now and again	most of the time	always	sum	never	seldom	now and again	most of the time	always	sum
1 I feel dejected and melancholic	38.2	27.3	25.7	7.0	1.8	100	38.2	34.9	23.9	2.9	0.1	100
2 I have no feelings	64.7	16.4	10.7	2.5	5.6	100	58.7	23.1	10.7	3.9	3.6	100
3 I am in an excellent mood	4.8	13.5	25.1	40.5	16.2	100	2.6	9.4	18.6	61.4	8.0	100
4 I am interested in many things in life	1.1	3.3	14.1	41.7	39.8	100	0.7	3.1	11.7	47.0	37.5	100
5 I feel restless and cannot sit quietly	35.0	30.9	22.0	7.4	4.7	100	36.2	36.3	19.5	6.1	1.9	100
6 I enjoy life	1.4	3.6	13.7	36.0	45.3	100	1.1	1.7	10.3	41.6	45.4	100
7 I feel there is nobody I am close to	49.5	24.8	11.3	5.4	8.9	100	32.5	33.9	16.9	7.6	9.1	100
8 I am glad to have achieved much in life	5.1	10.9	23.4	29.5	31.1	100	2.1	5.2	20.8	36.8	35.1	100
9 I am afraid of the future	30.9	20.3	29.2	11.0	8.6	100	40.7	29.0	24.7	4.2	1.4	100

** unpublished results, kindly supplied by P Potthoff, Medis-Institute, Munich

Table 4: German Unemployed of Nov 1981, 25 years or older, previously in employed, about 5-6 weeks after becoming unemployed: effects of demographic, biographi work-related, and unemployment-related factors on strains and on health, measured by reduction of variance in % of total variance (effects of splitting into two two subgroups according to first stage of tree analysis, AID 3 of OSIRIS)

Independent variables	Variable No.	included in final tree analysis
Demographic factors, work history, work orientation		
Age	1	
Sex/Marital Status	2	
Number of Members of Household	3	x
Structure of Household (married, with/without children)	4	
General Education	5	x
Occupational Education	6	
Unemployed more than once in the last 5 years	7	x
Over 6 months unemployed in the last 5 years	8	x
Past change in occupation (self-rating)	9	x
Past change in occupation for of health reasons	10	
Past vertical mobility (upgrading, downgrading)	11	
Instability of employment (number of work contracts within last 5 years)	12	x
Estimated time until interruption or end of working life	13	
Work orientation (rating of 6 statements according to personal preferences)	14	
Self-reported problems relevant to re-employment efforts (at time of registering unemployed)	15	
The Last Work Place Prior to Unemployment		
Occupational position (blue collar/white collar, differentiated according to qualification)	16	
Duration of last working contract	17	x
Period at workplace	18	x
Kind of dismissal (by employer, by employee, limited working contract)	19	x
Main reason for being dismissed (according to Labor Officer; including 'health')	20	
Health as main or additional reason for last dismissal (according to unemployed)	21	
Strain factor 5: Time pressure	22	
Strain factor 14: Social climate in company	23	
Index strain factors 6, 7, 11 (monotony, cramped conditions, dirty air/environment)	24	
Overall index of strain factors connected with last working place (1-16)	25	
Usually having been 'worn out' in the evening after work?	26	
Did the last job affect your health negatively?	27	

Table 4 cont/d

Global assessment of health status in the past 2 weeks (compare table 1) GAH	Common Complaints scale (11 selected items, compare table 2) CCS	Psychical Balance (9 items on depressivity; (compare table 3) PSB	Global Assessment of strains in the initial phase of unemployment GAS
2.8	6.8	0.6	0.5
0.6	1.2	2.6	2.4
1.3	1.0	1.6	0.2
1.5	1.3	2.4	0.1
0.2	0.4	0.3	0.5
1.2	1.4	1.4	0.6
0.1	0.1	0.1	0.1
0.6	0.8	0.9	0.2
0.5	0.4	1.0	0.5
4.6	3.4	1.6	0.6
2.0	1.9	1.1	1.0
0.3	0.2	1.8	0.9
1.3	2.8	0.2	0.7
0.1	0.8	0.3	2.1
8.5	11.0	3.4	0.8
0.8	1.5	1.3	0.8
0.4	0.7	0.4	0.8
0.7	0.5	0.5	0.8
0.8	0.8	0.8	1.9
4.9	4.1	3.4	2.3
7.7	8.9	3.6	0.1
1.5	1.4	0.9	0.3
1.3	1.5	2.6	0.3
3.0	4.1	4.7	0.3
2.7	2.3	3.1	0.8
2.8	6.6	1.8	1.3
12.7	20.6	2.9	0.6

Table 4 cont/d

Independent variables	Variable No.	included in final tree analysis
The First Weeks of Unemployment		
Re-employed 5-6 weeks later (about 10% of sample)	28	
Not re-employed 5-6 weeks later, but job in sight	29	
Difficulties seen by the unemployed finding a new job at all	30	
Subjective chance of finding an equally suitable job	31	
Do you badly need to find a new job very soon?	32	
Do you have great/moderate financial difficulties?	33	
Can you at least partially and for a certain time rely on savings of your own?	34	
Psycho-social strain 1: missing contacts with colleagues	35	x
" " " 2: I used the time of unemployment doing things I like	36	
" " " 3: more aggravation in the family than usual	37	
" " " 4: did not visit friends and acquaintances as often as before	38	
" " " 5: very anxious about getting a new job	39	
" " " 6: unemployment seemed to me not as bad as I thought before	40	
" " " 7: it was not easy to tell friends and acquaintances about it	41	
" " " 8: it was not bad to have more time for the family	42	
" " " 9: staying at home got on my nerves	43	
" " " 10: I often asked myself why it was me who got unemployed	44	
Index 1 Psycho-social strains 1-10 (weights 1-3 on each answer)	45	
Index 2 Psycho-social strains 1-10 (counting 1 for each definite answer)	46	
Health Indicators		
Are there chronic impairments lasting for several years?	47	
Did unemployment aggravate or relieve such chronic impairments?	48	x
G A H	49	
C C S	50	
P S B	51	
G A S	52	

* Not included in final tree analysis

Table 4 cont/d

Global assessment of health status in the past 2 weeks (compare table 1) GAH	Common Complaints scale (11 selected items, compare table 2) CCS	Psychical Balance (9 items on depressivity; (compare table 3) PSB	Global Assessment of strains in the initial phase of unemployment GAS
0.9	0.3	0.6	0.1
1.2	1.7	3.2	2.9
2.9	2.6	4.6	2.5
4.0	2.8	3.3	2.3
0.6	0.2	4.8	7.1
1.4	1.3	8.1	4.8
1.9	1.2	4.2	3.0
0.9	0.4	2.1	0.9
1.0	0.3	4.7	2.1
0.8	1.0	3.9	1.9
0.9	1.1	5.2	1.6
2.8	1.3	8.5	11.3
1.4	0.4	4.3	8.8
1.2	1.9	2.8	5.3
0.7	0.3	4.3	2.5
2.5	0.7	5.9	9.0
2.1	1.8	11.1	12.5
2.3	2.0	10.7	14.9
3.2	2.2	8.9	15.0
(23.1)*	(27.5)*	5.3	1.0
3.4	4.0	2.5	0.4
		9.5	1.5
(23.7)*		9.0	0.4
(6.9)*	(8.3)*		5.1
(1.7)*	1.3	5.7	

Figure 1 German unemployed of Nov. 1981; 25 years or older, previously in employment, 5 - 6 weeks after becoming unemployed: Global assessment of health status in the past 2 weeks as independent variable (GAH)

R = reduction of variance in % of total variance

$\bar{x}$ = group average of dichotomized variable:
1 in the last 2 weeks health status excellent or good
0 else

n = number of cases

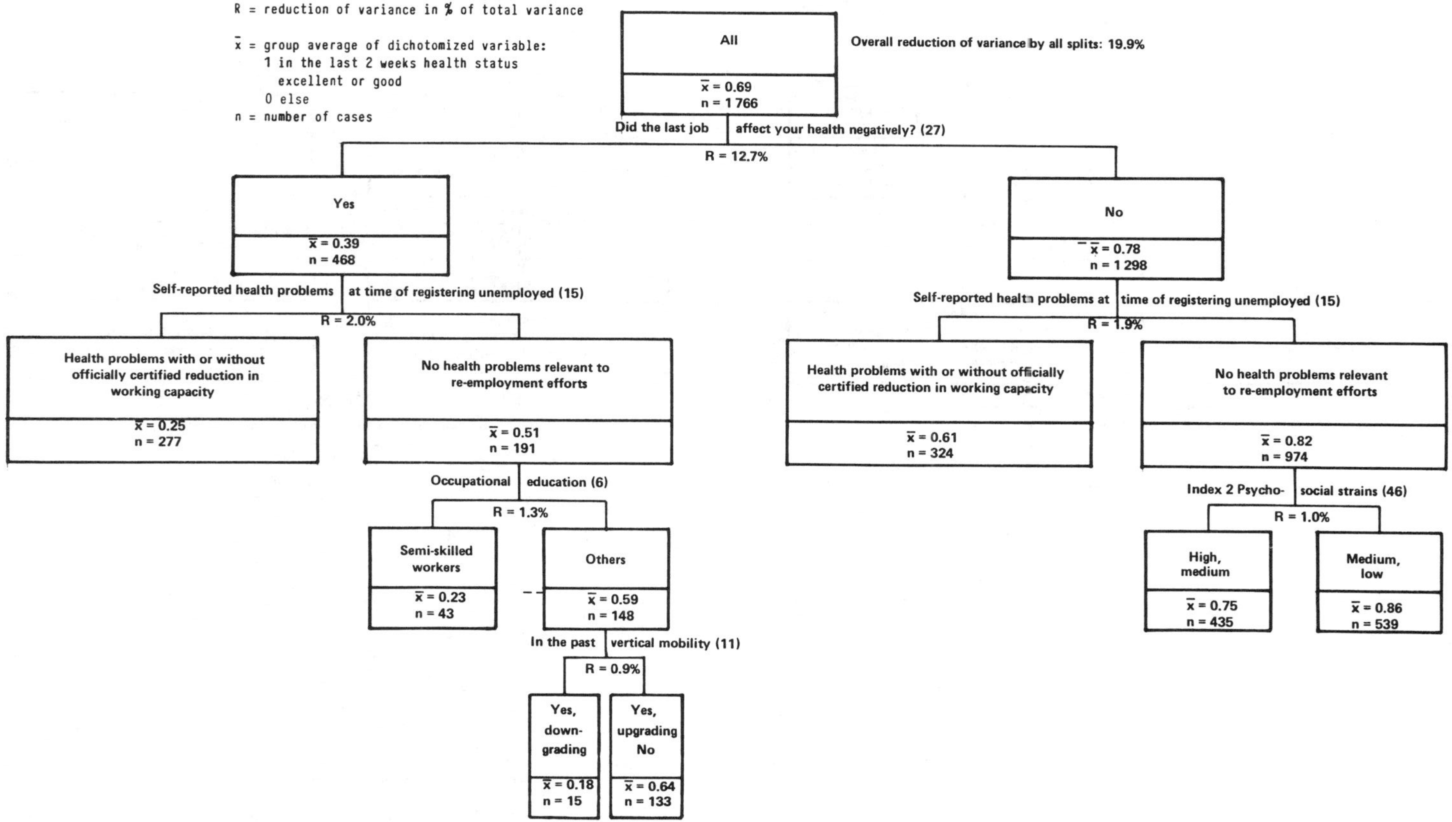

Figure 2 German unemployed of Nov. 1981, 25 years or older, previously in employment, 5 - 6 weeks after becoming unemployed: Common complaints (Index 0 - 33 on the base of 11 selected items) as independent variable (CCS)
Tree analysis

R = reduction of variance in % of total variance
x̄ = index value (group average)
n = number of cases

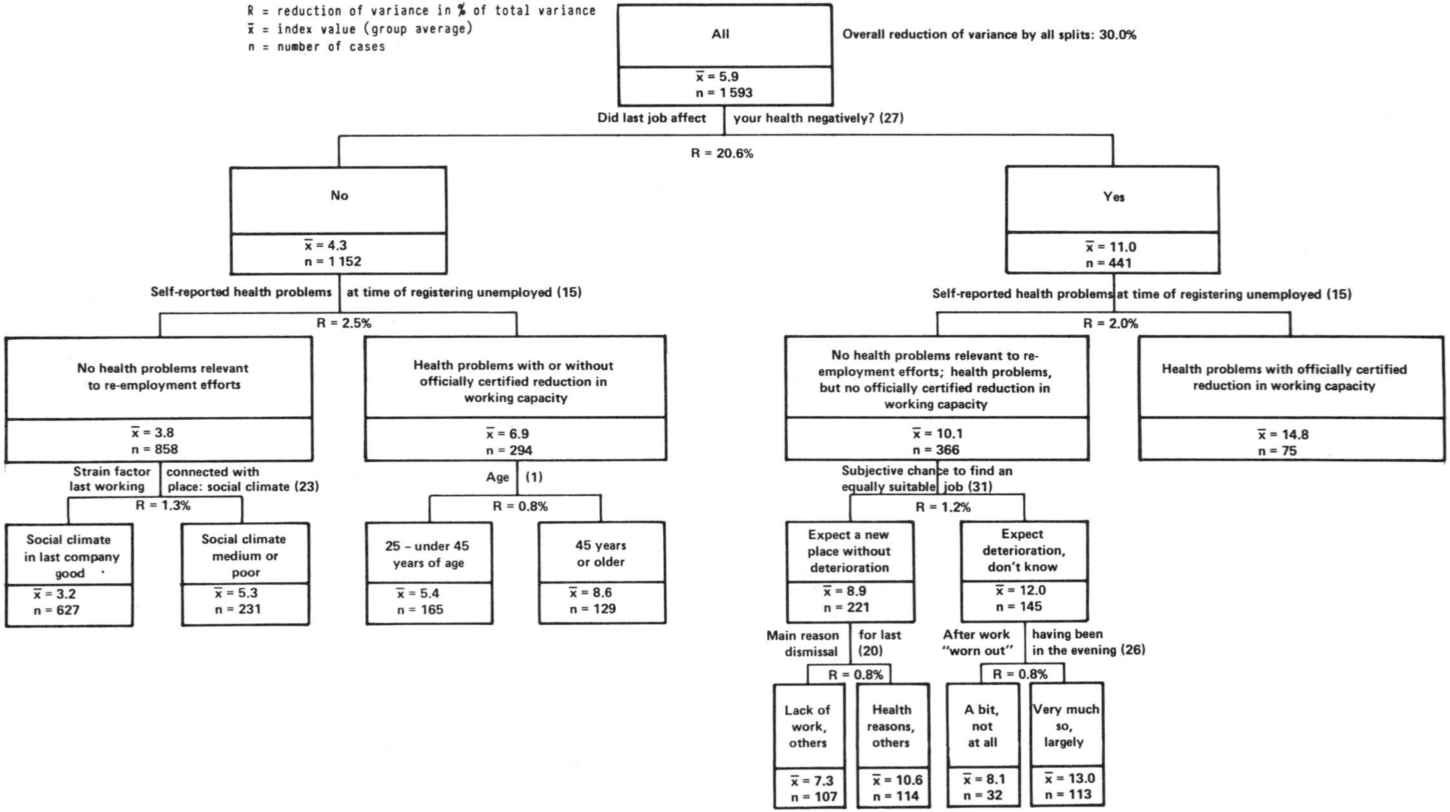

Figure 3 German unemployed of Nov. 1981; 25 years or older, previously in employment, 5 - 6 weeks after becoming unemployed
Psychical balance (index 0 - 36 on the base of 9 items) as independent variable (PSB)

Tree analysis

R = reduction of variance in % of total variance

$\bar{x}$ = index value (group average)

n = number of cases

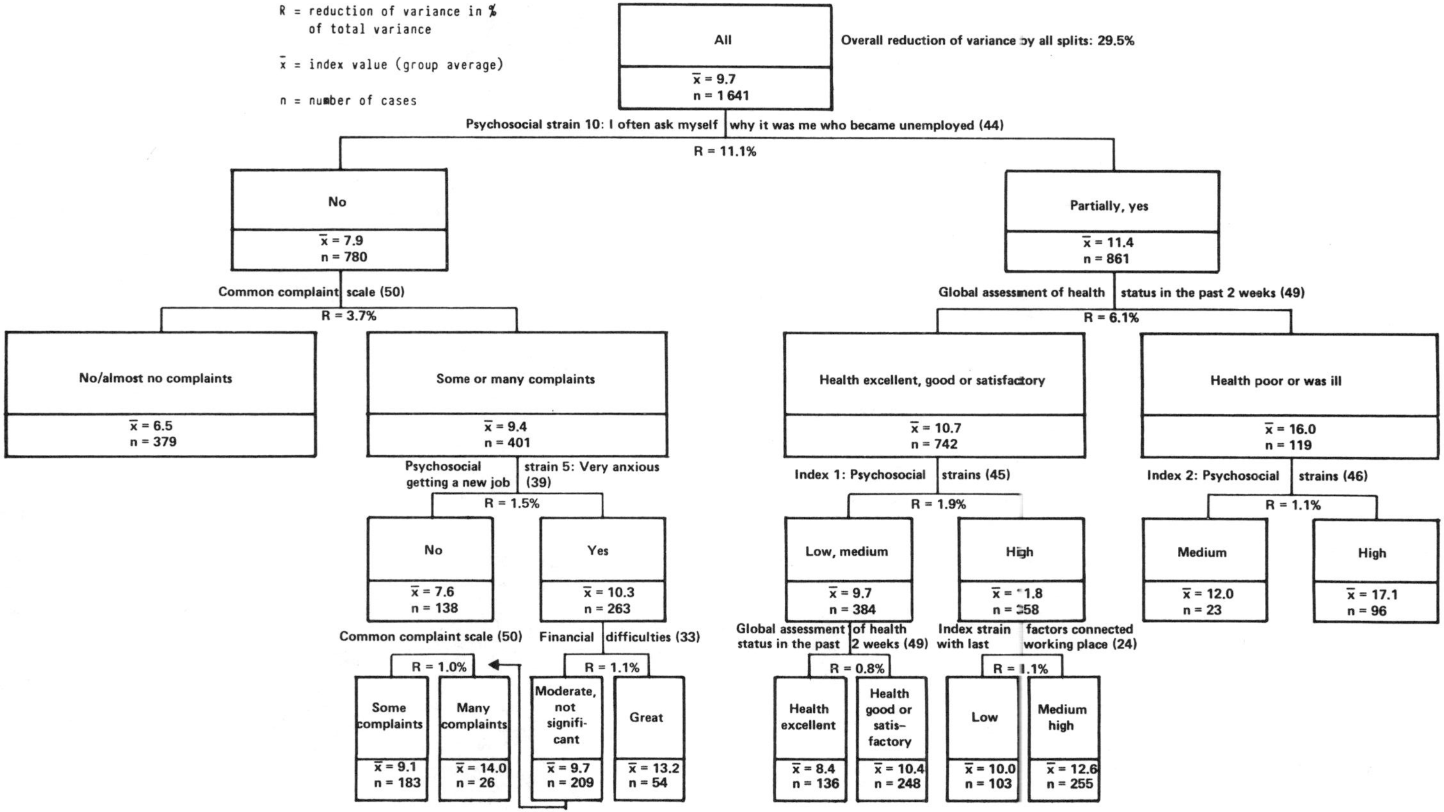

SOME RESULTS OF MEDICAL RESEARCH IN THE FRANKFURT/MAIN EMPLOYMENT OFFICE

Klaus-Dieter Thomann

In West Germany, as elsewhere, the unemployment problem is becoming more and more serious. In December 1982, over two million people were registered as unemployed. The official figures do not reveal the full extent of unemployment since they do not include vast sections of unemployed such as housewives, school leavers and persons formerly self employed. Over and above this, a relatively large section of the population has suffered occasional unemployment in recent months and has consequently felt the hardship of the social impact of unemployment. Although all present studies show that unemployment has a considerable effect on the well being and health of those affected, this problem has received little mention in the West German medical press.

This paper reports studies conducted in the Frankfurt/Main Employment Office since August 1981 which provide initial information on the effect of unemployment on health. In addition, the second part of the paper will feature a study on people attending training courses in centres for professional advancement. This study is in the initial stages and will examine the effect of unemployment and the attendance at such courses in relation to mental and physical health.

From August 1981 to November 1982, 170 studies were carried out for the Employment Office in Frankfurt/Main. It consisted of young people still attending school, or already unemployed, whose occupational maturity and capability was to be assessed. The largest group consisted of unemployed who had been referred to the medical service by the unemployment advisory board in order to obtain medical appraisal of their aptitude and suitability for certain occupations. On the basis of this expert opinion, the employment advisor, where possible, placed the persons concerned in suitable jobs. Aptitude refers to the subject's ability to take both physical and mental stress. A group of subjects was also examined, in whose case the question of whether or not they had been justified in giving up their job for health reasons was to be looked into. A final group was sent for investigation in order to size up whether their aptitude was adequate for a job on the employment market in general or if the social security should be recommended to provide a pension. The number of cases in which it was found advisable to provide pensions was however small, this being less than five. The group investigated was not compiled by the examiner, but resulted from random selection by the employment adviser. It was extremely mixed and consisted of both adolescents and 60 year olds unqualified labourers and university graduates (unemployed who had been without work for a few weeks and some who had not worked for more than four years). The prospects for the future of the various individuals concerned were also considerably diverse.

Of the 170 subjects examined, impairment to health which was in all probability connected with unemployment was only detected in 35, ie in more that 20%. the number itself is too small to allow any relevant statistical evaluation and, apart from this, the data have not been analyzed sufficiently to extract more detail. In the total number of persons examined, illnesses which had already been in existence prior to unemployment played an essential role, although only in a few cases had they given rise to the unemployment. Impairment to mental health due to being without work, a marked lack of perspective and somatization of conflict caused by unemployment were the main problems to the fore. The following cases are presented as examples.

Case 1

This subject was born in 1950 and is 32 years old. He attended school for eight years and then served a two year appenticeship as cook and a two year apprenticeship as waiter. He comes from a German speaking country and has been living in Germany for eleven years. He is married but has no children. He became unemployed in mid May 1982. The patient was examined four weeks later. At the examination, both the subject and his wife claimed that, when employed, his epileptic fits had occurred every three months, the maximum number of fits being one per month. Since becoming unemployed, the epileptic fits could not be controlled, despite massive stabilization with anti epileptics, and occurred daily. The physical findings revealed no peculiarities. The neurologist in charge had so far not considered unemployment to be an intensifying factor in pre existent epilepsy.

Case 2

This subject is 44 years of age and completed an apprenticeship in mining. After working for a long time in mining, he took jobs as transport worker or stacker and labourer in warehouses in, for instance, a large metal construction company in Frankfurt where he was employed for many years. He became unemployed for the first time in 1978 and, up to 1982, this was followed by four periods of unemployment interrupted only by periods of partial employment. His present period of unemployment has lasted for one and a half years. The patient is unmarried. His case history contains no specific illnesses. For about two years, he has been mentioning recurrent circulatory disorders and, for approximately ten years, has had relatively mild back trouble. He has also mentioned continuous headaches. The physicial findings revealed the patient to be severely prematurely aged and to have a chronic alcohol problem. In addition, he was considerably obese, had an enlarged liver, very pronounced acne, false posture of the spinal column and disturbed circulatory regulation. When questioned about his alcohol consumption, the patient stated that his drinking had increased in the last four years. When he had been permanently employed, he had drunk one or two bottles of beer per day, but he now consumes five to six bottles or more a day. He said: "What am I supposed to do when I don't have a job? I brood and can't sleep. How am I to get tired? When I drink alcohol, I become more tranquil and can sleep. What can I do?"

The patient, who showed every indication of alcoholism (with palmar erythema, enlargement of the liver and increased venous marking of the abdominal wall plus skin changes on the chest), had already left the house at 6.00 hours for the examination. The examination took place at 15.30 hours. This patient can be seen as a typical example of complete social uprooting with subsequent grave impairment to health.

Case 3

This patient is 38 years old and is married with three children. For a total of 18 years he was employed by the West German railway, first as a shunter and later as a cleaner. His case history shows him to have had a gastric ulcer in 1968 and hepatitis in 1970. In 1981, the patient was ill for four months with therapy resistant lumboischialgia and backache. Subsequent to this, his functional capacity no longer met his employer's requirements and he was dismissed on April 1, 1982. The first examination took place two months after the start of his unemployment and a second examination took place seven months later. While, at the first examination, the patient still had spine trouble and seemed slightly depressive, in November 1982 marked depression was evident in both the patient and his wife. The external situation of the consultation was already characterised by unemployment. Prior to being unemployed, the patient had earned approximately two thousand marks net. At the time of examination, he was receiving around one thousand two hundred and fifty marks. Although the interview took place on November 25, 1982, the family, for financial reasons, still had not turned on the heating in the apartment. The kitchen alone was heated by the kitchen stove. The patient and his wife stated: "All day long, we think over the unemployment situation and have no idea which way to turn. Everything seems pointless." Both the patient and his wife admitted that they were extremely despondent and frequently felt depressive. The husband claimed that he had often toyed with the idea of suicide, however, his family was a comfort to him and he would also like to provide for the family. Now that he was unemployed, he knew what it must be like "to be dead". The patient was being treated by a neurologist, was taking psychotropic drugs, but said explicitly: "The medication doesn't help". He was particularly affected by the discrimination on the part of the people around him. Friends and relatives had retreated. He alleged: "I feel they no longer want any contact with me because I might want money from them but I want absolutely nothing from them". When he had been employed, the situation had been entirely different. He and the family had had a lot of friends and colleagues. Now, he maintained "I feel treated like a piece of dirt". The 38 year old leaves the house only occasionally and only when something has to be taken care of. He is particularly downhearted because, having no money, he is, for example, not in a position to send his two elder children who live in Italy the fare for a visit over Christmas.

Case 4

This 54 year old patient, who had trained as a carpenter, became unemployed as the result of an accident at work in September, 1980. He was subsequently ill for 16 months. Afterwards, the patient was no longer able to achieve his full rate of output and was dismissed in February, 1982. He was first examined in March 1982. His case history contains nothing remarkable other than bronchitis in June and September 1981. During the final year of his illness, the patient had been considerably worried about his future, since two of his three children were still at home. The first examination was already very dramatic. The patient drew a number of job applications from his pocket and literally broke down and wept and was incapable of continuing speaking. His wife explained that this situation had been existent since her husband had received notification of the termination of his employment. He now smoked forty cigarettes a day where he had formerly smoked fifteen. He had become increasingly aggressive and in some instances violent towards her and the two children still at home. She herself dreaded returning home from her work at midday.

The physicial findings were normal, apart from marked enlargement of the liver and injuries to the right leg caused by the industrial accident. Reactive depression was what was most noticeable.

At a second examination in November 1982, the patient was thoracotomized subsequent to lung cancer being detected. The patient was informed of the diagnosis. Proceedings to obtain a pension were instituted. The future now seemed fairly "secure" to the patient and his wife. When questioned about how the situation after the loss of his job compared with that after he was discovered to have cancer, the 54 year old stated that, at the time he became unemployed, he had felt very very desolate and he had been at his wit's end. He now knew exactly where he was and he felt considerably better off at present than he had done previously. After he had lost his job, there had been a lot of quarrels and disagreements in the family. However, the situation had now quietened down. Although his desire to go to work and the impossibility of him getting a job continued to depress him, the fact that he had been provided with a pension had straightened things out. He could live with his cancer, but not with his unemployment.

Case 5

This 19 year old patient, who had finished school in June 1982 and who was now unemployed, was interviewed and examined for the first time at his home in September 1982, whereupon he immediately demanded a morphine injection. He was on a high dose of psychotropic drugs and had difficulty in articulating correctly. The entire living room was strewn with letters of application to the most diverse firms and with the corresponding letters of rejection. The young man was completely in despair and said over and over again in a disjointed manner that he had no work despite the fact that he was continually applying for jobs, that he did not know if he was to blame for the situation and that he simply could no longer see a way out. The patient seemed very depressive. However, he was still able to compose job applications on a typewriter. In addition to depression shortly after the start of his unemployment (after leaving school) the patient contracted prostatitis which, in his view, had led to impotency. Fear of being socially discriminated against by his environment and the fact that he felt himself to blame for the situation resulted, together with the prostatitis, in his becoming increasingly isolated. A few days later, he wrote a long letter in which he specifically stressed that he would very much like to work, but that his applications for jobs were always met with rejection. On receiving a letter of rejection, he always felt particularly lousy. His statements were continually mixed with dread of the future and the fear of not being able to establish a family. When the patient was examined for the second time at the end of November 1982, the situation had eased somewhat. He stated that, although he still contemplated suicide from time to time and often saw no sense in life, he had been able to discusss these problems with his neurologist and now had the prospect of professional training (a course to provide further professional training and jobs for unemployed). This prospect had shown the future in a somewhat better light and he had considerable expectations from this course. This case clearly shows how, alone through the hope of help and the prospects of finding a job at least for a short time, a critical mental situation can be eased.

The number of examples of this kind could be considerably increased. The common characteristic feature of the cases described is the combination of a pre existent instable state of health with the intense stress of unemployment. After a certain period of time, this unstable state of health becomes apparent in the emergence, encouragement or change in development of illnesses. Further studies and long term observations are necessary to enable the individual influencing factors to be correlated.

In conclusion, I would like to give a brief description of a study project planned for the near future. In the Frankfurt area, there are several vocational training centrs in which unemployed persons receive training for several months, in particular to maintain and supplement whatever qualifications they have and to take those concerned "off the streets".

When 26 people attending one of these vocational training courses (all unskilled or semi skilled labourers between the ages of 18 and 55) were interviewed for the first time, clear indications of the detrimental effects of unemployment were again noted. In group discussion, a markedly depressive mood was noticeable. The participants talked about the change in the rhythm of their life. During the day they had nothing to do and at night they could not sleep. Some of them took sleeping tablets and, on the next day, were indifferent to everything. One of the participants reported that, where he had formerly smoked twenty cigarettes a day, he now smoked fifty. Since his smoking had increased, he has had stomach trouble and has been eating less. Others complained continually of isolation with the most diverse effects. They now hardly had the courage to visit their neighbours, where the topic of conversation always centered around cars, holidays and other consumer goods which were no longer within the means of someone unemployed. Many of those interviewed claimed that formerly, in addition to coping with a job, they had had considerable reserves in capacity. Nowadays, they were scarecely capable of pursuing a hobby properly. It was no longer a relaxation for them, but had become a compulsion. Also, from what were they supposed to be relaxing?

I shall now deal with some results of the questionnaire. Those questioned had, on average, suffered a 40% loss in income compared to formerly. Eleven of the twenty six felt that they were in a poorer state of health since they had lost their job, seven considered their state of health not to have changed, and four considered theirs to be better. These four commented in particular that they had pursued their former occupation reluctantly. Nineteen worried about the future, while seven had no such fears of the future. In fourteen, this worry was also in respect of the family. Twenty one of the twenty six reported that they sometimes started to brood and felt despondent. More than fifty percent (14) stated that they at times felt that life no longer had any meaning (presuicidal). The unemployed claimed familial support by relatives and friends to be good (seventeen of the twenty six were able to discuss their problems with their relatives). Twelve of them, ie just less than half, claimed that the family understood their situation and helped them. Although twenty two of the twenty six stated that they were not to blame for the fact that they were unemployed, they at the same time indirectly attributed blame to themselves, since almost all admitted to feeling terrible when they were asked where they worked and then had to admit to being unemployed. Twelve alleged that they were considered by many people to be work shy and lazy. Approximately a third of the twenty six stated that there had been more rows in the family since their unemployment, and the same percentage remarked that they had become more irritable towards their children.

It is interesting that, of the twenty six questioned, only eight claimed to have become seriously ill since the start of their unemployment. Twelve answered this question explicitly in the negative. Only in four cases was the doctor visited more frequently subsequent to unemployment than prior to unemployment. Only five of those questioned had actually discussed their unemployment with their doctor.

The replies to the question on concrete symptoms contrast with this. Fifteen of the twenty six stated that, since being unemployed, there were more days on which they did not feel well than was the case prior to unemployment. The symptoms most reported were disturbed sleep (in 50%), headaches (in 11 of 26) and feelings of anxiety (in 11 of 26). Eight reported high blood pressure (contradiction of the question on visits to the doctor), five reported sweating and six palpitations. Three of the twenty six questioned had had more cardialgia since being unemployed. In addition, several complained of nervousness, complete weariness and depression. Five had noted an increase in their cigarette consumption and the same number reported that they were consuming more alcohol since becoming unemployed.

The results of this initial consultation give clear indication of possible impairment to health due to unemployment. To obtain more precise information on the effects of unemployment in this particular group and to examine the influence of possible factors, a long term investigation of persons attending courses in vocational training centres of this kind is scheduled to take place in the coming year. Interviews and examinations will be carried out on starting or prior to starting a course, during the course and few months after the course has finished. In these, the question of how far such courses have a mitigating effect on the impact of unemployment on mental and physical health will be investigated. In particular, the collective examined will be more accurately broken down according to case history, outlook, perspective, family situation etc. It is hoped in this way to obtain more material on the connection between unemployment and ill health and on the effectiveness of vocational training.

HEALTH STATUS, HEALTH SERVICE AND SOCIO ECONOMIC DEVELOPMENT OF PROVINCES IN POLAND

W. Cezary Wlodarczyk

If compared with the Western European economics the way in which the economic system in Poland affects the health, health services, and the well-being of the population is different in certain respects. There is no open unemployment and health policy is submitted to an extensive state planning system operating at both national and provincial level. Nevertheless, economic development and economic stress still generate potentially the strongest factors influencing health. This paper describes a preliminary analysis to identify such influences, and presents some tentative results.

In the main hypothesis it is assumed that some "natural" trends operating through social and economic trends and health resources may be stronger than purposeful decisions of health planners. Identification of these natural trends is of primary importance for health policy.

In the paper a threefold typology of areas covered by health policy interventions is put forward. This typology distinguishes:

a) long range decisions affecting an investment process carried out in provinces;

b) decisions shaping the distribution and allocation of health resources;

c) decisions concerning the productivity of health resources.

Cross sectional analysis, using official statistics, has provided the first and tentative results to test this hypothesis. Though the method applied (setting up of unconstrained computerized multi-regression equations) has failed in some cases, the evidence derived seems to confirm our hypothesis.

Part One
GENERAL BACKGROUND

One of the major problems facing the social and health policies in Poland is that of the differences between particular regions and areas of the country. This is quite natural. Each complex system faces the problem of internal differences between its subsystems. It is broadly believed that an advantageous development of the whole system is feasible only if its particular subsystems are harmonized(1). All those responsible for health policy, at global level, fully realize this:

> "There is a wide gap between the developed and developing countries in their health levels and in the resources they are devoting to health improvement. Moreover, within individual countries, whatever their level of development, analogous gaps are commonly evident between different groups of population."(2)

We think such awareness applies also to the national level; an attempt to overcome the disproportions often becomes the declared goal of social and health policies.

Recently this problem has been repeatedly raised in Poland. It was elaborated in the Parliamentary Document, accepted in 1973, specifying health care development trends up to 1990[3]. The need to overcome this problem was one of the essential arguments for enacting the health service reform in 1975[4]. It is also included in the activities schedule of the Ministry of Health, declared in 1982[6].

To illustrate the awareness of differentiated health needs and abilities to meet them official declarations should be supplemented with information on the discussions carried on during 1980-1982. Never before were health care activities subject to so severe criticism. However, what is interesting is that particular groups of experts called on by both volunteer and official representatives did not confine themselves to critical examination but formulated proposals for changes. This yielded a series of very interesting proposals for health service reform[6]. Furthermore, an attempt at a synthesis of particular proposals was undertaken and fully supported by the Ministry[7].

The work on the reform proposals, along with their essential effects, revealed numerous information gaps on disparities in the system, both in access to source information and in forms of processing and utilization of obtained information. Missing information often hampered genuine discussions based on factual knowledge.

Under these circumstances it was decided to enter on an analysis of factors determining the health status differentiation (health needs) of provinces and factors affecting the meeting of those needs. This project was meant as an attempt to use existing information sources with no attempt to carry out our own field studies.

Articulation of this idea was naturally inspired by the WHO's Managerial Process for National Health Development philosophy and its inherent holistic approach to health problems[8] as well as by research projects in which factors affecting health status are sought among socio economic factors within territorial units[a].

GENERAL RESEARCH PROJECT

Analysis unit

In our analysis the adoption of provinces as subjects of analysis was prompted by the managerial rather than health related viewpoint. The province is the unit of administrative division resulting from the 1975 reform and cannot be regarded as a territorial or social unit focussing the life of the population of a given area (at least for the time being).[9] Therefore it cannot be fully acknowledged as a complete set of social, economic and other factors affecting health status, as opposed to a local community, enterprise or family. Yet, we do believe it plays an essential role in the accomplishment of health policy.

(a) See papers presented at two WHO meetings in Copenhagen and Munich and in this book.

This results from specific relationships between the structures of representative authorities, administrative authorities and health care system management. This is illustrated in Table 1.

The multilevel system of relationships between representative, administrative authorities and health service management system contains just two common levels: central and provincial. That means that it is at those levels that essential strategic decisions on the health policy are made. This results from several premises. Firstly: very rarely are decisions made by health service managers on their own behalf (more at the central than at the provincial level); much more frequently they formulate decisions to be formally made by the authorities of relevant administrative levels. Secondly, health managers make their contribution to collective administrative authorities which enables them to raise health problems in decisions pertaining to other domains. Thirdly, the existing statistical system provides for elaborations, for provinces, of both health and socio economic information. Despite the well grounded criticism of information quality, the availability of information at this level does promote decision making. Consequently, it may be argued that for the third level of health care management, ie the district, mainly executive functions are left.

The arguments raised above confirm the usefulness of acknowledging the province as a territorial unit in relation to which, and within which, health policy is being made. On the other hand, they do not refer to the problem of identifying the subjects responsible for this policy, ie to identifying a group of organs of political, representative and administrative authorities making decisions affecting the health status of provinces' populations.

For our analysis, the outcomes of specific decisions, and not the precise establishment of authorship of those decisions, are significant. Health effects are usually a sum of very complex sequences of interacting factors and it is hard to reconstruct a uniform sequence of causal interrelationships enabling the identification of one originator. The common multiplicity of health phenomena is, in our country, strengthened by the complexity of decisional procedures applied and by obliteration of the units of responsibility between particular organs of authority. Consequently, our analysis is not an attempt to establish decison mechanisms related to health at particular provinces but an attempt at description and interpretation of correlations between certain phenomena. The attempt to establish "natural" correlations and dependencies relating to health at province level results from the assumption that health policy is rational only when based on reliable analysis of facts. After all it should be taken for granted that we'd better know than not know the realities.

TABLE 1*(10)

Levels	Representative Authority	Administrative Authorities	Health Service Management	
			Authority	Advisory Functions
Central Level	Parliament /Seym/	Government	Ministry	Scientific Board Institutes
Regional Level				Medical Academies
Province Level	People's Councils	Province Head	Province Chief Physician	Provinces Specialists
Preventive Therapeutic Area/District/			HCC/Health Care Complex/ Director	Consultants
Community	People's Councils	Community Head		

* In Table 1, political authorities/organs of Polish Unified Workers' Party/ have been disregarded. This sytem, functioning at all levels, may play an essential role in the formation and accomplishment of the health policy.

Level of analysis

The interacting systems mentioned so far include: interrelationships between socio economic status at the province and its inhabitants health status on the one hand and relations between health needs and abilities to satisfy them (which is, obviously, affected by the province's socio economic status), on the other.

In both sets of relationships mentioned above, the causative role is attributed to elements of the provincial socio economic status. Thus, those elements play a double role in the determination of health policy. Firstly, they constitute the health status determinant, resulting in both positive and negative changes. Secondly, they constitute a factor affecting the capabilities of health services to meet health needs. Those capabilities are related to the acquistion of resources, whether financial, staff or equipment.

In our opinion, understanding this double role is of primary significance for the making of health policy for provinces' requirements.

The double role of socio economic factors is part of a broader system of multilateral interrelationships. For purposes of our analysis, we have adopted a model of hypothetic relationships presented in scheme 1.*

The figure illustrates two aspects of the problem:

(i) the phenomena handled as "natural". The model presents both a direct** impact of socio economic status on health status, revealing at the same time the dependence of this status on decisions on investment development in a given province, decisions made in the macrosystem; and also indirect impact of socio economic status on health status, by affecting health service outlays, resources, their productivity and utilization;

(ii) intentional and purposeful phenomena. The model presents those types of decisions incorporated into health policy which interfere with the natural processes. The level of health expenditure, resources and productivity may be fundamentally influenced by health policy interventions.

For this analysis, we are distinguishing between three types of decisions through which health policy may affect provincial health status. Those are the decisions on:

investment process in the province;
health service resources distribution
health service resources productivity.

---

* This scheme includes an evident simplication while identifying health status and health needs. The complex problem of their mutual relationship is beyond the scope of this paper(11).

** Within the adopted model which is another obvious simplification.

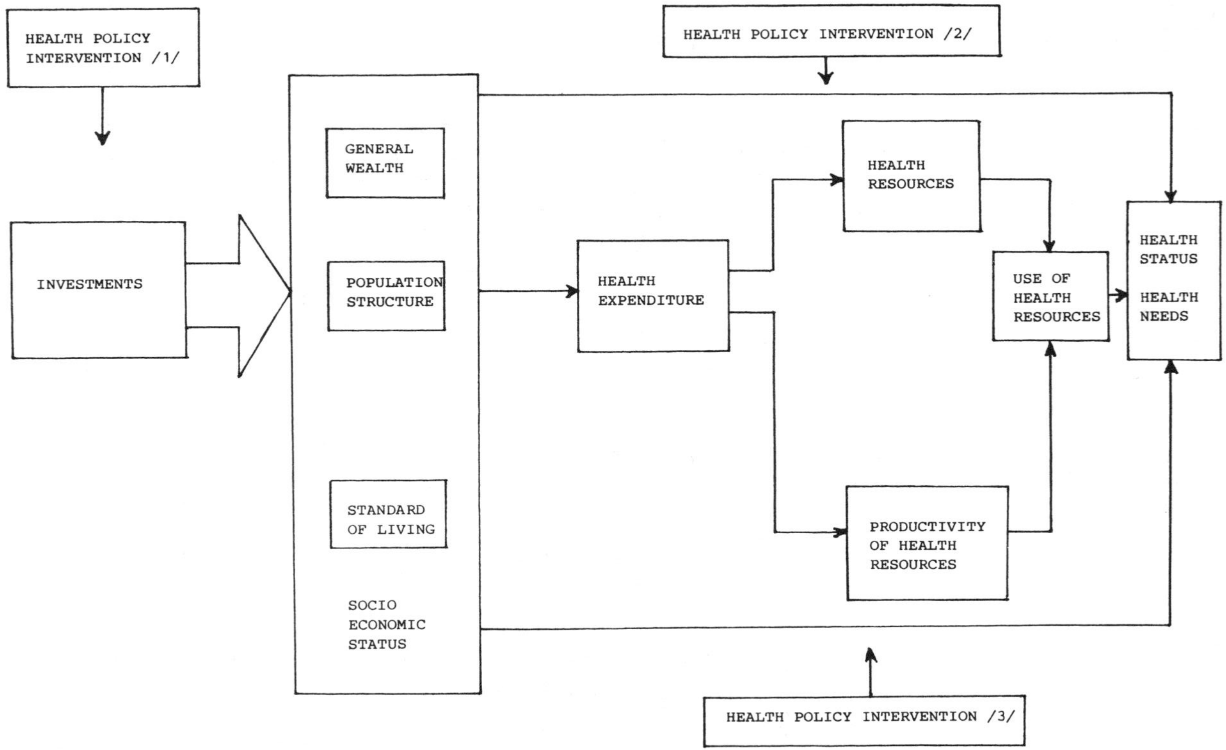

SCHEME 1. Determinants of health status (health needs) at a province level.

The most far reaching and comprehensive outcomes within the health situation may be attained by the first type of decision. The type and quantity of investments, along with the level of industrialization, evidently affect the natural and social environment, as well as behaviour. Comprising, indirectly, also hereditary aspects, they cumulate most of the factors which are known fundamentally to affect levels of health.[12] Thus, the factors that basicallycondition health status vary with decisions of this type. In its ideal and idealistic form, health policy would affect health status through those particular decisions. Yet, the possibilities of affecting health status by these, most effective, methods are usually considerably limited. Thus, although

> "the health care organizers realize that socio economic factors may more evidently affect health conditions than their own work"[13]

yet, they consider health service activity the basic tool to be applied in improving the population's health status. This is why such great significance is attributed to the decisions on health resources allocation and productivity.

Types of decisions

To clarify the conceptual basis of this we give a brief description of the types of decisions referred to. A stipulation should be made here that our typology does not pretend in the least to cover all types of decisions that may be involved in formulating health policy for the provinces.

Decisions on the investment process

Throughout post war development in Poland, decisions on investments have been governed by the conception of "socialist industrialization". Most researchers agree that this conception subordinated economic decisions to political decisions relating to social phenomena.

> "The primary value which industrialization is supposed to serve is the development of socialistic society."[14]

This general formulation is supplemented through specification of definite purposes resulting from the decisions on industrialization. These detailed goals include the following elements:

a) provision of a rapid rate of economic development;

b) raising the population's material and cultural level of life;

c) quantitative and qualitative strengthening of the working class;

d) full employment;

e) elimination of drastic differences in the level of socio economic development between particular regions.[15]

It is worth emphasising that the conception of socialist industrialization (especially in its early articulations) exhibits a certain automatism or explicit correlation between economic and social phenomena. Although this conception is subordinated to non economic goals, yet economic phenomena are regarded as the autonomous causative force. Under those conditions, the goals of industrialization, the health goals have been mentioned directly. Indirectly we might surmise their occurrence in what is called the living standard or qualitative strengthening of the working class. What is particularly interesting to us is that balancing of disproportions between particular areas is considered. We might suppose that "disproportions" include health status and health needs as well. It is certain, however, that health goals did not achieve significant priority, though their role was increasing with time and the notion of economic development was gradually replaced by that of socio economic development. However, they have never become the primary decisional premises, as expected in such a model of social policy where

> "if the adopted goals come into conflict, then health is considered more important than material progress."[16]

Decisions on resources distribution

According to the conceptions discussed so far, the requirements of personnel resources (and other health resources alike) may be evaluated at three levels:

a) analysis of demographic data;

b) setting up professional tasks and roles;

c) evaluation of health needs, based on mortality and morbidity data.[17]

The third approach is commonly regarded as most promising but most difficult at the same time. Various difficulties in interpretation of health needs carry over into the planning area. However, awareness of those difficulties should not (in our opinion) imply that such an approach not be used in decisional processes relating to resources distribution. What seems significant for a rational evaluation of decisional premises is a very precise definition of which health aspects are meant.

It should be stressed here that the choice of any methods determining requirements for resources is, in itself, a choice within the area of health policy. There is a conflict between the option of more equitable distribution of resources and the option of "preferential allocation of health resources to those in greatest social needs." In relation to the conflict between those options (between equality and justice) accomplishment of comprehensive health policy enhances the need for a clear choice from the area of politics rather than health policy.

What has been said so far refers to assumptions of rational health policy within resources distribution.

The processes of resources distribution are subject to various influences from broader social, economic and political phenomena. There are certain "natural" tendencies, for example, that richer regions are more apt to have health resources than the poor regions,[18] thus neither the postulate of "equal share" nor the one of the "just share according to needs" applies here.

Due to such tendencies any efforts of rational health policy are frustrated. However, the relatively easy attainment of resources in rich provinces may both hamper and advance the implementation of a rational health policy. It becomes a barrier if the amount of resources hitherto obtained is above the level of accepted needs. Further cumulation of resources deprives the poor regions (that are equally or more in need) of the possibility of obtaining them, intensifying the existing disparities. It may, however, be an advantage if those richer regions also exhibit a higher level of health needs. This is probable inasmuch as the wealth usually results from industrialization and relevant changes in the natural and social environment. If that is the case the socio economic development aggravates health needs but at the same time yields the possibility of better health care organization. Thus, in so far as health service resources strengthen health potential, everything that promotes their increase, thus, also the province wealth, may be regarded as a factor that is positive to health.

Decisions on health resources productivity

In the process of achieving health goals the problem of resources utilization must be tackled so as to assure maximum efficiency. In literature dealing with these problems the notion of a balanced model defining the relationships between needs, resources, their productivity and use may be encountered.[19] In this model it is assumed that correspondence of needs, resources and utilization, whether great or little, can be achieved.

This, however, is an evident simplification and the use of a gradual process seems advisable both due to features of the phenomena analysed and to a certain hypothesis related to health managers functioning.

This hypothesis assumes that apart from extreme cases of health needs of extraordinarily high level, in most cases the response to greater needs and/or higher use is either a high level of resources or high productivity. If this is the case, we could hardly expect a simultaneous increase in all elements of the model. Our opinion is rather that an increase in resources is accompanied by decreased productivity and vice versa.

A further consequence of the adopted hypothesis is the statement that the principles of health policy should comprise the criteria facilitating the choice between two options: one of them being directed towards resources and the other towards productivity With no such explicit criterion, the choice between the two options will be exploited by the "natural" tendencies on resources distribution. Thus, rich provinces will generally prefer the resources directed option, thereby leaving the efficiency option exclusively to the poor areas.

Types of decisions vs types of research

One of the premises conditioning the distinction between three types of decisions was diffentiation of information needs. Each of those types of decisions calls for different information, hence the differentiated research projects supplying the information.

1. For decisions on investments the data on the health aspects of socio economic processes are of primary importance. Each economic decision entails certain social effects, such as migrations or changes in lifestyle, which, in turn, affect health. (We are taking no account of the type of intermediary mechanisms here). Our belief is that the more precise the information on the correlations in that area, the more intense the persuasive force of health policy advocates. Provinces' socio economic characteristics are handled as causative factors, the population's health status as an effect. Such factors as health care expenditures, health resources and utilization serve as intermediary variables.

2. For decisions on resources distribution, identification of "natural" processes affecting allocation is the major problem. The features of provinces' socio economic situation are handled as the determinant of health resources level. Health needs (health status described by a set of parameters) serve as a criterion of correct (rational) resource distribution.

3. For decisions on resources productivity the major issue becomes the identification of "natural" processes influencing the choice of a strategy for health sevices delivery. At a given level of health need, the province's socio economic position is handled as a determinent of the efficiency of resource use.

Variables

The concepts in the model concerned are so general that their real meaning remains vague unless a proper operationalization is done. In the situation where numerous obstacles in access to reliable information exist, the danger that the empirical meaning of terms would stray from the meaning implied by theoretical requirements is very pressing. Trying to avoid this menance we adopted a "stage by stage" approach. It assumed that in the first stage of the study a set (module) of easily obtained data is built up only. This set serves as a base to tentatively operationalize concepts as well as to analyse some relationships among variables in order to assess the completeness of the data.

Concerning both definitional and explanatory requirements this analysis is to bring about a list of information lacking. The missing data will be supplemented progressively and subsequent modules will be included in further stages of analysis.

Therefore the set of information used in the first stage of the study is an obvious compromise between accessibility of data and exigencies imposed by the theoretical model. The results of this compromise are represented by the following list of variables:

Health status/health need/indicators

Hc_1 incidence rate of diarrhoea in children aged 0 - 2

Hc_2 measles incidence per 100,000 inhabitants

Hc_3 tuberculosis incidence per 10,000 inhabitants

Ha_4 sexually transmitted diseases incidence per 10,000 inhabitants

Ha_5 dysentery incidence per 100,000 inhabitants

Ha_6 viral hepatitis incidence per 100,000 inhabitants

Hm_7 infant mortality rate per 1,000 annual live births

Hm_8 total mortality rate per 1,000 inhabitants

Hm_9 cardiovascular diseases mortality per 1,000 inhabitants

Hm_{10} malignant neoplasms mortality per 1,000 inhabitants

Indicators of population structure

D_{11} density of population

D_{12} urban population ratio

D_{13} active earners per 1,000 inhabitants*

D_{14} proportion of active earners employed in industry and construction industry*

Indicators of province's wealth

W_{15} value of fixed capital per capita

W_{16} investment expenditure per capita*

W_{16} gross production of industry per capita*

* in socialist sector only

Indicators of living standard

L_{18} public roads, density per 100 km^2

L_{19} dwelling space per capita

L_{20} retail sales per capita*

Health expenditure (purposeful outlay)

P_{21} total outlay for health services per capita

P_{22} investment expenditure for health service per capita

P_{23} current expenditure for health service per capita

Health resources

R_{24} physicians per 10,000 inhabitants

R_{25} pharmacisits per 10,000 inhabitants

R_{26} nurses per 10,000 inhabitants

R_{27} hospital beds per 10,000 inhabitants

R_{28} rural population per rural health centre

R_{29} population per pharmacy

Activities of health services (Use and Productivity of health resources)

A_{30} cases of medical treatment in polyclinics per inhabitant

A_{31} cases of medical treatment in polyclinics per physician

A_{32} cases of hospital treatment per 10,000 inabitants

A_{33} cases of hospital treatment per hospital bed

A_{34} average stay in hospital (in days)

A_{35} occupancy rate per hospital bed

A_{36} cost of hospital treatment per case

A_{37} cost of medical treatment in polyclinics per case

---

* in socialist sector only

It seems that even before the first stage of analysis has been completed some obvious gaps in the data can be discerned, e.g. an age structure in demographic indicators or environmental factors in indices of living standard. The omissions reinforce the tentative character of this study.

Principles of interpretation

Our analysis used the principle of geographic measurement of variables as in cross sectional studies. This was due to the difficulties in acquisition of information illustrating time dependent variation of particular parameters describing the provinces position. The information obstacles result from two groups of causes. Firstly: the present borders of provinces were delineated in 1975, thus no statistics describing those regions can go beyond this limit. This poses a significant disadvantage for observation of long term trends (so important in analysis of the issues concerned). Secondly, many researchers allege that the variability of a considerable part of economic situation parameters results not from actual variability of economic phenomena but from numerous changes in methods of calculating particular indices.[20] Such an argument underlies some critical appraisal of our paper in which we have applied H Brenner's concept in our data analysis.[21]

The cross sectional analysis allows us to avoid these obstacles but at the same time limits the capabilities of casual interpretation of relationships analysed between the phenomena. Using this approach we may reliably certify the concurrence of phenomena. Their causal interpretation is rarely justified, except in the case of some rare theoretically confirmed relationships. Consequently, acknowledgement of a particular variable within a model as an independent variable would not justify regarding it as a causative factor. This reservation becomes particularly significant when only tentative results are analysed.

In further stages of research inclusion of the time factor through frequently repeated measurements will be possible. In this way, we should identify change in the system and the strength of causal relationships. Our intention however is not diachronic analysis but comparison of a series of results of synchronic analysis.

Part Two
RESULTS

The results should be handled as tentative findings for several reasons:

a) Selection of variables for analysis is of a preliminary nature. It is based on a "small" set of easily accessible data and is aimed at rendering the preliminary characteristics of relevant phenomena. This refers both to dependent variables and those handled as explanatory. The group of independent variables was very limited and involved only some of those commonly regarded in literature as most characteristic for particular types of phenomena: health situation, resources level and health system's activity level. Those variables do not yield complete characteristics of those types.

2) The results we have presented are based on the results of the first stage of statistical analysis, in which with several reservations, an econometric model was constructed by the selection of parameters at the required significance level. Thus the variables included in the model may be altered in further stages of the study.

3) Regarding statistical analysis at this stage a relatively low significance level has been adopted $p = 0,1$ (10%) (t statistics not less than 1.69). We have found a relatively large set of explanatory variables convenient and relevant for initial verification of the hypotheses presented above.

4) Despite the principle of random selection of explanatory variables in two cases they have been tentatively preselected. Firstly, variable Ha_4 (prevalence of veneral disease) was excluded from analysis as it exhibited strikingly strong correlations with a considerable number of variables; those correlations could hardly be sensibly interpreted. Secondly, following theoretical premises presented above health service activity variables have been excluded from the set of variables explaining parameters R(resources).

Determinents of health situation

Factors affecting tuberculosis incidence rate (Ha_3)

The model describing this variable assumes the following form:

$$Ha_3 = 0.147Hm_7 + 0.517Hm_g - 0.236R_{29} + 4.302$$

$R = 0.59$ (R - multiple correlation coefficient)

This equation does not confirm hypotheses of obvious and simple correlations between the socio economic situation and tuberculosis prevalence rate. None of the parameters of socio economic position of the provinces was included in the model at the significance level adopted.

None of the significant parameters of health service resources was included in the model either. Variable R_{29} (population per chemist's shop) should be regarded as accidental and insignificant. It should be noted, however, that tuberculosis incidence undergoes characteristic periodic fluctuations (the climax occurs every five years)[25] which cannot be directly allowed for in cross sectional analysis. In addition, our analysis involves neither the age structure of tuberculosis incidence nor of provinces population, which may be significant for interpretation of the relationships concerned. Hence the need of extreme caution in analysis of the model presented.

What is most interesting in this equation of health is some convergence of the province inhabitants' situation parameters. Infant mortality, death rate due to diseases of the circulatory system and tuberculosis yield a rather compact picture of the provinces health situation. There appears to be some health situation syndrome enabling relatively complex description of the provinces' health position.

The quality of approximation of the model is not particularly high ($R = 0.59$) though it exceeds the critical value.

<u>Factors affecting viral hepatitis rates</u> (Ha_6)

The model describing this variable assumes the following form:

$$Ha_g = 0.155\ Hc_2 - 0.913Ha_5 + 3.86Hm_7 + 4.369A_{33} - 51.539$$

$$R = 0.58$$

The rate of viral hepatitis incidence is usually associated with two elements:

general sanitary and health situation of a given area - type A

iatrogenic effects - related both to services recipients and providers (not sufficiently aseptic conditions in health service activities) - type B

Therefore, the factors conditioning the rate of the particular parameter concerned should be sought among the variables describing the socio economic position of the province and health service activities. The model is devoid of any factor related to the general position of the province. On the other hand health situation parameters inherent in the model yield a somewhat obscure picture. Two variables related to infectious diseases (measles and dysentery) have opposite signs, thus any syndrome of infectious diseases prevalence is excluded.

Instead, the model variable describing infant mortality rates confirms the former conclusion of a certain syndrome of provinces' health position. With all the necessary interpretative reservations, the presence of variable A_{33} (general hospital patients per bed) tends to confirm the hypothesis that there are possible iatrongenic effects of health service activities. Curiously the model contains a variable describing hospital effectiveness, ie a variable that is, in theory, regarded as best for interpreting the correlations found.

It should be emphasized that variable A_{33} contains the greatest variability loading* in the equation concerned, though the whole model achieves relatively low approximation value.

<u>Factors affecting the total mortality rate</u> (Hm_8)

The model describing this variable assumes the form:

$$Hm_8 = 0{,}001Hc_1 + 0.113Hm_7 + 1.014Hm_9 + 2.165Hm_{10} - 0.005D_{13} + 0.0005A_{35} + 1.142$$

$$R = 0.97$$

---

* It refers to the value of the partial correlation coefficient.

A very high approximation value of the model should be indicated ($R = 0.972$). Unfortunately, this high value results from a group of variables describing various mortality aspects, hence the conjecture that a purely definitional relationship is shown here rather than some formal relationship. In our opinion the method of automatic selection of variables adversely affected the results obtained. As variables of group Hm carry (in the equation described) great variability loading we could hardly manage interpretation of the other variables, though parameters included into the improved model will probably emerge from that group of variables.

Furthermore, the set of variables under analysis is devoid of age structure of the province inhabitants which may considerably distort the results.

Thus negative effects of variable D_{13} (the proportion of economically active population) may be noted only conditionally. The former part of the paper implied that this parameter should be regarded as an index of socio economic development of a province; now we might argue that these results suggest a positive effect of this complex factor upon the total mortality rates (increased level of activity is correlated with reduced total mortality rates). This conclusion is obviously interesting and thus should be subject to further analysis in subsequent studies.

Factors affecting infant mortality rates (Hm_7)

The model describing this variable assumes the following form:

$$Hm_7 = 0.555Ha_3 - 0.014W_{15} + 0.234W_{16} - 0.045L_{18} + 18.748$$

$$R = 0.62$$

We cannot deny we set the greatest hopes on analysis of the determinants of this variable. For, customarily, the infant mortality rate is regarded as a synthetic index of health situation, and thus the conditions affecting it are most significant for the issue we are analysing. The results, despite all possible reservations related to their temporary nature, confirmed our expectations to a great extent. The model includes two variables describing the general wealth of the province: W_{15} and W_{16} the value of fixed assets and the quantity of investment outlays per head. The first variable describes resources that have already been accumulated: "affluence" which is being utilized by inhabitants. The other variable describes the present "inflow" of resources, ie the process of accumulating resources to be utilized in the future. The level of affluence achieved appeared to be negatively correlated with the infant mortality rate: the higher the wealth the better the health situation.

At the same time, however, a positive correlation occurs between this index and investment outlays, thus: the greater the investment outlays the higher infant mortality rate, so the worse the general health situation.

The conclusions, formulated so far are further confirmed by one of the living standard indices (L_{16} - road density). According to our model the greater the road density the lower infants' mortality rate; so this aspect also of accumulated resources is positively correlated with health situation.

Our results are consistent with the hypotheses formulated and confirmed in different studies. These hypotheses assume that socio economic development (living standard) positively affects health status. At the same time the process of change, especially rapid fluctuations in the socio economic situation, results in adverse health effects.[26]

Curiously enough, the above hypotheses were formulated on the basis of analyses involving time variability (longitudinal studies) and have been confirmed in our cross sectional analysis. The attractiveness of the latter group of our results does not rule out the need to carry on further, more detailed, analysis of several variables specific for the phenomena concerned.

Determinants of resources distribution

Factors affecting the number of physicians (R_{24})

The model describing this aspect of health resources assumes the following form:

$$R_{24} = 0.934Hm_8 - 0.816L_{19} + 0.412L_{20} + 2.621R_{25} + 0.272R_{26} - 13.793$$

$$R = 0.93$$

The best predictors of the number of physicians seem to be two variables describing various parameters within health manpower resources: number of pharmacists (R_{25}) and number of nurses (R_{26}). This result is particularly interesting as it proves that resources may rarely be increased selectively through the growth of just one of their types. We might surmise there is a certain natural tendency to a simultaneous increase in the number of various groups of personnel.

This may impose significant limitions on substitutional handling of work done by various groups of health personnel, e.g. substituting nurses' for physicians' work.

The model includes two variables describing the living standard: the volume of retail sales (L_{20}) and the quantity of living space (L_{19}). The former variable has a plus mark. An increased living standard measured by this parameter is accompanied by an increased number of physicians. This link may evidence some mechanism inducing physicians to undertaking work under better conditions. Admittedly, physicians are more willing to take up a job at areas of higher living standard. However, this suggestion is qualified by the negative sign of the other parameter of the living standard. At the present stage of analysis we would be unable to submit any satisfactory interpretation of this relationship.

What continually underlines our analysis is the problem of the system's appropriate response to population health requirements. At this point of our considerations, this means the quantity of resources corresponding to requirements, which is consistent with the rule: the greater the requirements, the higher the level of resources. The model concerned involves a variable describing the level of total mortality rate (Hm_8), positively correlated with the number of physicians.

Despite all the necessary reservations about this study, this finding gives support to a certain optimism on the principles of resource distribution actually operating.

Factors conditioning the number of nurses (R_{26})

The model describing this aspect of health resources assumes the following form:

$$R_{26} = 0.017Hc_1 + 1.314Ha_3 - 0.423Hm_7 - 6.893Hm_{10} + 0.358L_{20} + 0.008P_{21} + 0.010P_{22} + 0.236R_{27} + 3.030$$

$$R = 0.93$$

The model concerned contains four variables describing health status, yet their role in terms of the postulate of rational resources distribution is obscure. On the one hand, two variables describing infectious diseases prevalence (Hc_1, Ha_3) are positively correlated with the number of nurses; at the same time two parameters of mortality (Hm_7 and Hm_{10}) are negatively correlated with that number. As parameter Ha_7 (infant mortality) is ascribed special significance as most representative for the health situation, then we cannot possibly infer anything about the accomplishment of rational distribution of nursing staff. This reinforces the conclusion that more precise measurements of health requirements are needed to improve the process of interpreting particular relationships.

The model concerned demonstrates that the number of nurses varies depending on health care outlays incurred in particular provinces. This refers both to total expenditure (P_{21}) and health care investment expenditure (P_{22}). Both these relationships confirm the premise that health service expenditure may be treated as a tool to allocated health resources. Our results seem to indicate that nursing staff is more susceptible to such allocation than physicians.

Two variables in the model described confirm the tendencies and relationships found previously. Firstly, the living standard measured by the level of the retail sales is positively correlated with the number of nurses. Secondly, the positive correlation of the test variable with the number of hospital beds (R_{27}) confirms the interrelatedness of various aspects of health resources.

Factors conditioning the number of hospital beds (R_{27})

The model describing this aspect of health resources assumes the following form:

$$R_{27} = -1.621Ha_3 + 1.84L_{19} - 0.027P_{22} + 0.040P_{23} + 0.716R_{24} - 14.778$$

$$R = 0.93$$

The positive correlation of current outlays (R_{23}) with hospital beds confirm the thesis of concurrence of high outlays and resources. The negative correlation with investment outlays may be understood as an attempt to overcome striking disporportions resulting from past decisions.

However, the hypothetical nature of interpretation of the problem should be stressed. The inclusion of the time parameter in the study should clarify the relationships.

The form of the model confirms the thesis (formulated previously) of interrelationships between the parameters describing particular aspects of health resources. The number of physicians (R_{24}) is a variable carrying a great loading of variability, in relation to the variable describing the number of hospital beds.

The role of variable Ha_3 (tuberculosis incidence) affords certain interpretative obstacles since it is high in areas with low health resource indices. High health expenditure in areas with low prevalence appears contrary to the postulate of rational resource distribution. However, tuberculosis prevalence may in this case be considered an index of socio economic position rather than health status. With the adopted broad definition of health such variations in the meaning ascribed to indices sometimes become justifiable. This hypothesis is consistent with the positive correlation of variable L_{29} (dwelling space) with hospital beds.

Determinants of health services activities

Factors affecting attendances at ambulatory services (number of consulations per inhabitant, A_{30})

The model describing this aspect of health care activity at provinces level assumes the following form:

$$A_{30} = 0.006D_{14} - 0.008W_{17} + 0.001P_{23} + 0.225R_{24} + 0.115R_{25} + 0.082R_{29} + 0.0008A_{31} - 0.0003A_{36} - 0.028A_{37} - 1.228$$

$$R = 0.96$$

Of numerous factors affecting the number of consultations, the model contains nine variables; the impact of two groups of variables is marked: first, health service resources, and second, various aspects of health service activities. The greatest impact is that of the number of physicians (R24) which carries on the greatest variability loading. The theory that the more physicians the greater the attendance at outpatients departments has, despite all possible reservations, some logical cause effect sequence.

Of the variables describing health service activities that of physicians' productivity (A_{31}), measured by the number of patients per physician, has the greatest impact. This relationship is entirely consistent with common sense expectations, though it calls for further analysis in view of the hypotheses formulated previously.

The costs per case of ambulatory treatment and hospital treatment are inversely related to attendances. The negative correlation with hospital treatment would have been comprehensible, had the resources been shifted towards outpatient care. But, the results presented in the model imply the reduction in costs of both inpatient and outpatient care. High costs of services cannot be reducing consultations in a system where patients do not bear the cost. Another economic variable in the model, current outlays on health care (P_{23}), is positively correlated with health service activity. This follows our expectations: the greater outlays, the higher the attendance rate. This would imply the category of consultation cost is rather a calculating than economic value, therefore its relationships may be of incidental nature.

Variable D_{14} (proportion of industrial and constructional workers) directly describes the proportions of population having easy access to the health care system within the occupational health service. Its presence in the model may be associated with increased rate of attendances at occupational health service facilities, though this is merely a tentative hypothesis calling for further verification. Industry itself (measured by the number of employees) positively correlates with increased attendance rate, whereas industry's contribution to provinces' wealth is negatively correlated. This would imply that wealthier provinces in this respect exhibit a lesser rate of attendances at outpatient health care facilities. Whether this results from better health status or from different attendances behaviour is an open question at this stage of analysis.

Concluding this fragment of analysis we might observe that the model contains no parameters of the population's health needs, all relationships being related to the area of socio organisational and economic factors.

<u>Factors affecting efficiency of ambulatory services physicians (number of consultations per physician A_{31})</u>

The model describing this aspect of health care activities assumes the following form:

$$A_{31} = -40.078Hm_7 + 0.808D_{11} - 0.556P_{23} - 164.735R_{24} + 394.510A_{30} - 5.128A_{35} + 7213,233$$

$$R = 0.96$$

The number of physicians at a province has a strong negative correlation with the effiency index: the more sparse are physicians, the greater the number of consultations they give. The "strength" and statistical significance of the correlation imposes a brutal conclusion: the more physicians the lower their efficiency at least in the crude numerical forms of this analysis. It is possible that efficiency in terms of health improvement <u>may</u> be better with longer consultations. The hypothesis that alternative strategies are required for satisfying needs, either through resources development or through efficiency increase, receives firm confirmation here.

The efficiency aspect discussed herein is positively correlated with the rate of attendances per province. The relationship found earlier is confirmed here but it should undergo more comprehensive interpretation. It must be pointed out that patients usually spontaneously apply to outpatient health care facilities, and productivity measured in this way is under clients', not physicians' control as a physician is usually obliged to admit all patients applying in a fixed time of service. Attendances per physician also increase with density of population (Variable D_{11}). It may be surmised that under the conditions of increasing urbanization spontaneous attendance increases due to greater accessibility. The impression that physicians' efficiency is coerced by the declared rather than real needs is enhanced by variable Ho_7, infant, mortality rate, appearing with a "minus" sign in the model, which is regarded the most significant health status index.

The conclusion, the worse the health status and greater needs the lesser physicians' efficiency, sounds crude, yet it seems to reveal a fact of major significance for social policy, even if (pursuant to the assumptions adopted) it is not considered a causal relationship.

This stage of studies yields one most striking result, ie the negative correlation between physicians' effiency and current outlays on general health care (P_{23}). That means that an increase in that category of expenditure is accompanied by reduced effiency.

Factors affecting the rates of hospital care (hospital patients per 10,000 inhabitants A_{32})

The model presenting this aspect of health care system activities assumes the following form:

$$A_{32} = -0.109Hc_1 + 6.869Hm_7 - 0.229D_{11} + 0.275P_{23} + 4,789R_{24} + 19.169R_{27} + 13.704R_{29} + 34,401A_{33} -0.075A_{36} -768.997$$

$$R = 0.98$$

As with the results described previously, a factor that is most strongly related to hospital care rates is one of the variables describing resources level (ie the number of hospital beds (R_{27}) and number of physicians per 10,000 inhabitants (R_{24}). The thesis: the greater resources, ie more beds and physicians, the more inpatients that seems to be well grounded. This is consistent with the occurrence of a syndrome of health resources level, affecting the environment as a relatively compact entity. The other parameter describing resources (R_{26}) seems also significant.

A strong statistical relationship occurs also between use of hospital beds A_{32} and treatment productivity, calculated as a number of patients per bed (A_{33}). The effectiveness so defined is positively correlated with the total number of patients, which seems a quite natural relationship.

Different signs accompany the two variables referring to economic characteristics. On the one hand variable A_{36} (hospital treatment costs) is negatively correlated with the rate of hospital care, perhaps due to the spreading of overhead costs; on the other current outlays are positively correlated, as expected.

At first glance the occurrence of variable D_{11} (density coefficient), with a minus sign, seems to pose interpretative obstacles. Usually this is thought to intensify spontaneous attendences, which stimulates the level of resources use and effectiveness.

However, it is possible that this trend refers to outpatient care exclusively and has no impact on hospital care. That would evidence that outpatient care constitutes a specific filter for patients "flow" to inpatient treatment. Thus the demand for outpatient care does not seem to affect significantly the rate of hospital care. What further enhances this conclusion is that the model is devoid of variables describing outpatient care activities.

The lack of the impact of patients' declared requirements on the number of beds does not mean that it is unaffected by real health needs. Certain foundations for the statement that in the situation concerned we are dealing wih an adequate response of the system to needs evidenced by the infant mortality rate (Hm_7), whose indicatory value had been confirmed earlier. A possible thesis is that the greater the health needs (worse health status), the higher the rate of hospital care, is highly optimistic, especially considering that this is the most expensive form of health service.

The unequivocally positive picture is somewhat marred by variable Hc_1 with a negative sign. However, as this parameter is regarded as a much poorer index of the health situation than Hm_7, we are assuming the above thesis is not generally shaken.

<u>Factors affecting the level of hospital care productivity (number of patients per bed A_{33})</u>

$$A_{33} = 0.003Ha_6 - 0.026R_{27} - 1.671A_{34} + 0.070A_{35} + 0.0004A_{36} + 22.280$$

$$R = 0.99$$

Though this equation looks quite well, reaching R = 0.99, definitional relationships seem to account for so high approximation level.

The highest variability loading is that of two variables describing hospital care effectiveness: average stay in hospital (A_{34}) and occupancy rate (A_{35}). (The relationship, the shorter the stay in hospital and the higher the rate of beds use, the more patients treated, may be regarded definitional only when all three interrelated parameters are considered cumulatively. When considered in pairs they may be handled as an empirical relationship which calls for reference to outside variables).

The dangers noted above do not occur when we are attempting to interpret the role of the other parameters occurring in the model. The thesis formulated earlier, of negative correlations between the level of resources and productivity, gets confirmed; number of beds (R_{27}) is negatively correlated with the number of patients per bed.

For the first time in the models produced a positive correlation appears between the effectiveness and treatment cost per case: the cost of one treated patient is positively correlated with the number of patients per bed. This indicates the possibility of intensifying work through increased outlays and not only through extensively increasing the number of beds.

However, taking into account the highly complex nature of variable A36 describing the costs of hospital treatment, we could specify in detail neither the mechanisms of the relationship described nor the possibility of its practical application.

We have previously noticed that the presence of group H variables in the model gives a tentative indication of how effectiveness may be adjusted to real health requirements. Justification of such statements varies with the type of health parameter involved in analysis. While searching for factors determinining the number of hospital patients (A_{32}) we mentioned adequate response to needs, indicated by the infant mortality rate. In the model described herein the incidence of viral hepatitis (Ha_6) is the requirements measure. This is ascribed diversified meaning; it is reported as a health status index and also an index of iatrogenic effects of the system. Under those circumstances the thesis on the response to requirements should be handled with particular caution. Firstly, a reservation should be made that perhaps some of the needs measured are themselves produced within the system; secondly, our analysis primarily indicates the association of the phenomena and in this case knowledge of the causal relationships seems indispensable to interpret the correlations found.

CONCLUSIONS

Naturally, fragmentary results permit merely partial conclusions which are an attempt at the precise specification of questions rather than rendering final responses. As we handled throughout only a limited set of variables, conclusions refer both to methodological and essential problems.

1. Results obtained by the method of automatic selection of variabes for the models cannot be evaluated explicitly. On the one hand, we have obtained very interesting models (eg Hm_7) and any improvement of those models would be relatively easy. On the other hand, in several cases, we have obtained unsuccessful models posing a great risk of definitional or apparent relationships (Hm_8, A_{33}). Apart from work resulting in an improved econometric value of the models, the set of variables included in the models may yield interesting essential conclusions (eg examining one variable of group A excluding the other variables of that group). Primarily, however, variables should be selected which are indispensable for attempts at interpretation made so far.

2. When the econometric form of some models is inadequate, analysis of essential results may seem untimely. Yet, in several cases the form of relationships found is so interesting that it really attracts attention.

2.1 In the group of health parameters some factors affecting infant mortality rates should be emphasised, as this is the most important index of health status at provincial level. The correlations between the health status measured by this index and provinces' socio economic situation have been confirmed explicitly. Furthermore, it has been confirmed that some indication of rapid economic change is accompanied by poorer health status.

2.2 In the group of parameters describing resource distribution the correlations between health resources and provinces' general wealth have been confirmed. However, in certain cases we found the interpretation difficult, when one of the living standard variables, L_{19}, played different roles in different models.

Neither is the role of health service outlays in increasing health resources clear, though it may be tentatively alleged that some kinds of resources, eg nurses, can be more purposefully affected than others. Though in certain cases the role played by the variables describing health status poses difficulties in interpretation, (eg Ha_3 in the model for R_{27}), yet, apparently, the process of resources distribution indicates the impact of health policy.

2.3 Models describing the conditions of use and productivity are least fair (despite very high approximation value, R from 0.96 to 0.99), therefore the conclusion relating to that group of results bear most reservations and are regarded as hypotheses for further studies. Firstly, attention should be paid to the role of health needs in conditioning the use of outpatient and hospital care; yet they constitute an important factor accompanying hospital care use. Secondly, the correlation between the amount and productivity of health resources is evident. It might be thought that those correlations are more significant than parameters of provinces general socio-economic situation. Thirdly, negative correlations between resources magnitude and productivity are striking. Even taking into account the reservation that aggregation of data at province level may underestimate the level of resources use, the correlations are too marked to be ascribed to statistical errors exclusively. And, finally, though the relationships between the level of health needs and productivity are not unambiguous (the role of Ha_6) the negative correlation between health status measured by variable Ha_7 and outpatient care productivity arouses apprehension.

3. Any general conclusions that might be valuable for health policy at provinces level would be resolved into two statements.

Firstly, the possibility of early intervention for health reasons, in the processes of provinces' socio economic development proves pertinent, as many parameters of such development clearly affect population's health status, especially the most sensitive index, the infant mortality rate. Secondly, it seems that, despite certain negative stereotypes, the distribution of health resources in aggregate matches the level of health needs better than the way the resources are applied. Although that does not mean that there are enough resources, yet the possibility of increasing productivity seems extremely important.

REFERENCES

1 eg Lundgren E F, Organisational Management, Cranfield Press, San Francisco 1974; Education of Managers in Health Services, Report on a Working Group, WHO, Copenhagen, 1978.

2 Formulating strategies for health for all by the year 2000, WHO, Geneva, 1979, p 7.

3 Indulski J A, Polish Experience in Country Health Programming (mimeo).

4 Indulski J A, Matulewicz M, Wlodarczyk C, Functioning of the health service in the new administrative structure (in Polish), Zdrowie Publiczne (Public Health) 86/11/1975.

5 Programme of Activities of Ministry of Health and Social Welfare (in Polish), Warsaw 1982, (mimeo).

6 Project of reorganisation of health service - version III, prepared by Polish Economic Society, Warsaw 1981; Indulski J A, Gdulewicz T, Szymborski L, Wlodarczyk C, Health Care in the Polish People's Republic: Attempts at Evaluation and Trends of Rationalisation, (in Polish), Zdrowie Publiczne (Public Health) 92/11/1981.

7 Basic principles of health and social service functioning in the reorganised national economy (in Polish), Warsaw, April 1982 (mimeo).

8 Managerial Process for National Health Development, Guiding Principles, WHO, Geneva, 1981.

9 See eg papers in Schwefel D, John J and Zollner H, 'The Effect of Economic Instability on Health', MEDIS, Springer-Verlag, 1983.

10 WHO, 1979 op. cit. p 14.

11 Lundgren E F, 1978, op. cit.

12 Lukaszewicz, A (ed), Problems of Planning and Socio-Economic Policy (in Polish), Polish Economic Society, Warsaw 1980, Part III, Problems of Shaping Socio-Economic Space.

13 Indulski J A, Wlodarczyk C, Organisational Levels in Health and Social Care, La Sante Publique, Bucharest, 2/1981.

14 Kalimo E, Health service needs, in, Measurement of levels of health, WHO, European series No 7, Copenhagen 1979.

15 Blum H L, Expanding health care horizons, Third Party Associates Inc, California 1976, from, Primary health care and working populations, Geneva 13-16 April 1982, WHO/OCH/82.2.

16 Kaprio L, Future of social and health service in Europe (in Polish), in M Sokolowska and J Holowka (eds), Social policy and health, Warsaw 1978.

17 Morawski W, Social industrialisation in Poland..., in W Morawski (ed) Management in society, Polish Scientific Society, Warsaw 1979, p 174.

18 ibid.

19 Illner M, The structure of social planning and the possibility of resolving social problems (in Polish), in, Sokolowska and Holowka (eds), 1978 op. cit. p 24.

20 ibid, p 27.

21 WHO Regional Office for Europe, Health services in Europe, vol 1, Copenhagen 1981, Chapter 5, pp 66-67.

22 Indulski, Gdulewicz, Szymborski and Wlodarczyk, 1981, op. cit.

23 White K L et al, Health services: Concepts and Information for National Planning and Management, WHO Geneva 1977, Chapter 5, Approaches to resources allocation.

24 Latuch M and Namyslowska M (eds), Social policy: Demographic Conditions, Tasks and Needs (in Polish), Kaiazka i Wiedza, Warsaw 1980.

25 Wlodarczyk W C, Szubert Z, Bryla M, An attempt to analyse some dependencies between economic and health status in Poland in the years 1959-1979, paper presented at WHO MEDIS-Institute Meeting in Munich, 11-13 September 1981.

26 J Kestrzewski (ed), Infectious diseases in Poland and their management in years 1961-1970, Warsaw 1973.

27 Brenner M H, Mortality and the national economy, The Lancet, September 15, 2/1979, pp 568-573.

JOB INSECURITY AND UNEMPLOYMENT: EFFECTS ON HEALTH AND WELLBEING AND AN EVALUATION OF COPING MEASURES

Sten Olof Brenner, Lennart Levi, Heikki Salovaara, Torbjorn Akerstedt, Robert Hjelm, Dag Sorbom, and Sten Tellenback

INTRODUCTION

According to current estimates (UN, ILO) the entire industrialized world is, broadly speaking, on its way toward record unemployment. In Europe there are already 13 million without work (including ten million in the Common Market countries), and in the USA there are about ten million. In the OECD countries, unemployment is expected to stabilize at around 25 - 30 million in the next three to four years, i.e. at a very high level. In the UN it is feared that by the year 2000 there will be over a billion unemployed in the world (1). Inevitably the situation in the world as a whole will have fundamental repercussions on the Swedish labour market as well.

Unemployment in Sweden

Sweden has long ranked among the industrial nations with the lowest unemployment. But even in Sweden the problems are great and probably growing. In August 1982, there were 166,000 persons who were directly unemployed, while 104,000 (152,000 in May) persons were participating in various labour board programmes. Many persons still able to work are going into early retirement, so many in fact that early retirement has become an instrument of labour market policy. In one year, unemployment among the members of the Unemployment Benefits Fund within the unionized sector has increased by 35%. Thirty-one thousand employees received notice of layoff in the first six months of 1982. Many times more live in continuous fear of being laid off. Nor are there any indications of a speedy upturn in employment. On the contrary, National Labour Board forecasts indicate a continued decline during the coming winter. The total number of job vacancies will probably decrease further. For many youths just out of school an indefinite period of unemployment must be expected. Growing unemployment is predicted for one branch of industry after the other. Thirty thousand industrial jobs are expected to vanish (in addition to the 50,000 that disappeared last year). Cutbacks in the public sector àre also now beginning to have tangible effects on employment. The unemployment rate among female municipal employees is now very high. The result could be an unemployment rate of a magnitude which, though perhaps low in comparison with that of Belgium and Great Britain, has not been experienced in Sweden since the thirties.

Nonetheless, surprisingly little is known of the effects of this situation on health and well being, or of the possible ways to prevent damaging effects.

The effects of unemployment

Much research has been done on unemployment in many countries, especially between the two world wars but the extensive social insurance system in our country is one of the reasons why the results of foreign research in these areas cannot be applied directly to the Swedish situation.

Janlert (Ch. 1) presents (in modified form) Everson's and Klausen's survey (2) of current literature on the medical effects of the various phases of a plant shutdown.

They discuss the following effects during the phases of notification, shutdown, unemployment and stabilization: increased uric acid level in the serum, increased release of noradrenalin, high blood pressure, increased drug consumption, more contacts with doctors, increased absence due to illness, more psychological symptoms, reduced general wellbeing, increased serum cholesterol, increased family problems.

The most up to date reviews in this area of research in Sweden are found in Meidner (3) , and Janlert (Ch. 1). According to Meidner, as yet there has been no multidisciplinary research directed toward investigating the effects of unemployment on health and wellbeing. Meidner thinks this is due to "the refusal to accept unemployment as anything other than a temporary misfortune" in an economic administrative labour market policy. Janlert also states that "Swedish studies are generally speaking non-existant".

At present, however, a few such studies are in progress or being planned at the following institutions:

- The Social Medicine Research Unit in Luleå, which is part of the Social Medical Institution at the Karolinska Institute (follow-up of 170 long-term unemployed construction workers as well as a questionnaire study of unemployed youth in a population of 1100 pupils leaving comprehensive school).

- The Varmdo-Nacka Project, Stockholm County Government (follow-up of thirty laid-off dock workers and their families).

- Institution of Sociology, University of Lund (repeated interviews with 40 dock workers on the Oresund docks and repeated questionnaires to 500 dock workers at the same dock).

A model for the relationships between insecurity, unemployment, stress and ailing health

Brenner's perspective together with Kasl's and Cobb's multidisciplinary studies at the individual level and other research, support the assumption that job insecurity and unemployment make major adaptational demands on individuals and groups and that the latter respond to these demands with psychological and physiological stress reactions that in certain individuals and under certain situations can lead to ill health. Such a sequence of events fits in well with the theoretical model for psychologically caused ill health that we presented a decade ago and have used since then as a basis for most of our research (Figure 1). The model is premised on the assumption that stress-inducing and hence health-impairing processes are caused by a poor fit between the demands made and possibilities offered by the environment and the individual's capacities, needs and expectations. The first-named factors in the present case consist in social situations which for the majority of people entail overstimulation or understimulation, role conflicts, role ambiguity, poor personal control over one's own situation, lack of structure, lack of predictability, and lack of meaning. It seems likely that job insecurity at work and unemployment are marked by several of these characteristics and hence constitute high-risk situations (Box 1 in our model).

Susceptibility to one and the same stress will vary from one person to another. High risk groups (Box 2) are probably those that are marred by:

- Certain personality traits (tendency toward depressive or agressive behaviour, low self-confidence, etc.)

- Poor perception of reality

- Inability to cope constructively with problems

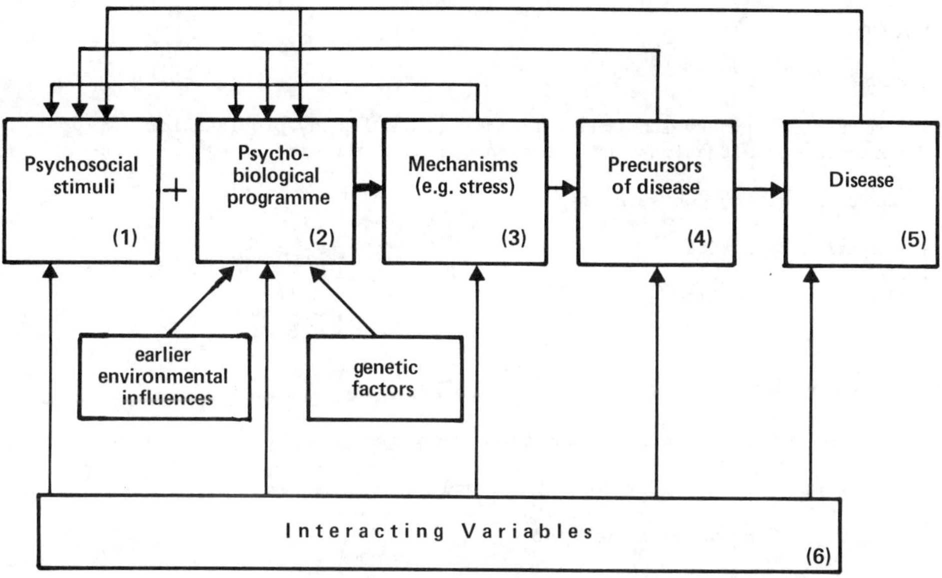

Figure 1 A theoretical model for psychosocially mediated disease. The combined effect of psychosocial stimuli (1) and the psychobiological programme (2) determines the psychological and physiological reaction mechanisms (3), e.g. stress, of each individual. These may, under certain circumstances, lead to precursors of disease (4) and to disease itself (5). This sequence of events can be promoted or counteracted by interacting variables (6). The sequence is not a one-way process but constitutes part of a cybernetic system with continuous feedback (from Kagan & Levi, 1975).

Exposure to high risk situations gives rise to reactions that could lead to disease (high risk reactions Box 3), particularly for high risk groups, but to varying degrees for other persons as well. These reactions include psychological reactions (cognitive and affective), behaviour (e.g. misuse of alcohol and tobacco, self destructive behaviour, sleeping-patterns), and physiological reactions (e.g. changes in the release of pituitary, adrenal and thyroid hormones, changes in the organism's defence mechanisms against infection). The course of events is modified by interacting variables (Box 6) e.g. social support or the lack of it, from family members, friends, workmates, etc.

With minor modifications, this general model can be applied to the range of problems with which this project is concerned.

In a recently published study by Hepworth (4), certain changes in the individual's psychosocial situation that seem to be caused by unemployment are described. These changes might give rise to psychophysiological stress reactions, which in turn could cause ill health. Thus Hepworth found that unemployment had a strongly negative effect on the subjective perception of being able to fill the day with activities. This perceived situation in turn was highly correlated with the occurence of ill health. See Brenner and Bartell (5 and 6).

METHODS

Groups

The multidisciplinary longitudinal observational study provides for a description of situations and reactions in the following cases:

- positions giving job security
- suspicion of notice
- the threat of notice
- notice of layoff
- layoff
- time between the layoff and becoming unemployed
- the transition from work to being unemployed
- unemployment of varying duration
- temporary or permanent resumption of work
- early retirement

The target groups for this study will thus be:

- employees who have gone through all stages in this sequence of events or some of them, and who thus may be compared with themselves retrospectively and prospectively.

- employees who have received notice of layoff but are still not unemployed (group comparison).

- employees who have not received notice of layoff and who may be expecting or do not expect to be unemployed (group comparisons with regard to different degrees of security or insecurity).

The intervention study provides for an evaluation of measures that may be reasonably expected to be of assistance in coping at three levels. For ethical and practical reasons, these measures are administered in the present project as a "package" without any attempt to distribute them among randomized subgroups (see below). On the other hand, a group of laid off persons who receive this action package is compared systematically with a comparable control group not receiving the package. This entails access to two groups who have both been laid off and for whom contamination effects can be kept under control as far as possible. Thus, the individual components in the "package" cannot be evaluated experimentally, although their effects can nonetheless be described, if less ambitiously.

Measurements

Technique or instrument	Variables	Groups
1. questionnaire	a) background data b) work conditions c) daily activities d) control over own life e) assessment of oneself and one's relations with others f) social medical indicators	all subjects in all groups
2. diary	a) quality of sleep b) emotional mood c) daily activities	all subjects in all groups
3. interviews	experienced fit between individual and environment	selection from Group 1 (about 30 persons)
4. tests	personality self-esteem perceived social support family relations coping mechanisms	all subjects in all groups
5. behaviour observations	daily activities	selection from Group 1 (about 30)
6. medical and physiological measurement	hormones immunological defense mechanisms blood fats etc. health data	all subjects in all groups or a selection from them (immunological defence mechanisms)
7. official registry data industrial health care center, health insurance office	background data	all subjects in all groups
8. economic registry data etc.	data on various economic and work conditions and health data	the unemployed in Olofstrom, Blekinge county and Sweden over the last decades

Statistical description and analysis

The present study is being carried out in five groups with repeated measurements before and after unemployment and intervention. The relatively advanced statistical analysis that this requires will be carried out in accordance with the procedures present in Jöreskog and Sörbon (7), in their project "Methodology in Evaluation Research", Lisrel V (Jöreskog and Sörbom, (8)); more conventional methods of descriptive statistics are also used.

SOME PRELIMINARY RESULTS

Reliability of the psychosocial measurements

Many items were included in the questionnaire and diary to measure the cognitive, affective and behavioural status of the participants. Some of the items were well-established scales, others were constructed for this specific study. By mixing old and new scales it was possible to evaluate the validity of the scales, as well as to assess their reliability. It is too early to judge the validity of all scales, but one of the necessary conditions for high validity, namely high reliability, is clearly at hand. See table below.

Table. Reliability of the measurements. Cronbach's alpha for a selection of scales.

Scale	Cronbach's alpha
Daily activities: variation	-
Daily activities: evaluation of	-
Trust in different parties	.88
Perspective on future	.71
Social support (workmates)	.91
Working conditions	.75
Social support (family)	.98
Social support (others)	.75
Goldberg's self-esteem scale	.83
Goldberg's General Health Questionnaire	.88
Psychosomatic complaints	.89
Sjöberg's Mood Scales (comparable to Present Life Situation	.94

Other types of scales included items on more specific aspects of the present situation and the view on the future prospects.

Internal validity of the measurements

By means of principal component analysis the internal validity of the various measurements was explored. The factor structures found were tested by confirmatory factor analysis (a special case of the general LISREL V model).

A strong, invariant factor measuring the psychological or affective state of the participants was established.

Variables	factor loading	t-value
GSE (Goldberg's self-esteem scale)	.728	- *
GHQ (Goldberg's general health questionnaire)	.834	11.1
Psychosomatic complaints	.536	5.9
Sjöbergs mood scale: week-days (SMW)	.681	8.7
Sjöbergs mood scale: holidays (SMH)	.700	8.7

* GSE was used as a constant to fix the scale. This means that no t-value can be computed.

The factor, called affective reactions, was replicated on the second measurement. Furthermore, the factor structure was shown to be invariant over the two measurements collected up to now.

The change in affective reactions from job loss to unemployment

The fact that the affective reaction factor was invariant over the two situations: (1) immediately before job loss, (2) two months after job loss, i.e. during unemployment, makes it possible to measure even minor changes in affective state between the two occasions mentioned. Such an evaluation was done with LISREL, an analysis on structured means. The analysis yielded a satisfactory solution with a small but significant difference in true factor mean between the two situations. The difference was in the direction of improved psychological state. According to the stress model this improvement is caused by a change from a totally unstructured and overstimulating situation (the uncertainty proceeding job loss) to a more stable and comprehensible situation (unemployment). However, in the long run, according to the stress theory, unemployment will lead to stress and impaired health and well-being due to understimulation and lack of meaningful activities.

Some preliminary interrelationships between measurement 1 (job loss) and measurement 2 (unemployment)

In order to explore and test the structure of the measurements of cognitive, affective and behavioural states/reactions LISREL analysis was performed:

1) on each measurement occasion separately

2) on the two occasions jointly, i.e. using a longitudinal model of analysis

In brief, a meaningful structure with satisfactory statistical properties (non-significant deviations from the assumed model) emerged.

A sub model is shown here to give an indication of the type of analysis performed and kind of structure found.

The model is illustrated in Figure 2 below, and the testing of the model and the resulting empirical model is shown in Figure 3.

As seen in Figure 2 it is assumed that the psychological reactions can be separated into three factors:

1) cognitive state

2) affective state

3) behaviours/reactions

For the moment no regard is given to physiological measures. In the assumed model the relationships within the variables (structural relationships) as well as the relationships between the two measures (process relationships) are indicated.

Figure 2 Assumed (theoretical) sub model

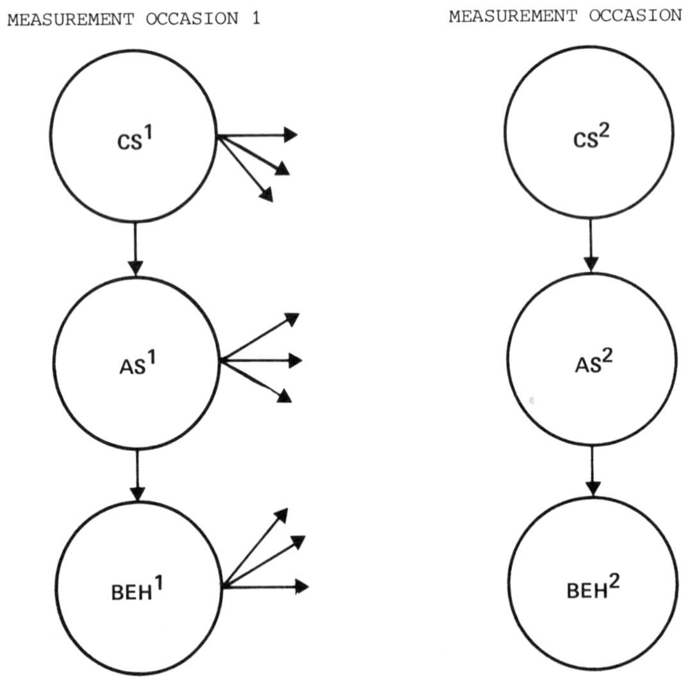

CS = cognitive state

AS = affective state

The assumed model was used as an input to LISREL together with correlations between the variables picked out to measure the theoretical constructs.

Theoretical construct (latent variable)	Measured variable(s) (manifest) variable(s)
cognitive state	perspective on future
affective state	see factor above
behaviour	sleep in minutes per night

The analysis resulted in the following empirical model, which was statistically satisfactory: See Figure 3.

Figure 3 An empirical model of psychological reactions to job loss and unemployment. Standardized structural coefficients. (P = .21) n = 90.

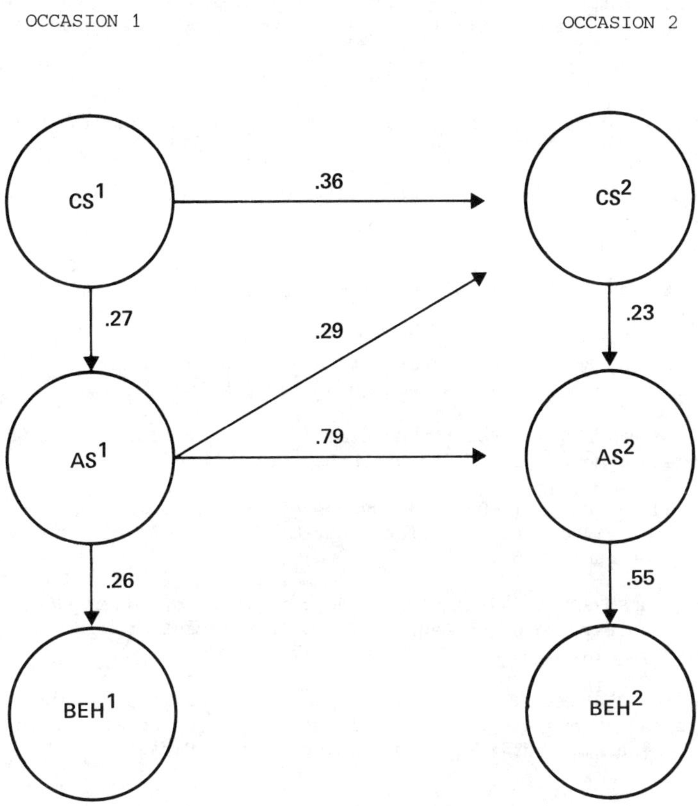

The analysis showed that some of the assumed relationships were empirically supported, while others were lacking. No unexpected relationships emerged.

In brief, the psychological state on occasion 1 explained a large part of the psychological state on occasion 2. A good predictor of affective state was the perspective on the future. The sleep pattern at occasion 2 was influenced by the affective state (better state gave more sleep).

A possible explanation of the weaker relationship between affective state and sleep at occasion 1 is the restrictions imposed on wake and sleep patterns by the work.

DISCUSSION

Some preliminary analysis gave meaningful and statistically satisfactory results.

Although no conclusions can yet be drawn concerning the effects of job insecurity and unemployment on health and well-being in this study, the results indicate that the complete study will allow such conclusions.

The additional information given by physiological and medical data could possibly sensitize the analysis to changes in health and well-being.

REFERENCES

1. JANLERT U (1981) Medicinska effekter av arbetslösheten. Läkartidningen 78:39:3374-7.

2. IVERSEN L, KLAUSEN H (1981) The closing of Nordhavn shipyard 1976 - the consequences for the workers in relation to employment, economy and health. Cardiff 1981 (Stencil).

3. MEIDNER R (1981) PM om forskningen kring arbetslöshetens individuella effekter. 1981 (Stencil).

4. HEPWORTH S J (1980) Moderating factors of the psychological impact of unemployment. Journal of Occupational Psychology 53:139-145:1980.

5. BRENNER S-O and BARTELL R (1982) Structural analysis of some psychological aspects of unemployment. Stress Research Reports No. 162, Stockholm.

6. BRENNER S-O and BARTELL R (1982) The psychological impact of unemployment: a structural analysis of cross-sectional data. Journal of Occupational Psychology (to be published).

7. JÖRESKOG K G and SÖRBOM D (1980) Simultaneous analysis of longitudinal data from several cohorts. Research Report 80 - 5, Department of Statistics, University of Uppsala.

8. JÖRESKOG K G and SÖRBOM D (1981) LISREL V. Analysis of linear structural relationships by maximum likelihood and least squares methods. Research Report 81-8. Department of Statistics, University of Uppsala.

ASSESSING THE EFFECTS OF UNEMPLOYMENT ON HEALTH SERVICES USE IN A SPECIFIC GROUP: A RESEARCH PROPOSAL

J. P. Auray, G. Duru, I. Dussuyer, J. Riondet, M. Terrenoire

INTRODUCTION

The present paper outlines an approach which looks in a restricted manner at the health unemployment relationship for a specific group using highly circumscribed data. It is contended that there is a need to develop such approaches in view of the many inconclusive resulted obtained by research on this subject (Ramsden and Smee 1981; Cook 1982, Fox 1975).

The proposal to be described attempts to overcome several methodological difficulties by (1) focussing on the socio-professional category of 'cadres' - employed in managerial positions; (2) selecting from this population a sample of unemployed 'cadres' (made redundant but with previous salary maintained); (3) comparing their health status (defined by health service use over the 2 year period before unemployment occured and the 2 following years, with the matched control sample.

One difficulty for research in this field is that relying on surveys or interviews of the unemployed is both time consuming and costly (the unemployed are not easily accessible) and the influence of the interview situation on self reports about health status cannot be ignored. Other problems arise when one tries to use data from existing records. In France while the National Census has relevant data on socio demographic variables and on employment, there is no link up to health statistics for the general population. Even if such a link up was feasible, and permitted, health statistics (those originating from the Social Security) have their own drawbacks. The French National Health scheme, while virtually insuring everyone for health care, only has data on its files of those who have requested reimbursement for a specific act or health service use[(a)]. It is frequent practice not to claim reimbursement on the day the health service was used, but at some later date. Since the records only contain the date on which Social Security payments were made and not the date when the health service was used, there is a displacement in time which can sometimes be for more than 6 or 12 months and can distort findings if a short period is studied. In addition, Social Security records are only kept for 12 months, thus making the study of long term effects impossible. Finally, and most regrettably, the Social Security has no data on pathology or diagnosis for individuals. This information remains confidential in the files of individual practitioners.

Most importantly however, we still do not know whether and how much of the ill health experienced by the unemployed is caused by their unemployment and how much is determined by conditions prior to job loss (Jahoda et al 1972). Instead of clarifying the causal issue, many studies appear to be perpetuating the ambiguities and it may be that the data relied on so far have not been sufficiently sensitive. Aggregate studies, in particular, may have exhausted their potential for clarifying the relationship (Brenner 1976, Stern 1981). Other approaches, more adapted to the difficult measurement issues involved, are clearly desirable.

(a) In France the individual pays the doctor or health service per act and subsequently claims reimbursement from the Social Security, justifying his entitlement by salary slip, unemployment card.

CONCEPTUAL FRAMEWORK AND RESEARCH DESIGN

Definition of the socio professional category "cadres"

Fortunately for researchers, there are specific groups in the population, who, wanting a more complete health insurance, join Private Insurance Schemes, providing supplementary coverage ("Caisse de retraite complémentaire") which centralise information on the utilisation of health services, together with information on employment. One such group are the "cadres" who, broadly classified as belonging to the middle class, generally represent top and middle level management. The work situation of the "cadres" can be characterised by a considerable amount of responsibility, and authority over others and by the amount of variety in their work which is only indirectly supervised from above. The "cadre" has generally considerable control over his work, the speed and the way it is organised and carried out; there is room for discretion and initiative as long as set goals are achieved. Incomes tend to be high[(b)] and jobs are secured by contracts. Opportunities exist for promotion and fringe benefits (expense account, company car). There is also likely to be a close link between their social status, their self image and their job.

To speak about "cadres" as a relatively homogeneous socio professional group is somewhat misleading. The term covers very real differences in job role, position and tasks (technical, managerial, production, administrative, commercial) both in the private and public sector and depending on the source of information used, large variations are obtained in the number of individuals defined as "cadres". Nevertheless, it has been suggested (eg Gourmelen 1981) that there are common elements a high symbolic value attachment to the job and inherent job frustrations.

As an intemediary between those who implement decisions and those who initiate and make policy and top managerial decisions, the "cadre" to whom authority is delegated, is often in an ambiguous position in the employment hierarchy. At the same time, high achievement needs and low job mobility often lead to a firm attachment to the company or business in which he is employed.

However, with the current economic crisis, "cadres" are finding themselves faced with job instability, just as workers lower down in the employment hierarchy are, and the hidden frustrations of the "cadres" job are now being revealed. Previously they could be contained or compensated for by increases in salary and fringe benefits. Although the rate of unemployment of "cadres" is below that of other socio-professional categories, there has been a noticeable increase in the proportion of "cadres" unemployed, from 2.1% in 1971 (job seekers registered with the Employment Ministry) to 3.4% in 1979, representing a monthly average of 63.000, compared with 6.9% for all salaried workers in 1979.

(b) In 1975, the average annual salary was 88.000 FF for "cadres superieurs" and 43.000 FF for "cadres moyens"; average annual salary for salaried workers was 29.000 FF and the basic wage 14.000 FF.

In a recent study (Gourmelen, 1981), conducted by the ANPE (National Employment Bureau) in which unemployed "cadres" were interviewed (2,046 responses were obtained by postal questionnaire response rate 58%); the profile of the unemployed "cadres" revealed their high education level, a long stable employment history, with few job changes. The last job was held, for 41% of the sample, for at least 5 years. A majority were unemployed for the first time (75%). Two sub-groups are specifically identified.

1) a minority of highly qualified young "cadres" (less than 30 years) who are either looking for their first job or who had lost a short term contract job and had experienced only short periods of unemployment.

   and

2) a second larger group composed of older "cadres" (24% were 50 or older who have been in stable employment for a long time with few job changes. Individuals in this group have generally lost their previous job as a result of economic dismissal and are experiencing their first spell of unemployment. Their chances of finding work are relatively small and they face strong competition from younger, better qualified "cadres" who are pehaps more diversified and better adapted to the demands of today's job market. Many had been unemployed for at least one year (23%).

The conclusion drawn from the study was that for the second group of "cadres" unemployment is severely penalized and it might be expected that for these older men, unemployment may be a particularly disturbing and stressful event as the change from active employment to sudden inactivity is likely to be without preparation arriving with little or no warning, and an event over which the individual can exercise little direct control.

While it is not necessary to identify the precise mechanism by which economic fluctuations exert an influence on health, it is appropriate, in a society where national health insurance schemes eliminate or minimise the need for individuals to pay for health service use, (and thus where modifications in available revenue as a result of job loss ought to have little influence on such use), to examine the hypothesis that when a high symbolic value is attributed to work as in the case of the "cadres" and when there is a sudden unexpected job loss there is a traumatic impact on health status and thus lead to health care consumption.

Unemployment, as the sudden loss of a job, due to external economic circumstances, can represent a situation which tests an individual's capacity to cope and adapt. In this way, unemployment and the reactions it provokes differ little from other life change events. Marris (1974), for example, has described "grief" reactions to a broad range of social changes whereby the individual attempts to develop some meaningful continuity between past, present and future relationships. Toffler (1970) has also summarised some of the findings on life changes requiring considerable adjustment and coping and which show correlations with illness indicators.

Gaulier (1982) in a French study has also identified such grief reactions among the unemployed. Feelings of painful loss, general depression, frequent symptoms of distress, a sense of helplessness, direct or displaced anger were noted and are very similar to the mourning reactions for a deceased person. He suggests that for the "cadre", the greater his job responsibility, the more the job loss represents a personal crisis for him and where subsequent inactivity may represent a form of "social death".

The present study will thus be looking at the health unemployment relationship within the relatively homogenous group of "cadres" for whom work may have similar high symbolic value, and where the rate of unemployment is still relatively low. It is also a group where environmental factors known to be associated with poor health status (low income, poor housing) are likely to be less influential.

Database

Cooperation has been obtained from a large Private Insurance Fund providing supplementary coverage for "cadres" in the Rhone Alpes region, allowing access to their centralized data bank.

The Fund specifically covers the socio professional categories of "cadre" and "assimilé"[c] and has records dating back 10 years on approximately 100.000 individuals who voluntarily join the scheme and pay its premiums to obtain supplementary health and social benefits. The Fund also provides benefits in case of disability, unemployment, retirement or death. The data bank has information available on the following variables:

TABLE 1

Description of variables

VARIABLES	NOTATION
Date of unemployment as defined by "mise en garantie de resource"	TMGR
Age at the moment T	AGE (T)
Family situation at T	SITFA (T)
Salary bracket at T	SAL (T)
Date of death	DATDE
Number of days sick leave before T over k years	JAV (T, k)
Number of days sick leave after T over k years	JAP (T, k)

(c) "Assimilés" refers to "contremaître", "agent de maîtrise", job categories that are just below that of "cadres" and representing office and white collar workers with some managerial responsibilities.

VARIABLES	NOTATION
Individual health services use before T over k years (p components)*	CAV (T, k)eR^P
Individual heath services use after T over k years (p components)*	CAP (T, k)eR^P

* Included are frequency and type of health service use and their cost.

Measurement of Unemployment

The definition of unemployment is important when deciding which unemployment statistic to use. In France, the National Census Bureau defines the unemployed as "those available for of a job" and includes first job seekers. A more restrictive definition is where the individual has been dismissed from a job. Again another definition is in terms of being eligible and receiving unemployment benefits. The National Employment Agency again relies on another definition: the unemployed are those who have registered as "looking for work".

The data on unemployment obtained from the Fund are likely to reflect quite accurately the occurence of job loss. As automatic deductions from salaries for the Fund's premiums stop upon job loss, the Fund makes up points lost for this reason so that retirement benefits remain unaffected by the unemployment. Selected for analysis in this study is a specific group of unemployed "cadres" those whose unemployment is covered by the legislation concerning "mise en garantie de ressources". What this roughly means is that when job dismissal occurs for economic reasons (factory closure, bankruptcy) to individuals who are 55 years or older, the government supplements regular unemployment benefits up to age of retirement to the previous income level.

Indicators of Health Services Use

As for the Social Security records, the Provident Fund unfortunately has no information about the pathology or diagnosis of the individual in relation to his use of health care services used. Details do exist as to the frequency and type of care or service. Thus we know whether the individual was hospitalised or went to a nursing home; whether doctors (GP or consultant), dentists, laboratory analysis, or nursing care were used; drug prescriptions or medical equipment purchased. In addition, a precise monetary value is placed on the different services used so that costs can be estimated and included in the analysis.

Using "medical consumption" or health services use as an indicator of the individual's health status may appear a simple and fairly reliable way of obtaining information about an individual's health. Although such recorded health information is not a true measures of actual health status. From previous studies (Brown, 1976), it is known that there are many social factors which motivate an individual's use of health services. It is also known that the socio professional category of "cadres" have general lower mortality and morbidity rates, compared to other categories. At the same time, they are high consumers of medical services. Thus Mizrahi (1981) found, using 1970 data on health service use across socio professional categories, that there were 3 groups with low health services use: agricultural workers, shopkeepers, skilled and unskilled workers, while white collar workers, "cadres", and professionals have high health services use. Use of specialised health services in particular correlates with the higher socio professional categories.

Given the very complete health insurance of the "cadres", that this group are likely to know their health care rights and use them, it can be argued that health services use as measured by frequency, type of act and cost are sufficiently sensitive to reflect changes in health status when unemployment occurs.

METHOD OF ANALYSIS

Samples, matched for age, family situation and salary, will be drawn from the population contributing to the Fund. Specifically one sample of unemployed "cadres" will be selected from those who have become unemployed, as defined by the "mise en garantie de ressources", during the period December 1979 and January 1980. The control sample will have been in continuous employment and in the Fund's data bank for at least three years before that period.

In each sample, we will measure the variables relating to the health services use of each individual during the two year period prior to December 1979 and for the two year period following January 1980.

It is proposed:

1. Firstly to test the hypothesis of homogeneity of health services use before the time of job loss as defined by "mise en garantie de ressources" and after this time for the unemployed sample. Individuals will thus act as their own controls. Significant differences will be tested by the usual non parametric statistical tests (Student matched and Wilcoxon matched).

   We will also examine the influence of the variables Age and Family Situation in the statistical variables being considered. For this purpose, a non parametric analysis of variance[d] will be carried out. The explanatory effect of age on health services use before and after the time of job loss will also be tested using a linear model.

(d) Kruskall-Wallis test.

2. A second approach designed to eliminate the effect of the passage of time on health services use, will be carried out on the matched samples from the unemployed (P1) and employed population (P2). We will first test for the homogeneity of health services use before December 1979, on sample P1 and on sample P2 and secondly, the homogeneity of health services use before December 1979, and after January 1980 over a two year period for sample P2. Finally, the homogeneity of health services use after January 1980 on samples P1 and P2 will be tested. As before, the statistical tests used will be the Student matched or, if the usual hypotheses of normality are rejected, a Wilcoxon matched test which does not make any assumptions about the variables or the distribution of standard deviations. However this test is less powerful.

Figure 1

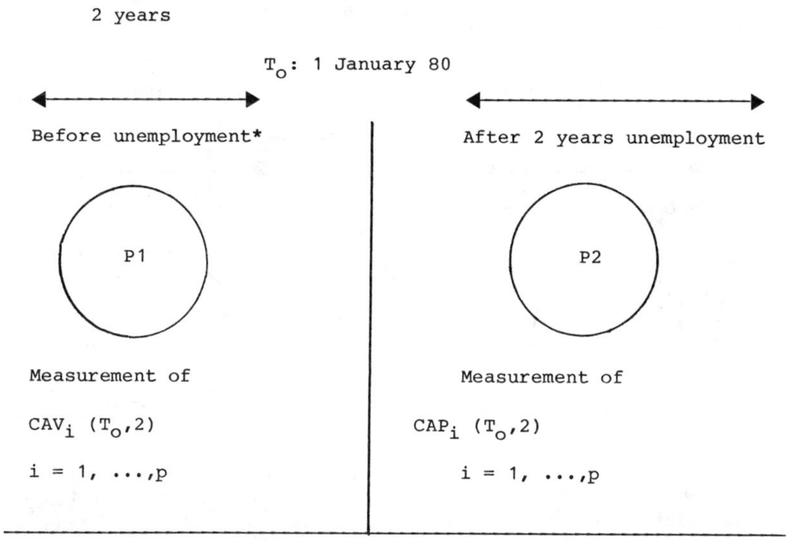

The following will be tested:

1. Ho: $E\,[CAV_i\ (T_o,2)] \quad = \quad E\,[CAP_i\ (T_o,2)]$

against:

H1: $E\,[CAV_i\ (T_o,2)] \quad \neq \quad E\,[CAP_i\ (T_o,2)]$

2. Non parametric analysis of variance using factors AGE, then SALARY.

---

* defined as "mise en garantie de ressources".

3. Linear model: $CAV_i\ (T_o, 2) = a\ AGE\ (T_o) + b$

$$CAP_i\ (T_o, 2) = c\ AGE\ (T_o) + d$$

Validation of the model is carried out by testing:

$$a = c \quad \text{against} \quad a \neq c$$

$$b = d \quad \text{against} \quad b \neq d$$

Figure 2

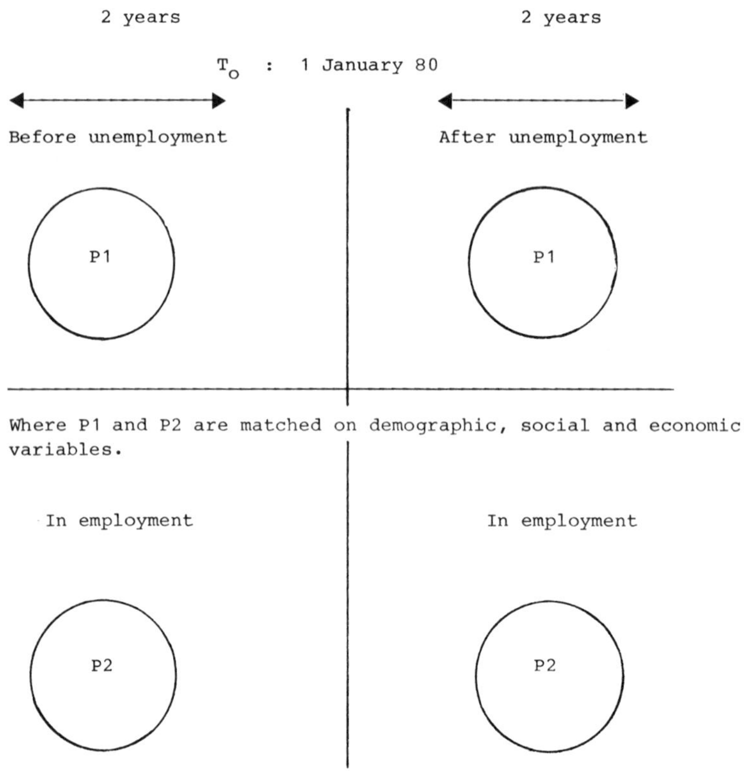

The following will be tested:

1. $H_o : E[CAV^{P1} (T_o, 2)] = E[CAV^{P2} (T_o, 2)]$

   against

   $H_1 :$ " $\neq$ "

2. $H_o : E[CAV^{P1} (T_o, 2)] = E[CAP^{P2} (T_o, 2)]$

   against " "

   $H_1 :$ $\neq$

3. $H_o : E[CAP^{P1} (t_o, 2)] = E[CAP^{P2} (T_o, 2)]$

   against " "

   $H_1 :$ $\neq$

NB

The notation $CAV_i (T_o, 2)$ designates the i^e projection of variable $CAV^i (T_o, 2)$; and the same applies for $CAP_i (T_o, 2)$

$CAV^{Pj} (T_o, 2)$ designs the i^e projection of variable

$CAV (T_o, 2)$ as measured on sample Pj,* J = 1, 2

* Description of medical facts.

Supplementary analysis could eventually be carried out on deceased individuals (information is available on cause and date of death) and on the group "assimilés" and on the group of self employed who under certain circumstances adhere to this Fund for "cadres".

CONCLUSIONS

As a contribution to the clarification of the complex unemployment health relationship, the proposal just described represents an attempt at empirically demonstrating whether unemployment, defined by "mise en garantie de ressources" has a measurable impact on use of health services in the specific socio-professional category of "cadres". We believe that it should produce precise, quantitative and statistically unambiguous results in response to our limited research question.

It is likely that from the findings obtained it cannot be concluded that unemployment has an influence on health services use ie no significant differences will be found for the same individuals before and after job loss nor between individuals who have experienced unemployment and those who have remained in continuous employment. The results may thus reveal the necessity for conducting further micro analyses, with more precise identification of subgroups among the unemployed and of mediating factors, such as social support.

References

Brenner, H., 'Mortality and the National Economy: A Review and the Experience of England and Wales', Lancet, September 1976.

Brown, G. W., Social Causes of Disease in an Introduction to Medical Sociology, (ed.) Tuckett, D., Tavistock publication, 1976.

Bugener, M., Horellou-Lafarge, C., and Louis, M. V., Chômage et Santé, Economia, Paris, 1982.

Combe, M., L'Alibi - Troubles Psycho-Physiologiques Consécutifs à Une Opération de Licenciment Collectif, Gallimard, Coll. Témoin, Paris, 1970.

Cook, D. G., et al, 'Health of Unemployed Middle Age Men in Great Britain', Lancet, 5th June 1982, 1290-4.

Fox, A. J., Golblatt, P. O., 'Longitudenal Study - Socio-Demographic Mortality Differentials', Series LS, No. 1, HMSO, 1971-1975.

Gaullier, X., L'Avenir à Reculons: Chômage et Retraite, Les Editions Ouvrières, Lyon, 1982.

Gourmelen, M., 'L'Emploi et le Chômage des Cadres vus par l'ANPE', Travail et Emploi, Avril/Juin 1981.

Jahoda, M., Lazarsfeld, P. F., Zeidel, H., Marienthal: The Sociography of a Unemployed Community, Tavistock reprinted, 1972.

Louis, M. V., Galland, O., 'Les Jeunes Chômeurs: Rapport Cordes', Travail et Société, 1977.

Marris, P., Loss and Change, Routledge and Kegan Paul, London, 1974.

Mizrahi, A., 'Le Profil Economique et Sociologique du Malade Francais', La Santé des Français, Cercles Universitaires, PUF, Paris, 1981.

Ramsden, S., Smee, C., 'The Health of Unemployed Men: DHSS Cohort Study', Employment Gazette, 1981, pp. 397-401.

Scott-Samuel, A., 'Out of Work, Out of Sorts', *The Health Services*, 29/10/82, pp. 12-13.

Servan Schreiber, J. J., *Le Défi Mondial*, Fayard, Paris, 1980.

Stern, J., 'Unemployment and Its Impact on Morbidity and Mortality', *Discussion Paper No. 93*, Centre for Labour Economics, September 1981.

Toffler, A., *Future Shock*, Pan Books, London, 1970.

Part III

Policy issues

RECESSION AND HEALTH - THE POLICY IMPLICATIONS

Stephen J Watkins

In Chapter 2 I have summarised the findings of extensive research on the links between recession, unemployment and health. The policy implications of these conclusions can be considered at four levels. In increasing order of desperation these are:

1. So to conduct the economy that recession is avoided.

2. So to structure the economy that unemployment does not occur even in recession.

3. So to arrange social policy that the health damage of unemployment is minimised.

4. To plan health services so that the health damage caused by unemployment is taken into account in the services available.

It is also necessary to consider in the same way the other processes whereby recession damages health.

Avoiding recession

After the Great Depression of the 1930s it was felt that the new techniques of Keynesian demand management would prevent unemployment happening again. The idea was that unemployment reflected a lack of demand in the economy and that the injection of money would create the necessary demand and lift the economy out of the recession. It was recognised that sometimes the economy responded to an injection of money by inflation (in effect destroying the money that had been injected by reducing the value of money) but it was thought that this would only happen when the economy was already running at maximum capacity so that there was no scope for growth. It was therefore thought that recession and inflation could not coexist.

The horrible discovery of the 1970s was that an economy which was in recession could still respond to an injection of money by producing inflation instead of growth. The reason that this should have happened is not known.

Some economists argue that recessions are necessary in order to get rid of inefficient units. If an economy avoids recession it builds up inefficiencies and rigidities until ultimately the point arises at which it is necessary to rid itself of them and recession cannot be avoided. Therefore if an economy is to be run without recession it must develop some other way of fulfilling this function.

Others argue that the problem is that people become accustomed to the mechanisms of demand management and become adept at the process of diverting the injected money into their own pocket. 'Investment Technology' is diverted into money market distortions, property markets etc, whilst workers expect pay increases without increased production instead of permitting money to be used to employ the unemployed. This group of economists see the solution in linking Keynesianism to pay policies and direction of investment.

Others believe that the problem is that the tendency grew up of being non-selective in the form that the injection of money took. Money spent on public projects or given to the poor is far more likely to create jobs than money given to the rich through tax cuts or returned non-specifically to industry since it will be spent rather than saved. Similarly, help given to industry by spending money on socially useful goods will be more likely to create jobs than money given in the form of grants to pay firms to make things that nobody wants to buy.

Others (the monetarists) believe that Keynes was wrong anyway and some (the supply side economists) believe that the answer is to remove controls from industry.

The application of their methods in Britain, America and Chile have served only to make the recession worse.

Another school of thought believes that either the limits of industrial productive capacity (the ecology school of thought) or the limits of need for industrial production (the Keynesian under-consumption school) has been reached but we have not yet changed our mode of thought so as to see economic growth primarily in terms of better public services more leisure and an improved quality of life. Keynes himself envisaged such a situation ultimately being reached, but not just yet.

The debate between these different schools of thought is an economic debate which is a little beyond the scope of this paper.

Can we abolish unemployment?

There are those who believe that full employment cannot be restored simply by the kind of tuning of the economy which is implicit in most of the economic thinking reviewed in the last section.

This includes those who believe, like Shearman & Jenkins (1979) or Draper et al (1979) that we are on the verge of a technological revolution which will abolish millions of jobs, just as the agricultural revolution freed people from agricultural labour and allowed an entirely new direction to economic growth. It also includes those who are just pessimistic.

It is not, however, necessary to accept that unemployment is therefore inevitable. If we have a surplus of labour then either we are producing all goods and services which we need, in which case we can share out the work and all have more leisure, or we are not producing all the goods and services we need, in which case the unemployed can be employed producing them. That is a simple, and inherently pleasant, choice which our society manages to turn into a tragedy.

More leisure could mean longer holidays, earlier retirement, shorter working weeks, sabbaticals during working life, secondment for sport or education or public duties or any combination of these.

More production could include the building of schools, houses or hospitals, improved staff ratios in education or the caring services, new developments in the caring services, the production of socially useful goods such as medical equipment or aids for the disabled, the expansion of public transport, work on projects designed to help the Third World, increased incomes for the poor so that they can afford to buy consumer goods which other people can be employed making, more support for the arts (which are a labour intensive industry), or more employment on environmental improvement.

If this approach were to be followed, a number of judgements would be required. The first judgement would be the extent to which the labour surplus is permanent and the extent to which it is temporary. To the extent that it is temporary the problem would be to find temporary socially useful work for those who were displaced whilst at the same time ensuring that they possessed the skills which they would need on reintegration into the economy. Industries which expected to recover might be encouraged to keep contact with the workforce by seconding them in rotation, or part time, to socially useful work. Training for skills expected to be in short supply when the economy picks up would be important. Use of spare industrial capacity for short term socially useful production would keep industrial units together. Socially useful work programmes would be designed around the skills of the people who are available and would be predominantly short term capital schemes which, whilst useful, could be run down quickly if demand picked up in areas of higher priority.

To the extent that the labour surplus is considered to be permanent quite different considerations apply. Permanent socially useful jobs could be created in the light of social priority, rather than suit the jobs to the skills available. People would be retrained for the skills that were needed. Draper et al (1979), argue that expansion of the caring industries could play an importart part in this job creation.

However, if the labour surplus is considered to be permanent, it also becomes possible to consider the extent to which increased leisure should play its part in the solution.

A programme of abolishing unemployment, therefore, would need to start from the following judgements:

a) What is the extent of the labour surplus? - this is not the same as the number of unemployed. On the one hand some level of unemployment will always exist, even in full employment, because of people who are changing jobs. On the other hand, a programme of abolishing unemployment would draw into the labour market many who are now included in the "hidden unemployed" and might facilitate job losses in industries where there is surplus labour which is being retained in a state of underemployment because the only alternative is unemployment.

b) To what extent is this permanent; - the initial tendency must be to err on the side of regarding it as temporary. As events unfold people can be transferred from temporary schemes to permanent ones.

c) What are the priorities as between encouraging leisure and creating jobs?

d) Having determined how many permanent jobs are to be created by social expenditure, in what sectors are they of highest priority?

It would then consist of three sets of programmes in the necessary balance and pursued to such extent that unemployment was reduced to that level which reflects merely the permanent level of people between jobs in full employment (ie long term unemployment would be zero).

The three sets of programmes would be:

1. Measures to encourage leisure. These could consist of grants to support job sharing, legislation to limit working hours, legislation guaranteeing a right to part time work without discrimination, legislation on holidays, pensions adjustments to encourage early retirement or sabbaticals (for example, allowing people to draw a certain number of years of pension before retirement age at whatever time they choose) and measures to increase leisure opportunities, such as support for sports facilities, legislation extending access rights to the countryside, education for leisure, health education programmes centred around the concept of leisure etc.

2. A programme for creating permanent socially useful jobs by expanding public services, expanding public capital programmes and providing public authorities with funds to spend on socially useful equipment to be manufactured by industry.

3. A programme of temporary measures. This would guarantee meaningful socially useful work to anybody on demand, and a special agency would be created to set up such temporary jobs. This agency would also be responsible for retraining (in the United Kingdom such an agency exists as the Manpower Services Commission). Industries could be given grants to second workers to this agency if they wished to keep contact with them through hard times. The agency could also be permitted to make earmarked grants to public authorities to buy goods from industries which have spare capacity.

I have not mentioned the cost of such a programme. In resource terms it would cost nothing since the resource it uses is one which would otherwise be wasted. In cash terms it may cost money, but the money would be redistributive (it would simply allocate to the unemployed their fair share of society's resources in return for their fair share of society's work (which they have always been willing to do). In a moral sense it may be argued that it doesn't matter what it costs. Whatever it costs must be recovered from the rest of the population in taxation and they have no right to appropriate it by creating scapegoats.

In a political sense it does matter, because there are limits to the willingness of members of any society to carry through redistributive measures whatever the moral imperative. It is arguable however, that such a programme would not approach those limits. Fear of unemployment is so widespread that large numbes of people, besides the unemployed themselves, have an interest in its abolition. Its effect falls upon school leavers in a way which gives many who have no direct interest in its abolition an indirect interest through their children. The products of the programme - leisure and improved public services - are themselves benefits to which people attach value. And many estimates exist which show that the cost isn't horrifyingly large anyway. Some which build in a large Keynesian multiplier effect even conclude that the cost is negative (Whiting 1980). When account is taken of the savings in unemployment benefit, the extra direct taxes and the extra indirect taxes Mukherjee (1976) calculates that the state recovers 90% of job creation expenditure in Britain and more in some other countries. This assumes that jobs are created at wage rates which have the same average as the national average wage. It may be that the jobs created would have a rather higher proportion than average of jobs of lower skill levels and would therefore, even without any exploitation, attract wages which on average were rather below the national average. However, it must also be borne in mind that not all of those taking advantage of such a programme will have been in receipt of unemployment benefit. On the other hand the Keynesian multiplier will create jobs in addition to those provided by the programme.

Taking all these considerations into account, it seems likely that there <u>would</u> be a net cost but it is possible to argue that it would not be a politically impossible one, especially if the genuine benefits derived from the programme are properly spelt out and the moral imperative stressed. Genuine benefits combined with small costs and a glow of moral satisfaction are politically saleable.

Sustaining the unemployed

The health effects of unemployment may be derived from two sources. One is poverty and the other is psychological. So far as the first is concerned there is no solution to poverty other than money. There is much evidence that unemployment benefit in Britain leaves many unable to meet a socially acceptable minimum living standard (see Popay Ch. 18).

So far as psychological effects are concerned the factors which have been shown to be important are social support, the strength of the work ethic, self esteem and time structuring.

SOCIAL SUPPORT - Our society has attached far too little importance to the preservation of systems of social support. This is not a problem only affecting the unemployed, but affecting many other areas of health as well.

There is a need for a public policy to conserve and develop social support mechanisms. Greenblatt et al (1982) advocate the use of impact statements to document the noxious effects of planing developments on community social support systems. The Study Commission on the Family advocates family impact statements. In the field of labour policy it would be helpful to move away from the concept that geographical mobility of labour is efficient, and recognise instead that the destruction of support networks is a hidden cost. The Barclay Enquiry (1982), has advocated more social service resources for community development.

More immediately, and more specifically for the unemployed are two possible measures. One is the use of unemployment centres (Winfield 1981; Popay 1981, both make important comments on this development). The other is the idea of giving the unemployed free access to recreation facilities and free use of public transport so that they need not withdraw into isolation due to lack of money.

WORK ETHIC - Warr's point about the inappropriateness of encouraging the work ethic in a group of people only a fraction of whom can find jobs deserves attention. The largest single area in which change is needed is in the administration of unemployment benefit which in many countries, including Britain, is still heavily tied to the seeking of work.

SELF ESTEEM - The enhancement of self esteem will almost certainly be best achieved by the combination of measures falling under the other categories. A specific problem, however, is the behaviour of politicians and press who find it suits their interest to attack the unemployed. In a free society such behaviour cannot be banned. But, it can be repudiated loudly and publicly by other politicians and by the caring professions.

The behaviour of public officials who insult the unemployed in the course of their administrative duties is another matter. It could be made clear that it will be regarded as a disciplinary offence. In Britain, the special staff allocated to investigate social security fraud could be transferred, on cost effectiveness grounds, to work on tax avoidance.

TIME STRUCTURING - The unemployed should be offered counselling in the use of their time. Martin (1960) describes "disorders of leisure" which prevent large sections of our society from making use of free time. Education for leisure is important and should be incorporated into schools and into health education programmes. Dauncy (1981) has produced a handbook for the unemployed which contains useful advice on how to survive the experience.

Planning health services to meet the health damage caused by recession

There is no totally satisfactory model available for health authorities to predict the health damage which the recession will have caused so that they may plan to meet it. Brenner's work is all that we have got and in broad terms is probably adequately accurate for the purpose.

Stress in the general community

Policies designed to abolish unemployment would also abolish fear of unemployment. Policies designed to make unemployment more tolerable would diminish those fears. As far as the more general stresses of recession are concerned it is doubtful if they can be prevented except at the level of economic policies designed to prevent recession.

Policies which built up systems of social support would build up the capacity of society to resist stress.

Policies which reduced the extent to which the stresses of recession were experienced as individual problems and increased the extent to which they were seen as problems of the whole of society would considerably reduce individual stress. Such a process is one plausible explanation for the improvement in health in Britain in the Second World War.

Working conditions

The labour market in recession becomes more adverse to those who sell their labour. This process is most serious in the areas where it can do the most harm (in declining industries, in poorly organised workplaces, and in non wage areas of bargaining).

Public policy could aim to compensate for this by consciously strengthening trade unions in recession, and by increasing the vigilance of public health and safety inspectorates.

This may be politically unacceptable without a quid pro quo from organised labour. If so, and if the price required were the acceptance by trade unions, of some diminution in their wage bargaining power in times of boom, then as a trade unionist I would regard the price as worth paying.

Technological change and declining industries

Cross (1981) describes a scheme where surplus staff in a declining section of a large multinational company were guaranteed employment and then assisted to find other jobs. In this way, the staff was reduced without stress to the individuals involved. Such an approach is clearly a long way from our normal approach to declining industries which is to resist their decline, even at the expense of accepting deteriorating working conditions, until closure becomes inevitable.

There will always be declining industries and we need to evolve methods of handling the problem which do not resist change, but which are prepared to slow it down and control it so that social costs are minimised.

Subsidies to unprofitable industries (except where the subsidy is designed to represent social benefits, as in the case of public transport) could best be used in this way.

Social audit

We have seen that industry is not an unmitigated benefit. The Thomas effect may not be of purely historical interest. Indeed the evidence that some work is more damaging to health than unemployment suggests that it is still of some significance. The Thomas effect would disappear when marginal health gains from increased economic activity outweighed marginal health losses, not when marginal health losses became insignificant. Moreover, since the mechanism for this achievement would be the diversion of some potential growth into social controls it is likely that just after the achievement of this equilibrium there would be a stage where ground was lost in recession and health damage reemerged. This underlies my previous comments on working conditions but is of much broader significance.

We have comparatively recently passed the point in our economic development where the Thomas effect disappeared and we should regard the social control achieved as something to be built on and preserved rather than as an historical victory. There is a need to review and systematise our systems of social audit of industry, that is, of reporting on the social costs and benefits of production over and above those reflected in the profits of the enterprise.

Even in the market economies social audit has been seen as a state responsibility. The state can carry out social audit by exhortation, by encouragement with taxes and subsidies or by regulation. Economists have tended in their theoretical accounts to prefer systems of taxes and subsidies which bring social costs onto the profit and loss account of the company. However, politicians have not been as enthusiastic and have preferred a system of exhortation or regulation. There would be constitutional problems in such systems of social cost accounting which would almost certainly mean operating a system of taxes and subsidies outside the normal tax system since it is too inflexible for the purpose.

Relatively little attention has been paid to other ways of making industry socially accountable. Some attention has been paid to the idea that pension funds should be controlled by their members and should take account of their interests as citizens as well as their interests as investors. Schumacher (1973) advocated that the state should give up its right to tax industry in return for an allocation of share capital carrying the same yield. He then advocated that the voting of these shares should be vested in social audit boards representing the communities in which the company operated. It is possible to envisage other variations (for example allocations of shares could be given to health authorities both as a source of income and as a mechanism for health related social audit).

Any western country which implemented both the democratisation of pension funds and the conversion of tax rights into shares would achieve a situation of social accountability of most of its companies. Whether it would then know what to do with that system is another matter. The political implications of such proposals, striking as they do at the very roots of the distribution of economic power, are likely to prove more important than their social policy implications.

Research needs

In a previous paper (1983), I have indicated the strategy which I think should be pursued in research in this area.

Little is to be gained by further studies designed simply to ask whether unemployment is bad for people. Priorities for research should be:

(a) studies designed to investigate intervening variables. The study under way by Westcott (1983) will be particularly interesting.

(b) studies designed to determine the relative importance of poverty effects and psychological effects. This is a methodologically difficult area. The difficulty is that the poverty effects and psychological effects of unemployment go hand in hand so that it is difficult to find two samples of unemployed people who are matched in respect of one variable so that the effects of the other can be studied. One suggestion which I made was that a group of families who had suffered a particular decline in income due to the unemployment of the male spouse could be matched with a group of families who had suffered the same decline due to the unemployment of the female spouse and the health of the employed and unemployed spouses compared. However, it could be that the stress of having an unemployed spouse is as great (or greater) than the stress of being unemployed oneself.

(c) a study using the Stafford, Jackson and Banks (see Ch. 2) design but looking at biochemical risk factors rather than mental health.

(d) if a situation arises in which a group of workers facing a partial closure of their workplace choose to allocate redundancies by a random method, the opportunity thus provided for a randomised experiment design should be taken, although this situation would be unusual and may be undesirable.

The most important areas for research however, are into the other aspects of the health damage of recession, such as stress or working conditions, which have been much less intensively researched.

REFERENCES

Barclay Report (1982), 'The Role of Social Workers', National Institute of Social Work, London.

Cross, M., (1981), 'Redeployment of Managerial and Professional Manpower: A Case Study', paper presented at KAI Workshop, Hatfield Polytechnic, May 1981.

Dauncey, G., (1981), 'The Unemployment Handbook', National Extension College, Cambridge.

Draper, P., Dennis, J., Griffiths, J., Partridge, and Popay, J., (1979), 'Micro-processors, Macro-economic Policy and Public Health', The Lancet, 17 February 1979, 373-375.

Greenblatt, M., Becerra, R.M., Sterafetivides, E.A., (1982), 'Social Networks and Mental Health: An Overview', American Journal of Psychiatry, 139(8), 977-984.

Martin, A.R., (1960) 'Mental Health and the Rediscovery of Leisure', paper presented at the 13th Annual Meeting of the World Health Federation for Mental Health, Edinburgh 1960.

Mukherjee, S., (1976), 'Unemployment Costs', PEP, Vol XLIII, Broadsheet 561.

Popay, J., (1981), 'Unemployment Centres - The North American Experience', Unemployment Alliance, London.

Schumacher,(1973), 'Small is Beautiful', Abacus.

Shearman, B., & Jenkins, C., (1979), 'The Collapse of Work', Eyre Methuen.

Watkins, S.J.,(1983), 'Recession and Health: A Proposed Research Strategy', in John, J., Schwefel, D., and Zollner, H., (eds) 'Influence of Economic Instability on Health', Springer-Verlag.

Westcott, G.M., (1983),'Proposed Research on the Effects of Unemployment on Health in Scunthorpe', in John, J., Schwefel, D., and Zollner, H., 'Influence of Economic Instability on Health', Springer-Verlag; and ch.10.

Whiting, E., (1980), 'Unemployment Costs', Financial Times, 24 November 1980 (letter).

Winfield, G., (1981), 'Psychology and Centres for the Unemployed: Challenge or Chimera?', Bull. Brit. Psych. Soc., 34, 353-355.

HEALTH EFFECTS OF UNEMPLOYMENT AND NATIONAL HEALTH POLICY IN FINLAND

Tapani Malkas

1. Introduction

Unemployment has for many decades been a difficult problem in Finland. Its fluctuation has followed international economic activity. After the general boom in the early 1970s, substantial unemployment has appeared again, which is similar in nature to the unemployment in other developed market economies.

During the last ten years Finnish health care has been developed actively. With the Primary Health Care Act of 1972 the main emphasis was shifted from specialised hospital care to primary care, and the material and personnel resources of primary health care have increased rapidly. Some of the important principles have been an emphasis on preventive activities, selecting the appropriate level of care, the elimination of regional differences, ready availability of services eg by offering service free of charge, and systematic planning. The responsibility for organising health services lies with the commune, while the state guides and controls development through partial financing.

At the same time most of the indicators describing the state of health of the population have shown a rather positive trend.

The discussion about the correlation between unemployment and health started in Finland at the end of the 1970s. Some research has been conducted in the field and there has been a dialogue between administration and research. The negative effects of unemployment are not denied.

This paper discusses the effects of unemployment on the health of the population as well as changes in health and social policy made to reduce the harmful effects of unemployment in Finland. It is then possible to consider how far further measures can be based on the knowledge which already exists.

2. Unemployment and consideration of health in social policy

During the boom period in the early 1970s, we were in Finland concerned about the adequacy of the labour force. The promotion of the population's health became increasingly important; special attention was paid to the health of the male population of working age. In 1972 a considerable reform of health policy was carried through in the passing of the Primary Health Care Act. This was connected with a rapid increase in resources for health care.

As economic development slowed down, the developmental plans were repeatedly cut to the extent that the spending on health care even decreased somewhat. (Siren 1982; see also Figure 1).

With the increase of unemployment and the end of labour shortage it is to be expected that health would not retain the same priority.

There are also signs that the value of health in social decision-making has decreased: eg in Finland an active health oriented smoking policy has been carried out, the roots of which lie in the period of boom and shortage of labour. A price policy reducing consumption has been striven for. However, this year when several jobs in the tobacco industry were threatened, the government lowered the tax for some tobacco products in an attempt to maintain the level of consumption and thus also of jobs. Such a retreat from the value of health seems to be a common phenomenon in the present situation, although it does not often show itself in such stark contrast. For example, the present increase in the number of occupational and traffic accidents may reflect a preference for economic productivity to better health.

Based on the above one can estimate that unemployment has had its consequences on the health of the whole population, partly from cuts in the health services, partly from the decrease of the value of health in decision-making in society.

3. Elimination from the labour market and health

There is mutual dependence between unemployment and working disability. When dealing with this phenomenon in the Nordic countries, the term elimination from the labour market has been used (Berglind 1972, Kjaer 1978). A person who has little or no chance of obtaining or maintaining a job on the open labour market, is considered to be eliminated from the labour market. Eliminating a person depends on their working ability and the demand on the market. Those eliminated from the labour market can be classified as disabled or unemployed.

The elimination of those classified as disabled for work or unemployed takes place through different channels, and the social security of these groups is different. Disability compensation is more secure and financially more profitable to the individual.

As the number of unemployed job applicants has risen, the number of people on invalidity pensions and the number of new invalidity pensions has fallen slightly, while the number on unemployment pensions has increased.(see Figures 2 & 3).

One can conclude that during a period with low employment the elimination from the labour market took place in a more restrained manner, on grounds set by society, of which the most central were state of health, age and work load. With increasing unemployment the number of those going on invalidity pensions decreased. The elimination was inappropriate from the point of view of health. The share of the young and healthy of those eliminated increased.

It can be assumed that for those working at the upper limits of their working capacity, with a weakened state of health, the ill effects of working will be accentuated whereas the health risks caused by the lack of work will be emphasised for the young and healthy. By analysing those who have gone on invalidity pension it has been proved that the health criteria involved in being pensioned have become tighter during a deflationary trend, although no such decision has been made (Notkola 1980).

Although the channels of elimination have changed, it can be assumed that those being eliminated are still partially the same persons. Weakened health is a factor increasing the risk of unemployment, and in a bad employment situation the partly disabled might as well choose to seek unemployment as disability benefits. This decreases, in principle, the health hazards caused by the change in the channels of elimination. It has been shown that an increasing number of people went on invalidity pension after long periods of unemployment, this being especially the case when the disability was caused by psychic disorders or musculoskeletal diseases (Gould 1982). There is however no way to know whether these persons would under other circumstances have become out of work. Prolonged unemployment can be considered as a worsening factor in cases of partial disablity (Kjaer 1978, Lahelma and Mannila 1981, Lehtinen and Vaisanen 1979).

Work is often especially important for the partially disabled. With the tightening of the labour market these people have found themselves in difficulties. The number of sheltered employment places has stayed the same, although the need for them has increased. The employment measures for those with restricted working capacity have decreased from the beginning of the 1970s to the end of the decade by one third, simultaneously with the increase in the number of disabled job applicants.

It can thus be observed that those being eliminated from the labour market during a period of boom are chosen appropriately from the point of view of health, but with the increase of unemployment elimination has been less appropriate. The shift to unemployment pension has been facilitated for the oldest age groups and financial incentives have been given to encourage the employment of young people. At the moment the possibility of lowering the pension age in heavy and stressful jobs is being discussed.

On the above grounds it is to be assumed that inappropriate elimination from the labour market has had its effects on the health of population, partly on those who are unemployed, partly on the employed. The role of regulatory measures has been weak.

4. Unemployment and Lifestyle

Long term unemployment shapes the life of any individual. It is quite commonly considered that the way of life of the unemployed shows traits unfavourable to health (eg Jahoda et al 1971, Rostila 1980), especially if adopted at an early age. Unemployment is, however, very widespread among the young.

In modern society the importance of diseases linked to lifestyle is increasing. Influencing the lifestyle of the population is an important aspect of Finnish health policy.

In Finland, studies have shown that the health habits among the young unemployed are worse than among other young people. On these grounds, it has been hypothesised that this group will have a worse state of health in middle age, when the diseases linked to life styles start to manifest themselves (Kannas and Hietaharju 1980). The observed differences can, however, also be due to the different social backgrounds, and are thus not necessarily connected to unemployment.

The results obtained on the use of alcohol have been contradictory. It seems evident that at least in the youngest age groups unemployment has not increased the use of alcohol. The reasons given are that the young are still under the influence of their home, unemployment slowing down the process of cutting ties, and also that they have little money (Jyrkama 1980). Thus it is not clear that the youngest, at least, are adopting a debilitating life style.

The so-called "social guarantee" has been adopted experimentally in some communes to solve the problems of youth unemployment. This system grants young people work or vocational traning after a certain period of unemployment. The labour authorities are in charge of the experiment, but the health aspect has been considered in setting the age limits and the maximum length of the unemployment. Applying these experiments more widely has been considered. If they succeed, the health disadvantages caused by youth unemployment could be considerably alleviated.

For people who have already been working long term unemployment means a lowering in the achieved standard of living and a loss of status. The widespread reduction in living standards among long term unemployed has been documented in Finland (Lahelma and Mannila 1981), and may influence the health of the unemployed and the members of their family through many different mechanisms. However, the primary health care services having been free of charge since 1981 and the substantial subsidies for other health services at least ensure that economic difficulties do not restrict the use of health services.

An investigation carried out among long term unemployed in Helsinki shows that quite a large number of the unemployed had lost their jobs for unexpected labour market reasons, such as closing of the plant or reduction of staff. Former unemployment did not predict the duration of unemployment. Researchers consider that long term unemployment is often the result of a vicious circle where at first various factors related to life situation, the personality and health lengthen the period of unemployment and then a long period unemployed makes it increasingly difficult to find a job. During that process different problems eg health problems, come to the foreground. If the development is not cut short, it easily leads to a final elimination from the labour market (Lahelma and Mannila 1981).

5. Unemployment and stress

No special studies have been made of mental or psychosomatic illness or increased use of alcohol etc in situations of mass redundancy in Finland, although the problem is certainly topical. Unemployment may also dissolve the social structures which facilitate adaptation to the situation (Jahoda et al 1971).

In a follow-up study of mental illnesses during a five-year period in Finland, no difference in incidence was found between those who had not been unemployed before the period and those who had been unemployed for a shorter time, while the incidence was greater among those who had long been unemployed (Lehtinen and Vaisanen 1979).

Experiments with special mental health services have been made, for instance, in Sweden to handle problems arising in connection with a plant closure. The Finnish health services have not been active in this matter. When a state-owned plant employing several hundred of workers was closed a couple of years ago, it was proposed to establish a special mental health service to take care of the problems arising in that connection. But the workers rejected the proposal. They did not expect any medical measures from society, but measures which would provide them with employment opportunities.

6. Conclusions

Awareness of the effects of unemployment on people's health has not yet achieved such a level that the Finnish health authorities pay particular attention to them in their national health policy. However, certain general principles, eg the diminishing of regional differences and free primary health care services, have improved the situation of unemployed people.

This paper has stressed the importance of research into the health effects of unemployment. However, there is already so much knowledge acquired through research that active health policy measures can also be taken. If possible, the actions carried out should be evaluated scientifically. On the other hand, the need for research has not decreased, since the problem of unemployment seems unlikely to disappear in the near future. The effects of unemployment on the health of the whole population and those unemployed have to be examined separately. Especially important would be long term follow-up studies, because health hazards caused by aspects of lifestyle develop after a long latent period.

It is important to ensure that the value of health remains stable in social policy even if the value of the labour force diminishes. On the other hand, it is important to demonstrate all the consequences of unemployment and their economic significance.

When health effects of unemployment are emphasised it would be unfortunate to medicalise the issue. Health care should not take too great a responsibility for the economic problem, which can by no means be solved through the action of health services. We must be careful not to label the unemployed as "ill" or "deviant" because this only remders their situation more difficult.

References

Berglind H, Utslagning eller bristande arbetsvilja? Ett forsok til begreppsanalsy. Socialmedicinsk tidskrift 1976, 2, 86-96. (Elimination from labour market, in Swedish).

Brenner M, Influence of social environment on psychopathology: The historic perspective. In Barret J et al (ed), Stress and mental disorder, 161-177. Raven Press, New York 1979.

Gould R, Unemployment and disability pensions. A paper presented at the Nordic meeting on Early Retirement Research in Copenhagen, 28-29 October 1982.

Jahoda M, Lazarsfeldt P, Zeisel H, Marienthal. The sociography of an unemployed community. Aldine Atherton, Chicago and New York, 1971.

Jyrkama J, Tyottomyys ja tyottomien alkoholin kaytto. Alkoholipolitiikka 1980, 3, 102-111. (Unemployment and use of alcohol among unemployed, in Finnish).

Kannas L, Hietaharju M, Tyottomista nuorista sairaita keskiikaisia. Sosiaalinen aikakauskirja 1979, 1, 37-45. (From unemployment in youth to sickness in middle age, in Finnish).

Kasl S, Gore S, Cobb S, Experience of losing the job: Reported changes in health symptoms and illness behaviour. Psychosomatic Medicine vol 37 1975, 106-122.

Kjaer A, Udstoding fra arbejdsmarkedet. Socialforskningsinstituttet, studie 36, Kobenhavn 1978. (Elimination from labour market, in Danish).

Lahelma E, Mannila S, Pitkaaikaistyottomyys Helsingissa. Tyovoimapoliittisia tutkimuksia 26, Helsinki 1981. (Long-term unemployment in Helsinki, in Finnish).

Lehtinen v, Vaisanen E, Psychiatric Morbidity and Need for Psychiatric Treatment in Finland. Kansanelakelaitoksen julkaisuja AL:12, Turku 1979 (in Finnish with an English summary).

Notkola V, The development of cause-specific disability pensions in Finland 1972-1978. Helsingin yliopiston sosiologian laitoksen julkaisuja. Working papers no 14, 1980.

Rostila I, Tyottomyys elamantilanteena. Tyovoimapoliittisia tutkimuksia 25, Helsinki 1980. (Unemployment as life situation, in Finnish).

Siren P, The growth of health expenditure in Finland in 1960-1980 and the prospects for curbingits future growth. Paper presented at the Expert Group Meeting on Economic Efficiency in Health Care Delivery, Turku 28-30 September 1982 (International Social Security Association, ISSA/RDS/EG/TUR/10).

Fig. 1 Expenditure on health
Total health expenditure, % of GDP
Out-of-pocket payments, % of private consumption

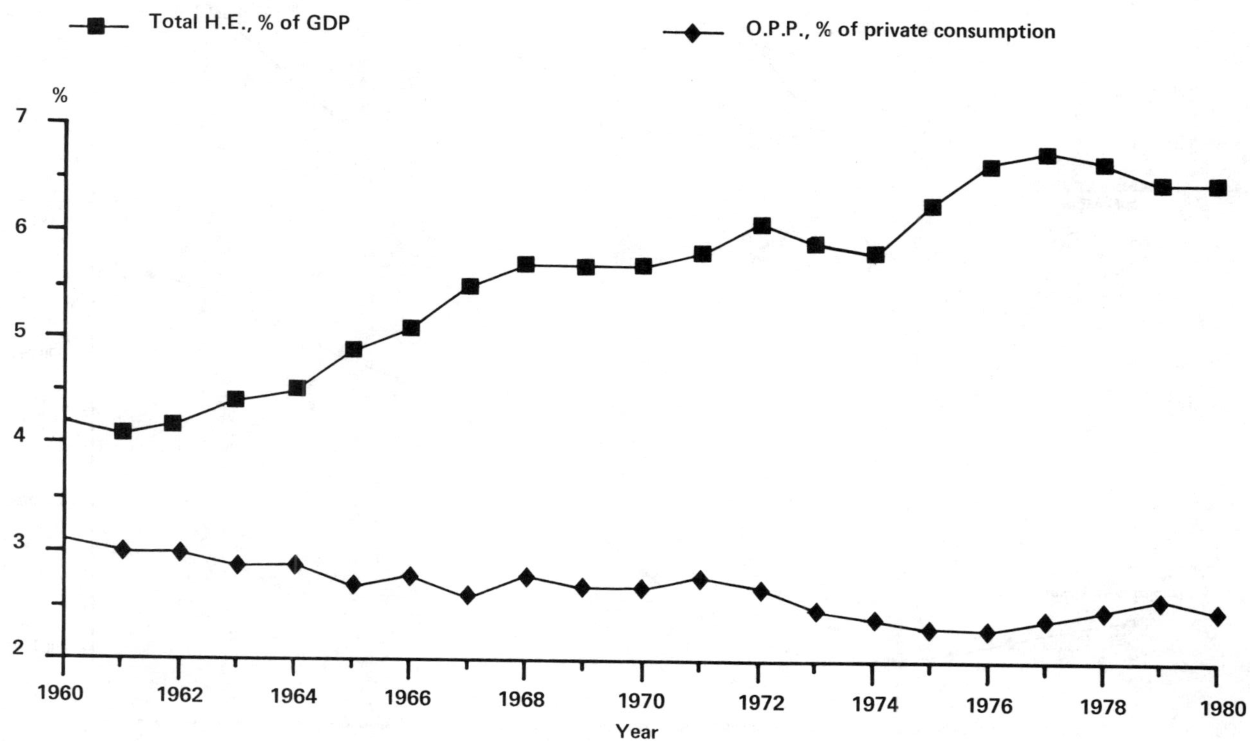

Fig. 2. The number of invalidity pensions, unemployed job applicants and unemployment pensions in Finland, 1965 - 1981

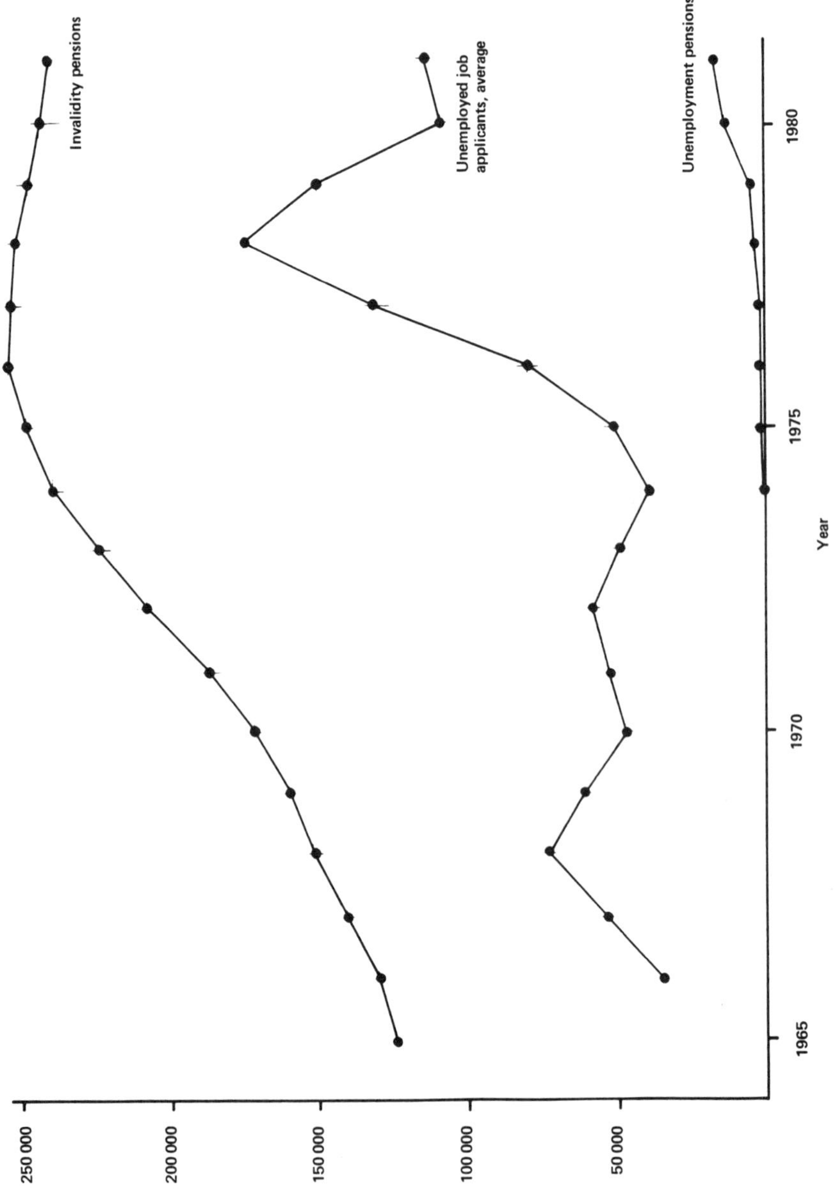

Fig. 3 New permanent invalidity pensions in Finland, 1970–1981 (social insurance institution)

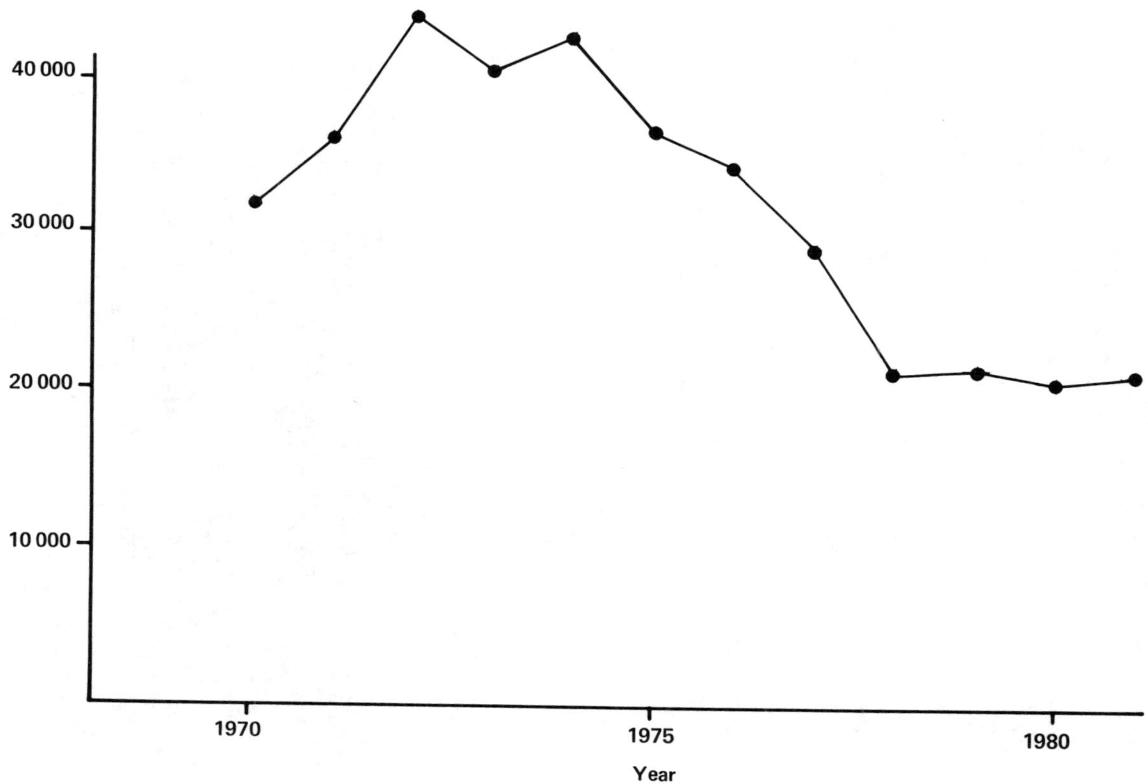

THE CONTRIBUTION OF PSYCHOLOGY TO THE REALM OF UNEMPLOYMENT IN THE COMMUNITY: INTERVENTION AND RESEARCH CONCEPTS

Thomas Kieselbach

1. Psychological impairment as a consequence of unemployment: Declarations from psychological associations and psycho-social institutions in the FRG

In a situation where the number of unemployed passed the 2 million mark in West Germany in 1982 and 2.5 million unemployed are already estimated for 1983, three West German Psychological Associations (The German Society for Behaviour Therapy (DGVT), the Association of Industrial and Occupational Psychology (VBAP), and the Section of Political Psychology in the Association of West German Psychologist (BDP) have turned to the public to point out the increase of psycho-social disorders which have been noted at the present time. If the prognosis for the future development of mass unemployment proves to be right, the number of people suffering from psychological disorders will definitely increase.

They underlined the fact that the figures of the official statistics do not nearly reflect the real degree to which the population of West Germany is affected by the problem of mass unemployment. In reality mass unemployment includes many groups which for different reasons have given up the search for employment and thus withdrawn from the labour market or other groups that are also not counted in the official system of registration of the Federal Employment Agency. Besides this the associations drew the attention to those who are secondarily affected by unemployment, that means the relatives, partners, and children of the unemployed who also may experience psycho-social impairment.

In the following I will quote some passages from this declaration because in my opinion such political statements made by professional associations which are confronted with the consequences of unemployment is quite a relevant way 'to give psychology away to society'.

The declaration first stresses the importance of work for the development of personality.

"The extent of psycho-social strain caused by unemployment depends especially on the significance which is attributed to work in our society.

The most important individual and social psychological functions of work in our society are:

- the individual realises his abilities in managing his work tasks and gains by this a feeling of personal competence
- the experience of possessing the necessary knowledge and abilities to perform a certain job constitutes the essential basis for the development of personal identity
- work represents an important field of social contact and is the basis of co-operative abilities
- by producing useful goods or services which are important for the maintenance and the future of society the working person experiences that he is of value for society

work gives to the employed a frame-work of social orientation which is essential for his self-assessment

even leisure time is considerably influenced by work contents and working conditions.

Only if this close connection between work and social status, self-esteem, and opportunities for psychological development is taken into account can a precise estimation of the individual and collective amount of damage which can arise from involuntary loss of employment be made.

The declaration states that numerous unemployed experience economic deprivation and social decline. At the moment only 60% of the registered unemployed in West Germany receive financial support from the government.

In addition the associations outline the manifold psycho-social damage on four levels. Corresponding to the epidemiological level the following effects are mentioned:

"increase of criminal offences, especially among youths

increase in drug addiction, suicide attempts, suicides and depressive symptoms

increase of psychiatric hospital admissions

increase of psychosomatic diseases

aggravation of numerous psychic disorders".

It has been pointed out that unemployment, on the individual level of the afflicted, may lead to:

"a loss of self-confidence, self-esteem and to a lack of confidence in others

depression, fatalism, and apathy as the last stage of discouragement in the long-term unemployed, which are connected with feelings of worthlessness and hopelessness

an increase of social isolation, and

the development of feelings of self-blame with respect to one's own family".

Besides that the consequences for the relatives of the unemployed are described as:

"increase of intrafamilial conflicts combined with withdrawal from social life

increase of developmental disorders in children of unemployed. a decline in school performance and in general a deterioration of family interaction (e.g. because of the loss of authority of the unemployed father)".

For those still employed, the experience of the social phenomenon of mass unemployment leads to fears of possible discharge, thus creating various social-psychological consequences. It is emphasized in the declaration that mass unemployment leads on that fourth level to:

> "an intensification of psychic pressure to work harder and to competitive behaviour causing a loss of solidarity among staff and to
>
> a tendency for people to renounce their right to sick leave when they are ill and not to seek necessary medical treatment".

The declaration further stresses that it is not the unemployed, but the economic and social system, which produces unemployment and therefore must be held responsible.

"The opinion of a part of the public that the unemployed themselves are primarily to blame for their situation - either because psychic defects led to their discharge or because a reluctance or unwillingness to work led to their failures to obtain a new job - gravely misrepresents the relationship between cause and effect.

"Individual causal attributions of this kind lead to a strengthening of the negative psycho-social consequences of unemployment in a striking way.

"The number of available jobs has dropped to a figure of 65,000 - leading to a relation of 30 unemployed to every job offered - and therefore for most of the unemployed there are no jobs at all, neither acceptable nor unacceptable ones.

"In view of this the dispute about what might be the percentage of 'scroungers' or 'work-shy' who 'live on social benefits' creates the impression that the reason for such a dispute is to shift attention away from the social causes of unemployment. This assumption is underlined by the observation that those internal causal attributions seem to increase in proportion to the development of mass unemployment as a constant factor in Western countries.

"It is our opinion that mass unemployment in the industrial nations in the long run results in psychic misery for large parts of the population and thus in severe long-lasting psycho-social effects which are very hard to repair - if not in fact irreparable.

"We think it a substantial simplification and limitation of the problem if political and economic measures to increase the number of jobs and/or to change the existing distribution of work should primarily be replaced by psychological advisory and training schemes.

"These interventions are at the moment definitely needed and can help to alleviate the psychic damage to the unemployed and their families; they are, however, conceptualized and executed from the perspective that the attendance in such programmes improves employment prospects.

This is only possible if the labour market provides enough employment possibilities. Curative psychological measures in the forefront of clinical-therapeutic interventions have in this respect the character of supportive help in critical life situations, which cannot be managed by the unemployed person without help from others. In the long run, they are, taken in themselves, isolated from real life and the everyday behaviour of the unemployed, and unable to prevent the development of psychic suffering or its recrudescence when unemployment becomes long-term.

"...The only measure promising success in the long run for the negative consequences of unemployment is the provision of work. It is necessary to change the present distribution of available work".

(Delcaration of 3 psychological organizations, 1.12.1982. In: Psychologie heute, March 1983). (1)

Other psychological associations as well as practitioners from various professions have come to similar conclusions. A group of psychologists working with drug addicts declared:

"The best therapy cannot prevent relapses if the client does not afterwards find vocational education or a suitable job. Even the most active and creative professional fails with his clients because of the limitations the social situation puts to his work", (Association of Drug Counselling Services in NRW, Deutsche Volkszeitung, 23.2.1978).

The German Society for Social Psychiatry stressed the economic significance of the psycho-social effects following prolonged unemployment:

"Our professional experience shows us that if nothing is done about unemployment in the near future, large parts of the population will become improverished and in miserable psychological condition. The resulting social costs arising through illness, physical and psychological damage, retardation, etc., will be much higher than the sums supposedly being saved through the present politics of austerity", (Newsletter of the German Society of Social Psychiatry, No. 8, 1982).

The failure of rehabilitation schemes taken for discharged psychiatric patients was documented at a meeting of representatives from rehabilitation centres and groups of relatives. There it was reported that it has become almost impossible to find jobs on the labour market for former patients. "Such a depressing and deprecating lack of prospects is leading to a high proportion of relapses", (loc. cit.).

2. Unemployment and political behaviour

Whereas the positions of the professional psychological organisations concerning the psycho-social damage caused by mass unemployment presented here are largely from the perspective of those affected, the relationship between mass unemployment and political radicalization has become a topic not only in broad areas of social science research, but also in the statements of politicians, albeit from the perspective of an internal, vertical control of the social system (SCHMID 1986).

I shall present in the following some examples which exemplify the socio-political consequences of mass unemployment. (2)

The President of the Federal Employment Agency, Stingle, evoked the Thirties when he announced the figures of unemployment in April 1982. He gave the warning that such a development might eventually occur again if the number of unemployed grew further. Previously, in 1976, he had stated in an interview:

"We can certainly take some credit for the fact that it has remained quiet in the streets. Perhaps this is because the payments of the unemployment benefits are made directly to the accounts of the unemployed ... If we had queues in front of the labour exchange, probably it would be different", (Handelsblatt, 4.3.1977).

Although it may appear rather naive, to make the cashless payments responsible for the fact that political discontent was not overtly expressed, it is evident that the memory of mass unemployment in the Thirties obviously evokes pictures of unemployed queuing in front of the labour exchange. There the anonymous unemployed became part of the social group which was a better basis for political action and agitation.

At the same time, in 1976, when the unemployment figures had just reached 1 million, the governmental representative for civic education of Schleswig-Holstein put forward his opinion that youth unemployment represents "a political time-bomb of the greatest danger" which has already begun to tick, "a time-bomb of dramatic upheavals against the establishment", (Frankfurther Rundschau, 12.1.1976).

Even a British government committee with a Conservative majority came to a similar prediction in 1981 after having investigated the economic and social situation of Wales:

"We are impressed by the conviction of some of our witnesses who stress the risks of serious social disorder if there were to be very high and chronic levels of unemployment, particularly among the young. Wales, if condemned to suffer the incidence of worklessness endured in the Thirties, is unlikely to respond with the apathy and despair that enveloped so many in those days", (First Report of the Committee on Welsh Affairs, July 1980, cf. OSMOND 1981, p. 127).

Much sociological and psychological research is also guided by the same idea about unemployment and political attitudes. They deal with the problems whether the grave personal experience of unemployment leads to questioning the legitimacy of the political and social systems or whether the experience of unemployment creates political extremism and radicalism (e.g. TUCKER 1940, AIKEN et al, 1968).

The political warnings of the social consequences of mass unemployment quoted have in common the underlying assumption that unemployment of millions of people brings about the danger of convulsions to the political system. Up to now there has been no serious social unrest. Collective actions against dismissals or against already existing unemployment have been the exception. So far the self-organization of unemployed in initiatives or 'self-help-groups' have found only little resonance, even the participation of the unemployed themselves is relatively low.

A possible sign of the changing situation among the unemployed in West Germany was the first national congress of unemployed which was held at Frankfurt in December 1982. Two hundred and fifty groups of unemployed from all over the country were represented. Altogether, 1,500 unemployed participated in the discussions of the workshops.

The most important topic of the congress was, how can the unemployed organize themselves in initiatives or in unions. The motto of the congress - "unemployed - but not defenseless" - was supposed to demonstrate that an active section of those who lost their jobs and therefore have been socially isolated, has begun to regain recognition as a social group. As yet, neither the trade unions nor the churches or psychosocial support systems have really taken up the interests of the unemployed. Therefore they have been forced to act largely outside the major political and social organizations. Despite these negative experiences, the participants of this first congress of unemployed made use of the historical lessons of the unemployed movements in the Thirties, and have rejected an autonomous organization which might favour a cleavage between those who have a job and their unions and those who don't have a job.

Furthermore, they refused to excuse the political parties from their responsibility for a political and social development which has caused mass unemployment.

At the conference it was very impressive to listen to stories of young unemployed who described changes in their way of coping with unemployment when they talked about the different stages they experienced.

It started with resignation and apathy after a long period of unemployment accompanied by the well-known symptoms such as feelings of uselessness, suicidal thoughts, alcohol abuse, over-sleeping, until they gave up searching for a job.

Only the identification with the social role of an unemployed and the contact with other unemployed persons in the self-help-group had a stabilizing effect upon them. Having taken up the struggle against the social causes of mass unemployment as their individual goal their psychological well-being improved significantly, so that they were able to cope better with the situation.

3. Psychological interventions in the realm of unemployment

A very central aspect of psychological research as well as intervention is a breaking down of existing social and individual mechanisms for the psychologizing of the problem of unemployment. On the scientific level through a confrontation

> with psychological theories which try to locate the causes for the loss of work or the lack of success in the search for employment in the psychic deficits of the person affected. Approaches which are expressed most clearly in the concept of 'work inhibition' (TIFFANY et al, 1970), but also in the simple social selection assumptions (ARNOLD & BERGLER, 1955).
>
> with the psychological implications of economic theories (as, for example, attempts at explanations using 'unemployment induced through social benefits', 'search unemployment' (among the too choosey unemployed) or the 'natural socket of unemployment' (WINDOLF, 1982, WITTMANN, 1980).

At this point I will make some remarks concerning the work of psychologists in the field of unemployment and how they handle this problem. I am going to talk about their approaches in three main areas:

in the labour exchange

in psychological advisory and training programmes, and

in psycho-social institutions.

3.1. Labour Exchange

The work of psychologists in the labour exchange in West Germany is presently concerned, due to institutional conditions, mainly with aptitude testing, which is subordinated to the needs of the vocational guidance department.

The diagnostic methods used by the psychological service of the Employment Administration are, as a rule, methods which have a positive, orienting value for the individual being tested, under the conditions of an open labour market and by use with people who are not in a psycho-social crisis. They were more frequently used for employees who wanted to change their employment or for those just starting in the labour market. Today, however, the great majority of those persons being diagnostically tested are unemployed. Many of them are in a crisis, which they sometimes cannot overcome without external support.

As a consequence, the function of psychological diagnostics under the condition of an extremely restricted labour market has changed. More and more, these psychologists are forced to follow the interests of the employers, not the job-seekers. As diagnostic selection is intensified, psychological work in the labour exchange has become more frustrating for a growing number of job-seeking clients. Furthermore, the intervention of the psychologist in the labour administration has the negative side-effect of supporting internal causal attributions on the part of the unemployed. I would like to illustrate this effect with an example from Martin Seligman (1975, p. 75).

Seligman describes in his book "Helplessness" the case of an employee who had been a successful manager in industry before he became unemployed. After a relatively short time he had already become withdrawn, apathetic, and made no further attempts to find new work. Even small disturbances strongly excited him. On the advice of his wife, he undertook a course of professional aptitude testing. The test results confirmed that he "had a low frustration tolerance, was unsociable, incapable of assuming responsibility, and that a routine, limited activity was best suited to his personality". The professional counselling agency advised him to become a worker on an assembly line. The advice gave him a shock. Nonetheless, the tests reflected his present condition. He considered himself to be incompetent, felt his career had been a failure and considered every little hindrance to be an unconquerable barrier; he considered himself to be incapable of decisions. Nontheless, this aptitude profile did not give a correct picture of his abilities; it instead reflected the process that had begun with his loss of work, the development of a depressive disturbance.

The intervention of the psychologist, based on the test diagnostics, led in this case to a confirmation of the bad test results and thus became socially effective; the results of unemployment were identified and accepted as individual deficits. Unless a way is found to reverse the consequences of a negative developmental process, psychological activity based on such a test,diagnostics will be rather a "contribution to the professional and social disqualification of unemployed people", (LAURITZEN 1982, p. 37), instead of making possible a re-integration into the labour market in the interests of the unemployed.

In this situation an active group of psychologists in the labour administration demands changes in their range of functions. They are striving for a change in the direction of advocatory work in favour of the unemployed and are asking for an engagement of the psychological service in promotion measures and psychological counselling of the unemployed. Besides that, they are making efforts to install and conduct programmes to train the personnel of the labour administration so that they can deal better with the psychological problems unemployment creates in their clients. These psychologists formed their own association in 1982, in order to strengthen their influence in realizing these goals. Already one-third of the psychologists in the labour administration is organized in the Association of Industrial and Occupational Psychology (VBAP). (3)

3.2. Psychological advisory and training programmes

Because of rising figures of unemployment in many Western countries, programmes are offered by governmental and private institutions providing advisory, qualificatory and psychological training schemes for unemployed. It is the primary goal of these schemes to improve the individual employment prospects of the participants. Besides that they intend to provide a psychological stabilization of the unemployed. The proposed main effect - to improve the employment prospects - is more and more unattainable, not due to the quality of the programmes, but rather mainly due to the economic situation. Analyses of the effectivity of qualification as well as psychological schemes show transition rates of only about 25% into normal jobs (SCHNEIDER 1981, HOFBAUER & DADZIO 1982). In Great Britain the transition rate varies from 10% (Short Training Courses), 18% (Project-Based Work Experience), 31% (Youth Opportunities Programme), to 36% (Work Experience on Employers Premises, v. Employment Gazette 1982, No. 10).

Concerning the second goal - the psychological stabilization - the findings were described to be far more positive. After the end of the programmes the participants were reported to be "more free, self-conscious and better informed" (SCHNEIDER 1982). The low success in improving the employment prospects must lead to the conclusion that the secondary effect - the psychological stabilization - has to be transferred to the centre of consideration for such programmes (BECKMANN et al, 1982).

Measures for the unemployed should be so conceived that they can really lead to the desired goals (KAPLAN, CASSEL and GORE, 1977, 48). Advisory measures of psychological training programmes for the unemployed from the employment administration should no longer aim exclusively at an improvement in job -mediation chances when the conditions of the labour market only allow a small number of the participants to find work after completion of the course. This can be demonstrated through the example of the implicit learning goals contained in the measures prescribed in Section 41a in the Work Promotion Law (AFG). These attribute the continued lack of success in the search for employment in part to a lack of ability in the writing of job applications and interviews as well as a low resistance to stress. Such assistance programmes contain the danger that those who remain unemployed after the course will tend to an internal attribution of failure, which can strengthen a negative self-evaluation with depressive reactions - although these measures no doubt pursue the opposite goal.

In order not to increase the psycho-social damage resulting from unemployment even further through such measures, they should be so planned that they contain as goals of equal importance psychic stabilization, the improvement of coping methods with continued unemployment and the initiation of mutual support systems among the unemployed (participation should naturally only be voluntary and without sanctions in the case of withdrawal).

But the perspective of lasting mass unemployment creates another dilemma for the psychologists who are involved in such programmes. Two psychologists who conceptualized and executed several training programmes for unemployed, described this dilemma as follows:

"The fact is irrefutable that having a large amount of structural and conjunctural unemployment, a well-trained participant who finds a job finally contributes to the dismissal of someone else whose abilities might be less. This means that more and more problematical, difficult-to-employ persons are losing their jobs. So far we have been successful in counselling the unemployed. Nevertheless this affects those, who are increasingly pushed aside, and therefore perhaps cannot be integrated into working life any more. So at last we have to ask the question how long our concept is realizable and does not contradict our goals", (SIEGRIST & WUNDERLI, 1982, p. 90).

3.3. Psycho-social Institutions

Epidemiological research has demonstrated the meaning of unemployment as a burden resulting from class society (v. FERBER, 1972). For the first time in West Germany a socio-epidemiological study has been published for the district of Northern Bavaria, which investigated the relationship between psychological disorder, job-related strain factors and unemployment (DILLING & WEYERER, 1980). A significant correlation was found between the "fear of losing one's job" and psychological disorder among employed persons, but the most significant association was between unemployment and psychological disorder. 60% of this group suffered from defects that needed professional treatment.

Many remarks by practising psychologists and their associations clearly stress unemployment as the phenomenon that burdens the psycho-social institutions to a great extent. Drug counsellors and psychologists in rehabilitation centres complain of a high proportion of relapses when their clients remain unemployed after a 'successful' treatment; school psychologists diagnose aversion to going to school in pupils whose most likely perspective is unemployment. Social-psychiatric institutions experience unemployment more and more as the main problem of their clients. But until now there has been no precise analysis of the extent to which psycho-social institutions are affected by this socio-structural problem.

An important contribution to psychological interventions in the area of psycho-social care is the de-psychologizing of unemployment for professionals and those affected.

Professionals in the psycho-social services frequently see that the unemployed who turn to their institutions, e.g. to a social-psychiatric service, do this with an addiction problem or a marital problem. Problems which result from unemployment are thus defined to conform institutionally and these are usually treated exclusively on the level of such institutionally conformative self-definitions. An indispensable aim of training and qualifying measures for professionals is that they must be put in a position to decode these self-definitions and, as far as possible, to relate them to the problem of unemployment.

Those unemployed, for whom the loss of work has led to a thorough identity crisis, easily fall into the temptation of applying psychologizing interpretations in dealing with themselves and their daily problems (KEUPP, 1982, p. 190f). This becomes clearest in the assumption of individual self-blame by the unemployed person himself. Such psychologizing interpretations can easily become self-fulfilling prophecies, when individual self-blame leads to a reduction in self-confidence and feelings of self-respect, to a stoppage of applications or a deterioration of self-presentation in job interview situations, thus resulting in a lack of success which is understood as a confirmation of personal deficits. Professional offers of help which break this circular process, undoubtedly have an important function here.

3.4. Functions and perspectives of psychological interventions

The adequacy of interventions of professionals working in the field of unemployment can be considered as a function of how far they are conscious of the economic and social-psychological meaning of mass unemployment. All these professionals are part of a social selection mechanism which functions in two different ways: first, people are excluded from the labour market (because of low efficiency or randomly in the case of mass dismissals), and second the most efficient and most psychically stable (or best socially adapted) unemployed are reselected and reintegrated in the labour market. As effects of this double filter process

- the forces of capital and labour are shifted in favour of capital

- the direct and indirect labour costs are decreased (also as an effect of artificially lowered illness rates)

- the level of demands of the employees and the unemployed concerning the quality of work is lowered

- the discussion about the 'humanization of work' becomes unimportant, and in general

- unemployment becomes a means of disciplinary punishment against political and union activities in the factories.

Only within this social framework can the indisputable positive influence of psychological interventions in the fields of labour exchange, psychological training schemes for the unemployed and psycho-social institutions be legitimated.

Attempts to conceive psychological interventions in the area of unemployment as primary prevention (in the sense of KAPLAN), create some difficulties. Since primary prevention of unemployment actually represents an economic and political problem, psychological attempts in the area of primary prevention easily fall into a dilemma.

CATALANO and DOOLEY (1980) solve this problem in that they introduce a differentiation between proactive and reactive primary prevention, whereby proactive prevention means legal measures for the avoidance or sanctioning of dismissals (as, for example, by the payment of the social costs of unemployment by the employer according to the causation principle, e.g. for re-qualification or psycho-social counselling and treatment), and reactive prevention stands for the early immunization of those already unemployed against the stress that is bound up with unemployment.

Extremely problematical attempts at primary prevention can however prove to be counter-productive in a political sense (as the example of MELKAS (1982)) in which a 'mental health centre' was opened next to a firm that was to be closed before the actual closing, in order to prepare the employees better for their dismissals. As a consequence, the professionals unintentionally found themselves in a conflict of interest with the employees, who were fighting for the preservation of their jobs).

When employees in general or employees who are concretely threatened with unemployment are informed of the consequences of unemployment in terms of psychological primary prevention, ambivalent reactions can be the result:

resistance to the dismissal may be strengthened on the one hand,

on the other hand, it can lead to a reinforcement of conformist behaviour, in the hope that one can thus avoid being individually affected by unemployment.

A way out of the dilemma of psychological primary prevention presented here is to some degree only to be found in a further development of prevention in the direction of a policy of empowerment ("empowerment" in the sense of RAPPAPORT, 1981).

Due to the limitations of an individualizing psychological intervention, but also due to the prevailing attitudes of (especially male) unemployed concerning the use of professional help in situations of crisis (cf. SPRUIT 1983), the embedding of psycho-social help within a context of political action appears reasonable, as long as it follows the goal of collectively increasing the control over one's living conditions (DOHRENWEND 1978). Here, the concern would be with the development of prevention which starts on the individual level, but which continues in the direction of a strategy of empowerment. In this way, the individual problems would be embedded in their social context, and collective solutions for collective problems would be sought. An important approach for overcoming the perspective which sees the unemployed solely as 'social victims' of the capitalist economy could be found in such a method.

Following this 'policy of empowerment' the psychological counsellor should advocate his clients' interest and should bring in his specific compentencies in a way that enables the unemployed to articulate and to realize his own interests. This means that the psychologist functions as a 'catalyst' (as WINFIELD 1981 described the contribution of psychologists in centres for the unemployed).

Such a policy of empowerment does not require a new psychological technique but a changed socio-political strategy, which aims at an alteration of the given political situation.

This strategy demands an extension of psychological competence in the following direction:

- primary and tertiary prevention have to be emphasized more

- a psychologist's qualification has to include knowledge about economic, socio-political and sociological questions and about how to co-operate with other professions

- the psychologist's responsibility is to be extended to the client's post-therapeutic situation. (4)

Preventive work in this form can, of course, be better accomplished in connection with political organizations, trade unions or self-help groups of unemployed than in psycho-social organizations.

The inclusion of the unemployed in trade union work could furthermore reduce the danger of a division between unemployed and employed and make a contribution to the maintenance of contact with former work-mates, at least in part, through common activities. Beyond this, both groups, the employed and the unemployed, could be brought to awareness that they could engage in a common struggle for common goals.

4. Concepts for research, education and intervention in the realm of unemployment: The Scientific Unit 'Work, Unemployment and Personality Development' (University of Bremen)

The previous considerations concerning psychological interventions in the area of psycho-social consequences of unemployment provide the basic assumptions for our on-going work.

The Scientific Unit was founded in 1982 with the objective of integrating different research areas on the 'socializing potential of occupational educational processes' and on 'humanizing of work' and to add new projects on the 'psycho-social consequences of unemployment'.

In the fields of unemployment research up to now, an empirical study has been carried out on coping strategies of unemployed psychologists (KIESELBACH, KLEIBER & SCHINDLER 1979, KLEIBER, KIESELBACH & SCHINDLER 1980) and a monograph published on the state of psychological research (KIESELBACH & OFFE 1979).

For the near future, we are developing the following concepts for research, education and intervention in the realm of unemployment.

4.1. Unemployment and psycho-social care

Experiences of professionals working in social-psychiatric services at Bremen substantiate the view that unemployment can cause psychic and personal distress in relation to which these institutions are quite helpless: neither qualitatively nor quantitatively are they able to provide help that would be adequate to the needs of their clients.

Analyses of the efficiency of institutionalized or non-institutionalized offers (from the closer social network or self-help-groups) will be carried out concerning the qualitative structure of differential coping attempts, self-disclosure and successful or unsuccessful help-seeking-behaviour.

These analyses could reveal deficits and obstacles as well as new intervention possibilities and thus supply basic information for the planning and development of more effective treatment and counselling steps.

Besides this, education programmes for the professionals working in these institutions will be developed, executed and evaluated.

Furthermore we are planning to provide existing self-help-organizations - as a form of concrete political counselling - with scientific knowledge and to support their work by supplying them with corresponding material.

On the other hand we intend to do some in-depth-interviews with unemployed who are active in those self-help-organizations to get a more precise understanding of the stage of coping with the individual experience of unemployment.

By comparing these results with the unemployed who sought help in the social-psychiatric institutions we will try to find out some mechanisms which are responsible for successful or unsuccessful coping attempts.

4.2. Counselling Strategies in the Labour Administration

An analysis of present counselling strategies and the development of more effective ones should enable the employees working at the labour exchanges to deal with the new demands in the field of job mediation and vocational guidance while being confronted with the psychic effects of unemployment in their clients.

Further investigation will focus on how the phenomenon of unemployment is cognitively represented in those counsellors and job mediators. There are three dimensions we consider as being important influences on how these persons deal with their job-seeking clients:

> Does the counsellor attribute the causes of unemployment predominantly to internal or external, to stable or variable factors?
>
> Does the counsellor regard the unemployment insurance as being an insurance against social risk not resulting from personal fault but from economic crisis or does he consider the insurance as being a benefit provided by the government that depends on the good behaviour of the unemployed person who wants to make use of it?
>
> Is the counsellor aware of the economic and social-psychological functions of unemployment mentioned above and what kind of self-comprehension does he have in relation to that?

On the other hand we will investigate how people, working in the labour administration are perceived by the unemployed. The results of this research will provide the basis for a necessary education and training of job mediators and counsellors, especially stressing the aspect of the psycho-social impact of unemployment and its consequences for the counselling process.

4.3. Education and intervention concepts

As a contribution to a policy of empowerment we plan to conduct seminars with unemployed union members in co-operation with the local unions. In this way we intend better to immunize them against the psychological stress of unemployment. The second goal we want to pursue in these seminars is to discuss the hindrances to an activation of the unemployed. (5).

For professionals in the health services and the employment and social administrations we are going to conceive and conduct information and educational courses about the results of medical and psychological research on unemployment to improve their interaction with the unemployed clients and to support the development of adequate intervention measures.

Some of these projects of the Scientific Unit will be executed as an integration of research- and education-project so that psychology students can profit from our work and thus get an education that is orientated towards practical and socio-politically relevant problems.

Footnotes

1. In April 1983 a more detailed declaration was published which was supported by 13 associations representing 40,000 professionals from different fields of psycho-social care: psychologists, social workers, occupational therapists and medical practitioners, v. Th. Kieselbach: Die individuellen und sozialen Kosten der Arbeitslosigkeit, in: JAHODA, M., Th. KIESELBACH & Th. LEIT-HAUSER (eds.): Arbeit, Arbeitslosigkeit und Personlichkeitsentwicklung. Bremer Beitrage zur Psychologie. No. 23, 1983a; also in: Frankfurter Rundschau, 9.5.1983.

2. cf. in greater detail: KIESELBACH 1983b, 1984.

3. This rather optimistic view concerning the possibilities of changing the conditions and content of work in the labour administration had to be qualified two years later. Attempts at establishing concepts of preventive psychological group counselling (v. GRUNAU 1984) have been realized but did not until now find the necessary support from the direction of the Psychological Service of the labour administration.

4. SHEPHERD (1981) for instance claims that clinical psychologists should engage more intensely in job mediating and in the creation of jobs for their clients to prevent relapses after a successful therapy.

5. In the meantime we have published a report on such a seminar: KIESELBACH & SCHINDLER 1984.

References

AIKEN, M., FERMAN, L. A. & SHEPPARD, H. L.: Economic failure, alienation and extremism. Ann Arbor, Mich.: Univ. Mich. Press, 1968.

ARNOLD, W. & BERGLER, R.: Psychologische Grunde der Arbeitslosigkeit alterer Angestellter. Luneburg, 1955.

BECKMANN, N., HAHN, K.D. & SCHELLER, H. J.: Theoretische Bergrundung und praktische Durchfuhrung von 4-Wochen-Kursen mit Arbeitslosen (nach 41a AFG). Paper presented at the Workshop for Political Psychology, Nov. 1982, Munich. In: MOSER, H. & PREISER, S. (eds.): Umweltprobleme und Arbeitslosigkeit. Gesellschaftliche Herausforderungen an die Politische Psychologie. Weinheim/Beltz, 1984, pp. 140 - 149.

CATALANO ,R. & DOOLEY, D.: Economic change in primary prevention. in: PRICE, R. H., KETTERER, R. F., BADER, B.C. & MONAHAN, J. (eds.): Prevention in community mental health: Research, policy and practice. Beverly Hills: Sage 1980, pp. 21 - 40.

DILLING, H. & WEYERER, S.: Behandelte und nicht behandelte psychiatrische Morbiditat in der Bevolkerung. Bericht an die Duesche Forschungsgemeinschaft. Munchen 1980.

DOHRENWEND, B.S.: Social stress and community psychology. American Journal of Community Psychology 6, 1978, pp. 1 - 14.

FERBER, C.V.: Gesundheit und Gesellschaft. Haben wir eine Gesundheitspolitik? Stuttgart: Kohlhammer 1971.

HOFBAUER, H. & DADZIO, W.: Die Wirksamkeit von Maßnahmen zur Verbesserung der Vermittlungsaussichten fur Arbeitslose nach 41a AFG. Mitteilungen fur Arbeitsmarkt - und Berufsforschung 15(4), 1982, pp. 426 - 433.

KAPLAN, B.H., CASSEL, J.C. & GORE ,S.: Social support and health. Medical Care 15 (5 Suppl.), 1977, pp. 47 - 58.

KEUPP, H.: Soziale Kontrolle. Psychiatrisierung, Psychologisierung, Medikalisierung, Therapeutisierung. in: KEUPP, H. & RERRICH, D. (eds.): Psycholosoziale Praxis. Munchen/Wien/Baltimore: Urban & Schwarzenberg 1982, pp. 189 - 198.

KIESELBACH, Th.: Die individuellen und sozialen Kosten von Arbeitslosigkeit. in: JAHODA, M., KIESELBACH, Th. & KEITHAUSER, Th. (eds.): Arbeit, Arbeitslosigkeit und Personlichkeitsentwicklung. Bremer Beitrage zur Psychologie No. 23, 1983a.

KIESELBACH, Th.: Arbeitslosigkeit und politische Orientierungen. Gewerkschaftliche Monatshefte 34 (12), 1983, pp. 802 - 820 (1983b).

KIESELBACH, Th.: Arbeitslosigkeit, Gesellschaftsbewußtsein und kollektive Interessenorientierung. in: MOSER, H. & PREISER, S. (eds.): Umweltprobleme und Arbeitslosigkeit. Gesellschaftliche Herausforderungen an die Politische Psychologie. Weinheim/ Basel: Beltz 1984, pp. 120 - 139.

KIESELBACH, Th., KLEIBER, D. & SCHINDLER, H.: Psychologenarbeits-losigkeit: Auswirkungen und Strategien ihrer Uberwindung aus der Sicht von Betroffenen. Ergebnisse einer empirischen Untersuchung. Mitteilungen der Deutschen Gesellschaft fur Verhaltenstherapie (DGVT) 11(4), 1979, pp. 742 - 763.

KIESELBACH, Th. & OFFE, H.: Psychologische, gesundheitliche, soziale und politische Probleme als Folge von Arbeits-losigkeit - ein kritischer Literaturuberblick. in: KIESELBACH, Th. & OFFE, H. (eds): Arbeitslosigkeit. Individuelle Verarbeitung und gesellschaftlicher Hintergrund. Darmstadt: Steinkopff 1979, pp. 7 - 140.

KIESELBACH, Th. & SCHINDLER, H.: Psychosoziale Auswirkungen der Arbeitslosigkeit und Hindernisse fur eine Aktivierung Arbeitsloser. Mitteilungen der Zentralen Wissenschaftlichen Einrichtung 'Arbeit und Betrieb' Universitat Bremen/ Arbeiterkammer Bremen. No. 11, 1984.

KLEIBER, D., KIESELBACH, Th. & SCHINDLER, H.: Ursachen, Erscheinungsformen und Auswirkungen der Psychologenarbeitslosigkeit-Zwischenergebnisse einer empirischen Untersuchung. in: MAIERS, W. & MARKARD, M. (eds): Leiber arbeitslos als ausgebeutet? Koln 1980, pp. 169 - 182.

LAURITZEN, G.: Bedurfnisse Arbeitsloser, von Arbeitslosigkeit Bedrohter und Unterqualifizierter an Fortbildung und Umschulung. Report to the Ministry of Labour (FRG). Unpublished paper 1982.

MELKAS, T. 'Health Effects of Unemployment and National Health Policy in Finland', paper presented at WHO Workshop on 'The Health Policy Implications of Unemployment in the Community', Leeds, December 1982.

OSMOND, J.: Wales: Will unemployment breed unrest or apathy? in: CRICK, B. (ed.): Unemployment, London/New York: Methuen, pp. 127 - 134.

RAPPAPORT, J.: In praise of paradox: A social policy of empowerment over prevention. American Journal of Community Psychology 9(1), 1981, pp. 1 - 25.

SCHNEIDER, H.: Erfahrungen mit 41a-Maßnahmen zur Verbesserung der Vermittlungsaussichten. Arbeit und Beruf 32(4), 1981, pp. 97 - 99.

SELIGMAN, M.E.P.: Helplessness. On depression, development, and death. San Francisco: Freeman 1975.

SCHMID, H.: Science and the control of social science. American Behav. Scientist 12(2), 1968, pp. 59 - 64.

SHEPHERD, G.: Psychological disorder and unemployment. Bulletin British Psychological Society 35, 1982, p. 127.

SIEGRIST, M. & WUNDERLI, R.: Probleme psychologischer Betreuung von Arbeitslosen. in: MINSEL, W.R. & SCHELLER, R. (eds.): Brennpunkte der Klinischen Psychologie, Vol. 4, Munchen: Kosel 1982, pp. 75 - 91.

SPRUIT, I.P.: To be employed, to be unemployed and health in families in Leiden. in: SPRUIT, I.P. (ed.): Unemployment, employment, and health. Leiden: Institute of Social Medicine 1983, pp. 137 - 177.

TIFFANY, D. W., COWAN, J.R. TIFFANY, P.M.: The unemployed. A social-psychological portrait. Englewood Cliffs: Prentice Hall 1970.

TUCKER, A.C.: Some correlates of certain attitudes of the unemployed. New York 1940.

WINDOLF, P.: Arbeitslosigkeit heute, Grauzonenbeschaftigung und informeller Sektor. Die neue Arbeitslosigkeit und die Grenzen der Sozialpolitik. Soziale Welt No. 3/4, 1982, pp. 365 - 399.

WINFIELD, I.: Psychology and centres for the unemployed - challenge or chimera? Bulletin British Psychological Society 34, 1981, pp. 353 - 355.

WITTMANN, W.: Die neuen Ausbeuter. Stuttgart: Seewald 1980.

RESPONDING TO UNEMPLOYMENT AT A LOCAL LEVEL

Jennie Popay

This paper describes a number of 'local' responses to unemployment in the UK and elsewhere. The examples have not been selected to be in any way representative of initiatives which exist. Rather, they reflect merely those responses I know about. Additionally, from those I am aware of I have chosen selectively to illustrate some major themes in relation to local responses to unemployment generally, and to unemployment and health and health policy in particular.

As will become evident, the responses described are diverse in their organisation, aims, objectives and activities. They include self-help groups, trade union and employer initiatives, action from within the Churches and statutory agencies, responses on the part of individual professionals, professional organisations and alliances of different groups. The activities involved are equally diverse and are clearly influenced by perceptions about unemployment and the 'needs' of people experiencing unemployment; by the priority attached to different 'needs' by those involved in the response; and by views about what is feasible at a local level in relation to unemployment.

1. Perceptions of unemployment and the 'needs' of the unemployed

It is possible to identify a number of different, but related, perceptions about who experiences unemployment and what the impact might be, which to a greater or lesser extent have influenced the development of local responses to unemployment.

Until recently unemployment - as an experience with adverse social and economic consequences - was largely viewed as an *individual* phenomenon, affecting mostly men. While women were seen to be capable of losing their jobs, it was widely argued that the experience would be less traumatic because (a) they could fall back into the role of housewife/mother and therefore experience a reduced loss of status and identity and (b) wives were commonly assumed to work merely for pin money.

Clearly, unemployment is not an individual experience. The unemployed are members of families and there is indeed evidence that unemployment is in fact concentrated in certain families. [1] Unemployment and its social and economic effects will therefore be experienced by the families of the unemployed and in some cases the whole community - a perspective which informs some, but not all of the local responses to unemployment. The position of women as unemployed workers is too complex to go into detail in this paper. Suffice it to say that the adverse health status of many women at home with young children, documented by Brown, Harris and others, suggests that the experience of being a housewife/mother may have much in common with the experience of unemployment. [2]

It is also increasingly evident that women's contribution to family income is keeping a large number of two parent families out of poverty, as well as an increasing proportion of female headed one parent families. [3] Women's unemployment is therefore increasingly recognised to be as important for individual and family wellbeing as male unemployment, and is the focus of a growing number of local initiatives. [4]

Remaining for a moment with the perceptions of who experiences unemployment, it is apparent from much media and public discussion that there is what could be described as a 'hierarchy' amongst the unemployed, with some groups being seen as deserving of greater priority than others. The situation of women has already been noted. There is similarly a view that older workers should make way for younger workers [5] and ethnic minorities and disabled people for example, may be seen as less deserving than others. Such a hierarchy is reflected to some extent in responses to unemployment with a large number of initiatives being directed towards young people, for example.

Moving on to the possible impact of unemployment, there is a growing realisation that for many individuals and families unemployment leads to a considerable fall in material living standards.

Many local initiatives have therefore focussed specifically on financial issues (such as information, advice and advocacy in relation to benefit entitlement) budgetting issues and debt management and local campaigns to obtain concessionary charges for the unemployed.

To varying extents and in different ways local initiatives have also attempted to alleviate the social impact of unemployment, to compensate for the loss of the 'latent consequences of employment'. [6] Activities in this sphere range from attempts to find or create alternative paid employment, to attempts to provide companionship and meaningful activities, such as education, leisure pursuits, skill exchanges etc. Some initiatives teach job search techniques and provide information and advice on employment services and training opportunities. Some of the educational activities - such as courses on low budget menus - are also focussed on mitigating the social impact.

As concern about the possible adverse effects of unemployment on health and wellbeing has grown, there has also been a parallel questioning of the role of health and social services, which has lead to some initiatives in this sphere.

Finally, it should be noted, that for many people, unemployment is primarily seen as a political issue. Some of the local initiatives, reflecting this view - have wider political objectives. There is a concern to promote local and national discussion about the extent and impact of unemployment and to agitate for change in policy at both national and local level.

2. Responses at community level

At this stage I had intended to attempt a classification of local initiatives according to the 'needs' they aim to meet and their structure or organisational base. However, while providing a tidy presentation, such a classification belies the adhocery and diversity of the reality. I therefore intend merely to describe some of the initatives of which I am aware, which I feel to be of interest, and which illustrate some general issues.

3. TUC unemployed workers centres

In November 1980, following a conference of affiliated unions, the TUC launched a campaign to organise services for the unemployed. [7] The TUC initiative has two equally important facets: the formation of a network of unemployed workers centres co-ordinated by the TUC and supported by individual unions, trades councils and regional councils; and a call to affiliated unions to do all they could to retain unemployed workers and to recruit non-unionised unemployed.

A number of principles were agreed. Any effective organisation had to be locally based, providing centres where unemployed people could come together and work with people still in employment, on a common basis. The centres would provide for short term needs, such as advice and counselling. They would give information and support, as well as education, representation and recreation. They would also meet longer term needs of campaigning for jobs and employment creation.

The centres were encouraged to develop their own identity and structures and unpaid regional organisers were recruited from amongst retired and unemployed union officials, who work with local trades councils. By the summer of 1982, there was a paid national development worker and 140 centres in operation. About 50 of them are full-time, usually staffed by long-term unemployed people, funded by the Manpower Services Commission. Part-time centres are open one or two days a week and both types of centres are housed in premises provided by local authorities, in community centres or labour party rooms. [8]

The extent to which the unemployed are actively involved in establishing and or running TUC centres varies and has caused some controversy in the past. However, they are now always represented on management committees and are involved to differing degrees in organising activities at the centres.

The composition of the management committees of TUC centres varies considerably, but a decision to raise funds for paid workers from the Manpower Services Commission programme, does dictate the composition to some extent. There are some who feel that the use of public funds and the accountability this entails, may unduly restrict more 'political' activities. However, others argue strongly that the benefits of having full-time workers far outweigh any restrictions imposed in this way. Clearly, this issue is not restricted to TUC centres and undoubtedly, as Table 1 shows, TUC centres are involved in a wide range of activities.

Table 1

ACTIVITIES IN TUC CENTRES

(from TUC Bulletin No 4)

Set out below are examples of the range of activities undertaken by different TUC Centres for the Unemployed.

INFORMATION	Materials provided by public, voluntary and trade union bodies
ADVICE AND COUNSELLING	'Surgeries' with local authority officials Referral services Legal advice
EDUCATION	Classes on adult literacy and numeracy. Courses on TUC campaigns, eg 'Unemployment: the fight for TUC Alternatives' Workshops on pottery, printing, photography. Readers Groups, linked with libraries, books donated by local groups.
ARTS	Drama groups. 'Keep fit' sessions. Discos, particularly for the young unemployed.
REPRESENTATION	Campaigning for free use of leisure facilities and travel. Providing meeting rooms and facilities for young people on YOP and Union Representatives. Arranging surgeries with full time union officials and direct union representation before tribunals.
ORGANISATION	Preparing newsletters for distribution at supplementary benefit offices. Organising 'outreach' work to make contact with the unemployed at home. Organising visits to workplaces and trade union branches for school and college leavers. Providing facilities for unemployed womens' groups and unemployed blacks' groups.
CRECHE FACILITIES	Childrens' books and toys. After school collection service.
COOKERY	Imaginative cheap meals provided at low cost.
SPORTS	Mainly five-a-side football fixtures at present, for the young unemployed.

4. Other self help initiatives

In the past few years an increasing number of existing community groups have shifted their focus to include employment and unemployment issues, whilst a variety of other self help initiatives have arisen either spontaneously, or based around for example, church groups, isolated plant closures, polytechnics, womens groups etc.

The 'Church Action with the Unemployed' campaign, for example, began earlier this year. [9] As with the TUC initiative, local groups are encouraged to create their own identity. The Church campaign is primarily aimed at the provision of information for local groups about practical action on three fronts: 'pastoral care' which could include self help groups, aimed at facilitating coping mechanism amongst the unemployed; work experience schemes aimed at improving employability; and job creation aimed at providing alternative permanent work. Table 2 is extracted from one of their pamphlets and gives some examples of initiatives under way.

5. Some difficulties faced by self help initiatives

The number of self help groups is unknown, but increasingly there are calls for the formation of networks to help establish and maintain unemployed workers groups and to share experiences and skills. The TUC publishes a regular bulletin, which is received by all TUC Centres and some of the 'independent' groups; local areas, such as Liverpool, have organised their own regular conferences of people involved in local initiatives; a British Unemployment Resource Network has now been established and publishes a regular newsletter. [10]

It almost goes without saying that many self help initiatives face immense practical difficulties. Funding, for example, is a constant problem and for some of the groups even finding a place to meet may present formidable barriers to their development - issues which I have discussed in some detail elsewhere. [11]

Perhaps two of the most difficult problems facing self help initiatives organised around unemployment, relate to the difficulties of actually contacting the unemployed and of establishing a community of interest among the unemployed and between them and the employed. The familiar process within community action, whereby small successes may lead to involvement in bigger and bigger campaigns, is not clear in the case of unemployment. Either the unemployed are unemployed or they are not. If they secure a job the motivation to remain in a group may dissipate quickly. Activities can be organised around intermediate targets, such as concessionary fares on local public transport, better treatment at local social security offices, or appropriate further education classes, but the essential contradiction still remains. Similarly, trade unions and the employed, concerned as they are with the world of work, have considerable difficulty relating to and/or accepting responsibility for working with the unemployed.

Table 2

PRACTICAL ACTION: WHAT YOU CAN DO

THREE MAIN ACTIVITIES

PASTORAL CARE
(Coping with being out of work)

* Start an unemployment group. Identify the special needs of unemployed people in your locality.
* Open a centre where people can meet for helpful counselling and advice.
* Adapt church premises for use as a drop-in or resource centre for action, information, leisure and recreation.
* Join with others in setting up self help groups.
* Promote discussion in your congregation on the changing role of work in life.
* Make unemployment the subject of a sermon or an article in your magazine.

WORK EXPERIENCE
(A better chance to get jobs)

* Sponsor a scheme under the Manpower Services Commission (MSC) 'Youth Opportunities Programme'. Provide young people with work experience on employers' premises. Set up a training workshop. Devise a project of benefit to the community. Get money and help from the MSC.
* Sponsor a scheme under the MSC 'Community Enterprise Programme'. Provide those adults who have been out of work for longer periods with temporary work of community benefit. Money and help are also available from the MSC.
* Note that these MSC Special Programmes do not create permanent jobs and are in a sense palliative. But they do offer training and experience which can help people, especially young people, to have a better chance of getting jobs that are available. Insist on high quality schemes that give real training.

FIND OUT WHAT OTHERS HAVE DONE

JUST A FEW EXAMPLES

1. On Merseyside three Church of England parishes have grouped together to convert part of one of their churches into a centre for the unemployed offering counselling, a library, newspapers and light refreshments. It is the base for an MSC scheme organising community projects in support of the elderly in the area.

2. On Teeside the Churches are involved in sponsoring care teams, each with a supervisor supporting six or eight unemployed school leavers. The teams are funded through the MSC Youth Opportunities Programme and their work includes gardening and decorating for the elderly, and helping to care for children.

3. In Northampton a group of Christians has formed a workers' co-operative. It is engaged in a warehousing operation, purchasing whole foods in bulk, packaging them and distrbuting them to retailers. Premises are shared with a sheltered workshop, set up as a charity by a group of local businessmen to provide temporary jobs for people recovering from nervous or mental disorder.

4. In South Wales, when a major redundancy was impending at the local steel works, the Newport and Gwent industrial mission realised that existing counselling provisions were inadequate. They promptly initiated action together with other interested groups. They set up a 'network' and published a list of the names and telephone numbers of all available counsellors and the skills they could offer. Network members contacted each other for help with referring people to the most appropriate counsellor. They continue to meet regularly to share experiences and exchange views.

..../cont'd

Table 2 (cont'd)

JOB CREATION
(New jobs and permanent work)

* Join with others to create a new job administering your Churches or maintaining the premises.
* Start a neighbourhood Co-operative to go gardening and odd job work, to clean windows and cars, to go shopping and do housework for people.
* Start an Industrial Common-Ownership enterprise. Join with others to use redundancy money as start up capital.
* Start a new business using existing local resources and skills.
* Ask the Department of Industry and the MSC what loans and grants are available to finance these activities.
* Persuade employers to take on extra people.

FIND OUT WHAT OTHERS HAVE DONE
(cont'd)

5. The Liverpool industrial mission team has set up a Youth Opportunities Programme scheme for girls, based in the Skelmersdale Ecumenical Centre. It offers basic training in general office procedures and simple reception and office work. Trainees are providing office services for a variety of Church and community groups.

6. In Scotland, Garthamlock parish has set up a part time drop in centre for young people out of work. After a slow initial response, it became clear to the minister that the centre would only succeed if they young people organised it themselves. They now have a thriving Garthamlock Recreation Club with its own elected president and treasurer. The congregation has welcomed the arrangement and is financing the cost of heating and lighting, and the minister helps as club secretary.

Many of the people concerned with these initiatives point out that it is often only the activists who are involved. The unemployed do not flock into the centres, for example, and there has been a growing emphasis on outreach work. There is also an emphasis on making contact with some of the more neglected groups amongst the unemployed. The TUC centres and others have, for example, been encouraged to establish creches, in order to attract unemployed women. There are now a growing number of groups specifically for women. Indeed, it has been noted by some commentators that these groups are amongst the most active. One particular development has been the growth of a campaign to encourage women to sign on for unemployment benefit. There is also a campaign to establish women's right to work outside the home. This involves the publication of a newsletter and organised demonstrations and marches. As with many local/community based initiatives it is difficult to give an indication of the scale of support for these campaigns.

The level and nature of involvement of the unemployed themselves in the management and activities of centres and other initiatives is vitally important if they are to be perceived as relevant and appropriate. Ian Winfield, a psychologist, has recently argued for example, that activities are often based on 'the assumed needs of the unemployed'. Rarely, if ever, do decisions appear based upon the genuine canvassed needs of the unemployed themselves! [12]

Once formed the aims of the groups or other initatives, are frequently the focus of debate. Many people involved are deeply concerned that centres should not become drop in welfare rights centres, whilst there has been considerable controversy recently associated with the concept of volunteering in relation to unemployment. There is recognition of the danger that such initiatives could become preoccupied with trying to teach the 'non-coping' unemployed how to cope with unemployment. In focussing on the unemployed in this way, the risk is that the mass of evidence showing that unemployment affects many members of the community besides those who lose their jobs, may be ignored. Additionally, there is also the possibility that some initiatives may be inadvertently colluding with the widespread tendency to blame the victims of unemployment for their own plight. This may arise if the primary focus is on inadequacies amongst the unemployed and tactics to change them.

6. Health and social services and unemployment

The scale of unemployment is such as to pose a major challenge to health and social services and the professional groups working with them. Social workers, health visitors, general practitioners, health education officers and many other groups, need to reassess their own theory and practice in relation to large scale long term unemployment and their role in relation to other sectors of the statutory and voluntary services.

The beginning of this process is already apparent in this country. In the past year or more there have been many meetings on unemployment, directed at particular professions. In July 1981, for example, the British Association for Counselling held a national conference on counselling and the unemployed person and in the summer of 1982, the Libraries Association held a meeting on Libraries and unemployment.

There have been many meetings organised for example by local Community Health Councils and aimed at both informing individual professionals, and the public, about unemployment and its impact and encouraging them to think constructively about how they might respond both in everyday practice and more specifically.

Whilst many UK initiatives in this sphere have been on a one off basis, a project in Ohio, in the USA, illustrates a more structured approach to both health and social service professionals training and the development of support networks.

Ohio public interest campaign displaced workers project: The Ohio Public Interest Campaign (OPIC) is "a state wide non profit organisation of citizens concerned with the economic problems in Ohio. In particular with the industrial exodus of firms out of the industrial states and the economic and fiscal problems generated for the state". The campaign is sponsored by individuals, and groups from a diverse range of backgrounds, including trade unions, religious groups and local politicians.

In 1981 the campaign obtained funding for a 'Displaced Workers Project'. [13]). The project has two goals; to help human service workers (that is social workers, counsellors etc) to better understand and more effectively respond to the special needs of the displaced workers and their families; and secondly to facilitate the development of workers support groups to help moderate the impact of the crises. In this way they hoped to prevent or ameliorate the economic social, psychological and health problems associated with unemployment.

The project involved the training of two groups of people, professionals working within state social service agencies (so that they can go back into their organisation and provide in service training to improve staff effectiveness in serving the unemployed and their families) and unemployed workers. The unemployed were to be trained to develop a network of self help groups amongst unemployed workers.

The training objectives were:

1. To provide information and analysis about the social and economic context and personal and family impacts of plant closure.
2. To provide information about community resources so that staff and unemployed workers can make more effective use of them.
3. To provide the structure, facilities and resources for a support group of displaced workers that will be on going.
4. To provide the structure and resources to aid these support groups to establish additional groups for other unemployed workers.

The training was to be through a series of workshops and at the end of the workshops OPIC staff would work with the trainees in the field.

The information available to me relates to an early stage of the project and primarily to the progress of the unemployed workers groups, an initiative I have discussed in some detail in an earlier section of the paper. But it may be worth making a few comments about the stability, organisation and activities of the support groups which formed. OPIC became involved in plant closures in different ways. In some cases, individual workers or union officials approached OPIC, in other cases, OPIC initiated plant meetings prior to a closure. Although many meetings were held, primarily providing information, only one 'plant specific' group continued to operate in the summer of 1981, based on a Church.

More frequently, members of these groups joined city wide groups, and in each of the six cities involved in the project, 2/3 on going groups existed. The groups had been involved in a range of activities including:

- surveying local job placement and training resources and publishing a directory
- surveying unemployed workers about their situation and needs
- preparing a directory of community agencies providing services for the unemployed
- exploring the feasibility of worker control of closing plants
- organising in support of state wide plant closure legislation

In one case the workers had successfully organised the reopening of a hose manufacturing company, saving 150 jobs and in mid 1981, the company had been operating profitably for two years.

This project is unusual combining as it does individual ameliorative activities, attention to social service provision and state wide advocacy around the issue of unemployment and large scale plant closure. It also received funding from a federal agency. However, whilst providing an interesting model, it would clearly be necessary to have more information about recent progress.

Linwood Employment Initiative Group: there are undoubtedly examples of innovative responses on the part of health and social services in this country. The Employment Initiatives Group in Linwood in Strathclyde is a case in point. Established in response to the imminent closure of the Talbot factory at Linwood, the group comprised representatives from the Chief Executives office, from the education department and from the social work services group within the Strathclyde Regional Council. In addition there were representatives from the Renfrew District Council and social work staff. [14]

Initially, a welfare rights presence was established within the factory before the closure, and plans were made to collect information on the number and type of enquiries made there and elsewhere in the area and on the assistance offered. Information was also to be collected on the use of health services and the uptake of free school meals for example. It was envisaged that such information would increase understanding of the nature and extent of the impact of unemployment in the area, as well as forming a basis for more appropriate and sensitive service planning. It remains to be seen what has been achieved in relation to these aims.

There are, of course, many other examples of individual health and social service professionals, responding in their own way to unemployment in a local area and there is much to be learnt from the experiences of places like Consett and Corby. Without question, health and social service workers have a critical role to play in relation to unemployment, given the isolation so often experienced by the unemployed and the family perspective such workers frequently have. Also of use is the contact health and social services may have with the unemployed and their families, who may be failing to take advantage of both statutory and voluntary support services. The implications of unemployment for health and social service workers is however, still a relatively neglected area and one which demands urgent attention. The role and responsibilities of the education service is another enormous field which I have not commented on. Undoubtedly there is much happening, but one of the most important challenges facing education in relation to unemployment is the need to reach the many isolated unemployed who have no contact with formal agencies. The Open University Department of Community Education is developing initiatives in this sphere.

7. Social responsibility and plant closure at a local level

So far I have not mentioned any responses initiated by employers but they do exist. With the closure of the steel works at Consett, for example, the British Steel Corporation set up an enterprise trust which has been concerned with retraining and job creation, albeit on a small scale. To date they have been responsible for the creation of only a few hundred jobs. Pilkington Glass is also responding to unemployment in a similar way by encouraging the development of small enterprises, but it is American examples which I wish to comment on here, for they provide interesting and unfamiliar (at least in Europe) models of 'social responsibility'.

Office of Employee Services: Pennsylvania: The Office of Employee Services (OES) was established by Court Order in April 1979. [15] It was to design and deliver services to 1 700 state employees who would lose their jobs when the residents of Pennhurst Mental Hospital were relocated in community facilities following legal proceedings. The OES was dissolved just nine months later in January 1980 as a result of a Court of Appeal ruling that 'relief for employees was not reasonably related to facilitating the rights of the retarded'. A final report was prepared giving an account of the establishment of OES, information on the employees and the communities in which they lived, an analysis of the effects of the closure, a description of the office, and the findings, conclusions and recommendations. Clearly, there is much that is very specific to the Pennhurst closure or to any situation of deinstitutionalisation and the initative was very short lived. However, the model, and some of the findings, conclusions and recommendations are of more general interest.

Following a court decision to transfer patients from Pennhurst, the court order also called for the preparation of 'a plan to provide opportunities for alternative employment to each employee ..... including employment in community programmes and otherwise'. After extensive consultation with for example trade unions, state and local government officials and employment agencies, the court ordered in April 1979 that the plan 'to provide information and services to Pennhurst employees' be implemented. It was to last for three years and the Office of Employee Services was to implement the plan. An 'Employee Information and Service Centre' was established at Pennhurst with the following goals:

1. To insure that all employees of Pennhurst were continually informed regarding the implementation of the Court Ordered Employee Plan

2. To act as a liason between the court, the Pennhurst employees and their unions. This role included performing an ombudsman function on behalf of employees.

3. To identify and define areas of employee needs and provide programs and services accordingly.

4. To the extent possible, to facilitate for each employee a transition from their present employment situation to their new role. This included attempting to minimise the negative effects of job loss, dislocation, disruption and the uncertainties and ambiguities inherent in this situation.

In additon to the Information and Service Centre, four professional staff were hired to provide job placement, counselling education to training and to mobilize community support.

1. A Coordinator of Job Placement would locate and develop jobs in state agencies, in the private sector, and in community based service settings for the developmentally disabled.

2. A Coordinator of Counselling Services, assisted by an Employee Planning Counsellor would help employees prepare individual plans designed to assist them in moving toward new jobs, new careers and new life styles eg retirement.

3. A Coordinator of Education and Training would develop programmes designed to prepare for work in community living arrangements established for mentally retarded citizens; prepare for high school equivalency examinations; develop basic skills; up-grade skills; and prepared for entrance into new careers.

4. A Coordinator of Community Services would mobilise community resources to provide mental health, social welfare, and other community support services.

Though short lived the Pennhurst programme report does contain some valuable insights and identifies potential problems for such an initiative. There was for example, a reluctance on the part of employees to seek help from the resource and job information centre.

Much of the initial activity of the office was focussed on individual counselling concerned with educational, employment and personal issues. This involved a number of different elements. There was, for example, a plan for priority placement of Pennhurst employees in state vacancies and plans to develop close contact with the private sector to stimulate job creation. Unfortunately the OES had no opportunity to implement this part of the plan.

The Employee Protection and Community Stabilisation Act: This piece of legislation being championed by the Pennsylvania Public Interest Coalition in 1981, had the explicit aim of promoting social responsibilty on the part of industry. Although clearly not directly transferable to other countries, this legislation does contain innovative elements.

At least 12 states including Ohio, Michigan, Connecticut, Maine, Wisconsin, Massachusetts and Pennsylvania, had passed or were considering legislation to reduce the extent and consequences of plant closure in the Northeast and Midwestern states of America. The details of the Bills vary considerably, but the most comprehensive involves sections covering: severance pay to all employees equal to one weeks pay for each year worked; continuation of health insurance benefits (for a limited time); payments to a Community Readjustment Fund of around 10-15% of annual payroll, to be used to foster local social services, community economic development and local industry. In Pennsylvania, the Bill included a clause requiring an 'impact statement' to be undertaken by the company involved, giving the number of workers affected and the potential economic and social impact on the community concerned. If the Bill were to be passed, a newly created Bureau of Employee Protection and Community Stablisation would investigate to determine whether the closures were economically necessary or justified and to develop alternatives to the closures. Since this paper was first written, the economic situation and the rate of plant closure in the USA, as in the UK, have deteriorated rapidly. There has been little success in relation to extending social responsibility along the lines identified in this legislation. Nevertheless the model these bills provide is still of interest.

The ability of British local authorities to undertake such activities is much more limited than American states, and not all aspects of such legislation would be appropriate, but the idea of increased social responsibility on the part of employers and the introduction of a social costing of unemployment are laudable objectives. That we need some of the detailed provisions is exemplified in the appallingly short notice of redundancy given to many workers in both the private and public sectors. Similarly, whilst we do have a redundancy scheme, its paltry provisions are illustrated by the findings of Bill Daniels' recent survey of the unemployed [16] where around 90% of the sample of 8000 unemployed received no redundancy pay or less than £500 and a mere 5% received pay in excess of £2 000.

8. Conclusions

This review of local responses to unemployment has ranged far and wide and inevitably many important initiatives will have been missed out from what is essentially a very subjective selection. Unfortuntely by their very nature local initiatives are difficult to catalogue and whilst some individuals and groups are attempting to distribute information, there is a need for a more systematic process of information exchange in this sphere.

There will also be many activities being pioneered within individual initiatives, in the sphere of education and counselling for example, which I have not described. I have deliberately chosen not to provide detailed descriptions of specific projects but rather to illustrate a range of responses to give a feel for the potential scope of local responses, to point to the different but equally important contributions which can be made by different groups within a community; and to demonstrate that local responses face a number of difficulties, both technical and more fundamental.

Potential scope: As I have noted, local responses include activities intended to develop individuals' ability to 'cope' better with the social, economic and psychological consequences of unemployment; to provide both general education and specific training; and activities aimed at providing employment, either directly through job creation or indirectly through job search techniques etc.

Who is involved: I have noted in relation to this question, that many local initiatives have been struggling with the issue of involving the unemployed. In the early stages of the TUC initiative for example, much controversy surrounded the composition of the management committees, which have now largely been resolved. But there are still very real difficulties associated with the relationship between the unemployed and the employed both within the labour movement in general and within the centres in particular. Professionals working within local authorities, health authorities, educational institutions and other outside institutions do have a contribution to make, but great care needs to go into clarifying what that contribution might be.

There are also difficulties associated with making and maintaining contact with the unemployed. Many of the self help groups recognise that they are catering for only a very small proportion of the unemployed, an issue which is of relevance to initiatives other than self help groups. It is likely that those unemployed most involved with any of the responses that I have been discussing are not those most in need of support.

A recurring problem for many of the initiatives which do actively involve unemployed people is the turnover of membership, as the most articulate members are often the first to find work, indeed membership of the group may enhance this possibility. However, it perhaps does not need to be said that in today's unemployment situation this 'problem' becomes less signficant!

Some of the responses I have described involved a strong role for employers, whether public or private, in relation to the social costs of unemployment. In particular, in the provision of social and psychological support, training and retraining and even job creation. Corporate responsibility on the scale illustrated by the example from Pennhurst Ohio, is not common in this country (and indeed it did not last long at Pennhurst!). We certainly need to look more closely at the way in which such responsibilities may be developed and what form they should take.

The activities of a number of local authorities in the UK, notably Newcastle, Leicester, Sheffield and the Greater London Council, are related to the issue of corporate responsibility. Through a range of activities, in particular through local enterprise boards, these authorities are attempting to take greater control of their local economies, but these are early days and little can be said about progress in these areas. Such wider initiatives do however bring me to my final point.

The Wider Context for Local Responses to Unemployment: In my view the present research on the links between unemployment and ill health demonstrate the need for a policy response now. But what that response should and can be is problematic. Research in this country repeatedly stressed the financial difficulties facing the unemployed, particularly those with larger families. Though concessionary charges for public facilities and other activities do have a role to play here, the potential for action at a local level is limited in this sphere.

Many of the unemployed do feel a need for social support and training etc, and here local responses have a very important role to play. However, some of these responses are by their very nature looking at the unemployed as an individual with little or no social context. This focus may have at least two implications:

1. The family of the unemployed may receive little or no support, a situation which may have adverse effects on health and wellbeing.

2. Individualistic activities perhaps best described as 'teaching the non-coper to cope', may predominate.

The history of voluntary and state services in health, no less than in other spheres, suggests that providing individual counselling and advisory services tends to be easier than actively pursuing policy change designed to remove the problems which make the individually oriented services necessary. The latter services are of course valuable and necessary. The problem for many local responses, is striking an acceptable balance (that is acceptable for some of the workers concerned) between providing this kind of service and taking part in the broader political debate.

Yet unemployment is more than just a challenge to the communities experiencing it, indeed if the responses are restricted to such communities, this will merely serve to reinforce existing inequalities in society, for those communities bearing the burden of unemployment are also most frequently the most disadvantaged in many other ways. Active involvement of professionals and the employed in the shaping of the broader political debate in relation to both income support and employment policy is essential if local support services are to be effective in the long term. And both are legitimate concerns of health policy.

References

1 These issues are discussed in a recent report from the Study Commission on the Family. L Rimmer and J Popay, Employment Trends and the Family, 1982, available from 3 Park Road, London, NW1 6XN

2 Brown G and Harris T, Social Origins of Depression: A Study of Psychiatric Disorders in Women, Tavistock, London 1978

3 Study Commission on the Family, Family Finances: An Interim Report from A Working Party, 1982

4 See for example National Council for Voluntary Organisations, Information Sheet No 6, Community based employment projects for women

5 Unemployment Alliance, Briefing Paper No 3, 1982 Older Workers, NCVO

6 Jahoda M and Rush H, The Psychological Consequences of Employment and Unemployment, Science Policy Research Unit Paper, 1980

7 This discussion is based on a longer paper prepared for the Unemployment Unit which discusses the TUC and other initiatives in the context of a similar Canadian initiative in the late 1970's. J Popay Organising the Unemployed: Some Reflections on Canadian Experience, Unemployment Unit, London, 1982

8 A recent discussion of the TUC centres was included in the Journal 'Voluntary Action', Summer 1982, available from NVCO, London

9 More information can be obtained from Church Action with the Unemployed, PO Box 576, Aston, Birmingham, B65 QL

10 More Information from: A Howell, Job Change Project, Birmingham Settlement, 318 Summer Lane, Newtown, Birmingham, B19 3RL

11 Op cit, ref 7

12 Winfield I, Psychology and Centres for the Unemployed: Challenges or Chimera?, Bulletin of the British Psychological Society, 1981, 34, 353-355

13 Details of this project are available from OPIC, 1120 Chester Avenue, Suite 340, Cleveland, Ohio 44114, USA

14 Details taken from a paper presented to the Social Work Service Group, Scottish Office, Seminar, March 1982

15 Final Report of the Office of Employee Services, January 1980, Office of the Special Master, 649S Henderson Road, King of Prussia, P A 19406, USA

16 Daniels W W, The Unemployed Flow, Stagel Interim Report, Policy Studies Institute, London 1981

RESUME

Introduction

La troisième réunion dans le cadre de l'Etude sur l'influence du développement économique sur la santé a été organisée en collaboration avec le Nuffield Centre for Health Services Studies (Centre Nuffield pour les Etudes sur les Services de Santé). Les participants, venus de huit pays, ont recherché les faits établissant un lien entre le chômage et la mauvaise santé. Ils ont pris connaissance des rapports sur plusieurs projets de recherche en cours, et ils ont discuté de leurs implications pour la santé et la politique liée à la santé.

Examen des travaux de recherche actuels

La recherche sur l'état des individus en chômage (c'est-à-dire au niveau de la microstructure) indique régulièrement qu'un chômage de plus de quelques semaines de durée cause un stress physiologique, qui fait monter la pression artérielle et aggrave le risque de maladies cardiaques.

En outre, ce n'est pas seulement l'état affectif des chômeurs qui se détériore, avec les changements correspondants du métabolisme; on constate également une tendance accrue aux troubles psychiatriques, comme en témoignent l'augmentation du nombre d'admissions dans les hôpitaux psychiatriques en période de chômage aigu ainsi que l'élévation du taux de suicides et de pseudosuicides par rapport à la moyenne. Les causes paraîssent en être les difficultés financières et l'interruption des relations proches, qui résultent d'un chômage prolongé.

La recherche au niveau national et en coupe transversale (c'est-à-dire au niveau de la macrostructure et au niveau intermédiaire de structure) prouve elle aussi que l'on observe plus de morbidité et de mortalité chez les chômeurs. Mais elle montre également que la santé de ceux qui ont un emploi peut aussi souffrir du fait de l'aggravation du stress de tensions au travail, de la détérioration des conditions de travail et de la peur du chômage. D'autre part, des groupes qui ne sont pas compris dans la main-d'oeuvre, tels que les nourrissons et les personnes âgées peuvent subir les répercussions du chômage sur la famille et de la détérioration des services sociaux et des réseaux d'aide sociale. On a démontré que la tendance à la recherche d'aide en général, et non pas seulement le recours aux services de santé, augmente en période de récession et d'instabilité économique.

Un volume important de recherche indique, comme on l'a vu, que l'aggravation du chômage et de l'instabilité économique provoque une augmentation sensible des troubles de la santé mentale et se répercute aussi non seulement sur la santé physique des travailleurs mais aussi sur celle de leurs familles et de la collectivité en général.

Il faudra réaliser d'autres études épidémiologiques, en coupe transversale et longitudinale et au niveau de la collectivité pour faire apparaître de quelles manières le changement économique cause les effets précités, particulièrement en ce qui concerne les rôles relatifs de la perte de revenu, de la pauvreté et de l'impact psychologique de la condition de chômeur. Il faudrait mettre l'accent sur les groupes sociaux et démographiques qui sont les plus vulnérables aux effets dislocateurs, en rattachant les informations socioéconomiques, démographiques et relatives à la santé.

Incidences des résultats de la recherche sur les politiques

Politique économique. On peut conférer aux décisions économiques une plus grande efficacité sociale si l'on tient pleinement compte des coûts sociaux, tels que l'érosion de la capacité de travail, et les coûts pour les services de santé et les services sociaux entraînés par le chômage et l'instabilité économique. Il faut en même temps souligner que n'importe quel emploi n'est pas nécessairement préférable au chômage : le travail a ses risques et coûts sociaux propres, particulièrement lorsque les conditions de santé et de sécurité, et les normes de protection de l'environnement sont relâchées au nom de la relance de l'emploi.

Politique de l'emploi. Dans la mesure où il y a des limites au nombre d'emplois qui peuvent être créés, il est préférable d'organiser un partage des possibilités d'emploi disponibles plutôt que de concentrer un surcroît d'heures de travail et de stress sur ceux qui ont déjà un emploi. En outre, il est possible d'organiser un travail socialement utile pour occuper temporairement la capacité disponible. L'emploi de travailleurs en-dessous de leur niveau de capacité et autres formes de sous-emploi ne sont pas des solutions viables.

Politique sociale. On peut limiter les dommages que le chômage cause à la santé en réduisant la pauvreté parmi les chômeurs et les autres groupes qui souffrent de l'instabilité économique, et en veillant à ce que les décisions des pouvoirs publics ne disloquent pas les réseaux d'aide sociale. Il est à la fois nécessaire, ce qui est parfois contradictoire, de favoriser, surtout chez les enfants, le sentiment de dignité lié au fait d'avoir un emploi et d'atténuer le sentiment de honte chez les chômeurs. Les organismes qui sont chargés, dans plusieurs pays, de conseiller les chômeurs ont besoin de capacités supplémentaires en temps de récession à cause des sommes accrues qu'ils ont à verser en espèces.

Politique des services de santé. Les services de santé peuvent être planifiés en vue de faire face aux besoins accrus dans le domaine de la santé résultant de la récession. Par une meilleure identification et quantification des charges imposées aux services de santé par les bouleversements économiques, on peut améliorer l'utilité et l'efficacité de ces services. Les activités d'organes non gouvernementaux, tels que les groupes d'auto-assistance, les syndicats et les églises ont un rôle constructif à jouer tant en matière de santé que de politique sociale.

Recommandations

1. Les gouvernements devraient tenir compte des implications étudiées plus haut du chômage et de l'instabilité économique en général sur les politiques.

2. Les gouvernements devraient promouvoir ou patronner la recherche sur les liens de causalité entre l'instabilité économique et la santé, et obtenir des informations sur la santé des groupes socialement les plus vulnérables de leur pays.

3. L'OMS, par l'intermédiaire de l'Institut d'Informatique médicale et de Recherche sur les Services de Santé de Munich, devrait continuer à servir de centre d'information pour la documentation, pour les ouvrages non publiés et non traduits, ainsi que pour la recherche en cours.

4. L'OMS devrait, en collaboration avec l'un des centres participant à l'étude, réunir un quatrième atelier dont les travaux seraient axés sur la santé des groupes sociaux plus particulièrement vulnérables à la récession et à l'instabilité économique.

KURZBERICHT

Einleitung

Die dritte Tagung im Rahmen der Untersuchung über den Einfluss der wirtschaftlichen Entwicklung auf die Gesundheit wurde in Zusammenarbeit mit dem Nuffield Centre for Health Services Studies abgehalten. Die Teilnehmer aus acht Ländern untersuchten, inwieweit ein Zusammenhang zwischen Arbeitslosigkeit und schlechter Gesundheit besteht, nahmen Berichte über eine Reihe von zur Zeit durchgeführten Forschungsvorhaben entgegen und erörterten deren Auswirkungen auf die Gesundheit und die Gesundheitspolitik.

Überblick über den gegenwärtigen Stand der Forschung

Untersuchungen über die Erfahrungen von einzelnen Arbeitslosen (d.h. auf der Ebene von Mikroanalysen) haben durchweg gezeigt, dass eine über einige Wochen hinaus andauernde Arbeitslosigkeit zu physiologischem Stress führt, der seinerseits Bluthochdruck sowie eine Erhöhung des Risikos einer Herzerkrankung mit sich bringt.

Ausser der schlechteren Gemütsverfassung - mit einhergehenden Veränderungen der chemischen Abläufe im Körper - bei Arbeitslosen, treten in stärkerem Mass Symptome von psychischen Störungen auf, was in einer Zunahme der Einweisungen in psychiatrische Kliniken in Zeiten grosser Arbeitslosigkeit und in einer überdurchschnittlich hohen Anzahl von Selbstmorden und Suizidversuchen seinen Niederschlag findet. Es scheint, dass das auf den finanziellen Druck und den Abbruch enger Beziehungen bei anhaltender Arbeitslosigkeit zurückzuführen ist.

Untersuchungen auf Landesebene und Querschnittstudien (d.h. auf der Ebene von Makroanalysen und auf der mittleren Ebene) haben den zusätzlichen Nachweis für einen übermässigen Anstieg der Morbidität und Mortalität bei Arbeitslosen erbracht. Andererseits ist es aufgrund solcher Studien wahrscheinlich, dass auch die Gesundheit der erwerbstätigen Bevölkerung durch erhöhten Arbeitsstress, schlechtere Arbeitsbedingungen und die Angst vor Arbeitslosigkeit beeinträchtigt wird. Überdies leiden vermutlich auch die nicht Erwerbstätigen, wie Kinder und ältere Menschen unter den Folgen der Arbeitslosigkeit für die Familie und unter der schlechteren sozialen Versorgung und Sicherheit. Es wurde nachgewiesen, dass es in Zeiten der Rezession und wirtschaftlichen Unsicherheit eine allgemein stärkere Tendenz gibt, um Hilfe nachzusuchen, und zwar nicht nur im Bereich des Gesundheitswesens.

Aus diesem Grund haben zahlreiche Untersuchungen gezeigt, dass eine hohe Arbeitslosenquote und eine Verschlechterung des Wirtschaftsklimas nicht nur bei den Arbeitslosen, sondern auch bei deren Familienangehörigen und in der Bevölkerung im allgemeinen zu einer beträchtlichen Zunahme von psychischen Störungen führen und sich ebenfalls nachteilig auf das körperliche Befinden auswirken.

Es sind weitere epidemiologische, Querschnitts- und Longitudinalstudien sowie Erhebungen auf Gemeindeebene notwendig, um deutlich zu machen, unter welchen Gegebenheiten wirtschaftliche Veränderungen die beobachteten Auswirkungen haben, vor allem was die relative Bedeutung von Einkommenseinbussen, Armut und die psychische Belastung durch Arbeitslosigkeit anbelangt. Der Schwerpunkt der Forschung sollte, durch eine Koppelung von sozialökonomischen, demographischen und gesundheitsbezogenen Informationen, auf die am meisten krisenanfälligen sozialen Gruppen und Bevölkerungsteile gelegt werden.

Politische Auswirkungen der Untersuchungsergebnisse

Wirtschaftspolitik: Wirtschaftspolitische Entscheidungen können eine stärkere soziale Gewichtigkeit erhalten, wenn die Sozialkosten, wie beispielsweise die durch Arbeitslosigkeit und ökonomische Instabilität nachteilig beeinträchtigte Arbeitskapazität und die Folgekosten im Gesundheits- und Sozialbereich, voll und ganz berücksichtigt werden. Gleichzeitig muss unterstrichen werden, dass nicht jede Art der Beschäftigung der Arbeitslosigkeit vorzuziehen ist: Arbeit bringt auch Gefahren und Sozialkosten mit sich, besonders wenn die Gesundheits- und Sicherheitsvorschriften sowie die Umweltschutzbestimmungen im Namen der Arbeitsförderung gelockert werden.

Beschäftigungspolitik: Insoweit als der Schaffung neuer Arbeitsplätze zahlenmässig Grenzen gesetzt sind, sollte man lieber die vorhandenen Arbeitsmöglichkeiten aufteilen als den bereits Erwerbstätigen mit grösserem Stress verbundene Mehrarbeit aufzubürden. Ausserdem können sinnvolle Beschäftigungsmöglichkeiten im Sozialbereich zum vorübergehenden Einsatz der vorhandenen Überkapazitäten geschaffen werden. Eine Beschäftigung der Arbeitskräfte unterhalb deren Qualifikationen oder sonstige Formen der Unterbeschäftigung sind keine brauchbare Lösung.

Sozialpolitik: Gesundheitsschädigungen infolge von Arbeitslosigkeit können durch eine Verminderung der Armut unter den Arbeitslosen und unter anderen Bevölkerungsgruppen, die unter der Verschlechterung der Wirtschaftslage leiden, eingedämmt werden sowie durch die Sicherstellung, dass das Netz der sozialen Sicherheit nicht durch staatliche Massnahmen gefährdet wird. Es besteht die zweifache - gelegentlich im Widerspruch stehende - Notwendigkeit, einerseits, besonders bei Kindern, zu betonen, dass die Tatsache, eine Arbeit zu haben, das Selbstwertgefühl hebt und andererseits unter den Arbeitslosen Schuldgefühle wegen des Arbeitsplatzverlustes abzubauen. Die zuständigen Beratungsstellen für Arbeitslose in einer Reihe von Ländern brauchen in Zeiten der rückläufigen Konjunktur zusätzliche Kapazitäten, um der steigenden Anzahl von Ratsuchenden, die sich mit finanziellen Problemen an sie wenden, zu helfen.

Gesundheitspolitik: Es kann eingeplant werden, dass die Gesundheitsdienste den infolge der Rezession gestiegenen Bedarf an Gesundheitsversorgungsleistungen befriedigen. Eine gezieltere Ermittlung der Art und des Umfangs der aufgrund einer Wirtschaftskrise auf das Gesundheitswesen zukommenden Belastungen kann zu einer grösseren Relevanz und Kostenwirksamkeit dieser Dienste beitragen. Der Tätigkeit nichtstaatlicher Stellen, wie beispielsweise Selbsthilfegruppen, Gewerkschaften und Kirchenverbände, kann eine sowohl gesundheitspolitisch als auch sozialpolitisch konstruktive Rolle zukommen.

Empfehlungen

1. Die Regierungen sollten den vorstehend aufgeführten politischen Begleiterscheinungen der Arbeitslosigkeit und wirtschaftlicher Instabilität generell Rechnung tragen.

2. Die Regierungen sollten Untersuchungen über die kausalen Zusammenhänge zwischen wirtschaftlicher Instabilität und der Gesundheit fördern und Informationen über die Gesundheit der sozial am meisten anfälligen Gruppen in ihrem Land sammeln.

3. Die WGO sollte über das Institut für medizinische Informatik und Systemforschung in München weiterhin als Austauschstelle für Schriftgut, sowohl für unveröffentlichte und nicht übersetzte Werke als auch für Veröffentlichungen über laufende Forschungsvorhaben fungieren.

4. Die WGO sollte in Zusammenarbeit mit einem der an der Studie beteiligten Zentren ein viertes Arbeitsseminar organisieren, wobei das Schwerpunktthema die Gesundheit derjenigen sozialen Gruppen, die besonders anfällig für wirtschaftliche Rezession und Instabilität sind, sein sollte.

РЕЗЮМЕ

Введение

Третье совещание в рамках Исследования влияния экономического развития на здоровье было организовано при содействии Центра по изучению служб здравоохранения (г. Наффилд). В совещании приняли участие представители восьми стран. Они рассмотрели данные о взаимосвязи между безработицей и нарушениями здоровья, отчеты о результатах, полученных в ходе проводимых в настоящее время научных исследований, обсудили их значение для деятельности в области здравоохранения и в смежных с ним секторах.

Рассмотрение результатов, полученных в ходе проводимых в настоящее время научных исследований

Изучение состояния здоровья безработных (т.е. исследования на микроуровне) со всей очевидностью показало, что безработица, продолжительность которой составляет более нескольких недель, вызывает физиологический стресс, обусловливающий повышение кровяного давления и увеличение опасности развития сердечно-сосудистых заболеваний.

Наряду с негативным воздействием на общее состояние здоровья, в результате которого происходят соответствующие изменения в организме, безработица вызывает появление психопатологических симптомов. Подтверждением тому служит увеличение в периоды роста безработицы числа пациентов психиатрических клиник; кроме того, в эти периоды регистрируется больше самоубийств и попыток самоубийств, число которых превышает обычные средние показатели. Очевидно, что эти явления вызваны финансовыми затруднениями и разрывом отношений с близкими, что имеет место в периоды длительной безработицы.

Проведение национальных и поперечных исследований (т.е. на макро- и промежуточном уровнях) позволяет получить дополнительные данные, свидетельствующие о повышении уровня заболеваемости и смертности среди безработных. Эти данные также говорят о том, что в связи с дополнительными стрессами на производстве, ухудшением рабочих условий и опасением потерять работу здоровью работающего населения также наносится ущерб. Более того, группы, не относящиеся к трудоспособному населению, такие, как дети и престарелые, по всей вероятности также испытывают воздействие, которое оказывает безработица на их семьи, а также последствия свертывания деятельности социальных служб и учреждений социальной помощи. Данные исследования также показали, что в периоды спада и экономической нестабильности в большей степени, чем обычно поведение человека характеризуется желанием найти поддержку вообще, а не только в медико-санитарных службах.

Таким образом, многие исследования говорят о том, что высокий уровень безработицы и экономическая нестабильность вызывают значительное повышение уровня психических заболеваний и, кроме того, отрицательно сказываются на физическом состоянии как безработных, так и членов их семей, а также населения в целом.

Необходимо и в дальнейшем проводить эпидемиологические, поперечные, продольные и коммунальные исследования в целях получения более конкретных данных о воздействии экономических перемен на здоровье, в частности, это касается таких факторов, как относительная роль потери заработка, бедности и психологического стресса, испытываемого безработными. Следует уделить особое внимание тем социальным и демографическим группам, которые наиболее подвержены воздействию негативных экономических факторов; для этого необходимо сделать сравнительный анализ социально-экономической, демографической и медико-санитарной информации.

Воздействие на политику результатов научных исследований

Экономическая политика. Решения в области экономики могут иметь более благоприятные социальные последствия, если они будут приниматься с учетом всех социальных факторов, таких, как например, снижение работоспособности и рост расходов на медико-социальные службы, вызванные безработицей и экономической нестабильностью. Одновременно следует подчеркнуть, что не все виды производственной деятельности лучше безработицы: работа характеризуется своими собственными вредными факторами и социальными издержками, особенно если во имя обеспечения занятости нарушаются санитарно-технические нормы и гигиенические стандарты внешней среды.

Политика занятости. Возможности создания дополнительных рабочих мест ограничены, и поэтому более целесообразно распределять имеющуюся работу среди большего числа нуждающихся в ней, чем увеличивать рабочее время и подвергать дополнительному стрессу тех, кто уже трудится. Кроме того, можно специально создавать рабочие места для временно безработных, используя их в общественно полезных целях. Нельзя считать правильным такое решение проблемы, когда квалифицированных рабочих привлекают к работе не по специальности или используют какие-либо другие формы неполной занятости.

Социальная политика. Ущерб, наносимый здоровью человека безработицей, можно свести к минимуму, если, во-первых, уменьшить бедность среди безработных и других групп населения, страдающих от экономической нестабильности, и, во-вторых, обеспечить принятие решений, от которых не страдали бы системы социальной помощи. Существует двуединая, иногда противоречивая, необходимость развивать, особенно у детей, чувство собственного достоинства, основанного на том, что у них есть работа, и в то же время снижать чувство собственной вины у тех, кто находится без работы. В ряде стран учреждения, ответственные за оказание консультативной помощи безработным, в периоды экономического спада нуждаются в дополнительных кадрах, поскольку спрос на эти службы увеличивается в связи с увеличением обращаемости к ним безработных, которые претендуют на получение пособия.

Политика здравоохранения. Медико-санитарные службы можно спланировать так, чтобы они удовлетворяли дополнительные потребности в медицинском обслуживании, обусловленные экономическим спадом. Более точное определение обЪема той нагрузки, которая ложится на медико-санитарные службы в связи с неблагоприятной экономической обстановкой, может способствовать повышению адекватности этих служб и их экономической эффективности. Мероприятия, проводимые неправительственными учреждениями, такими, как группы самопомощи, профсоюзы и церковь могут играть конструктивную роль как в области здравоохранения, так и в области социальной политики.

Рекомендации

1. Правительства должны учитывать вышеупомянутые последствия безработицы и экономической нестабильности в целом при разработке соответствующих политических решений.

2. Правительства должны поощрять или субсидировать научные исследования по установлению причинных связей между экономической нестабильностью и здоровьем, а также собирать информацию о состоянии здоровья наиболее уязвимых в социальном плане групп населения в своих странах.

3. ВОЗ с помощью Института медицинской информатики и изучения служб здравоохранения в Мюнхене должна и впредь выступать в качестве банка данных о неопубликованных и непереведенных материалах, а также о результатах проводимых в настоящее время исследований.

4. ВОЗ в сотрудничестве с одним из участвующих в исследовании центров должна созвать четвертое рабочее совещание для рассмотрения конкретных проблем охраны здоровья социальных групп населения, которые подвергаются особой опасности в связи с экономическим спадом и нестабильностью.